The Clinical Handbook of
PEDIATRIC
INFECTIOUS DISEASE

Second Edition

Edited by Russell W. Steele, MD
Professor and Vice Chairman of Pediatrics; Division Head of Infectious Diseases,
Louisiana State University School of Medicine, and
Children's Hospital, New Orleans, Louisiana, USA

The Parthenon Publishing Group
International Publishers in Medicine, Science & Technology

NEW YORK   LONDON

CIP data available on request

ISBN 1-85070-342-6

Published in the USA by
The Parthenon Publishing Group Inc.
One Blue Hill Plaza
PO Box 1564, Pearl River
New York 10965, USA

Published in the UK and Europe by
The Parthenon Publishing Group Limited
Casterton Hall, Carnforth
Lancs. LA6 2LA, UK

Copyright © 2000 The Parthenon Publishing Group
This edition published 2000
First published 1994

Typeset by Speedlith Photo Litho Limited, Stretford,
Manchester, UK
Printed and bound by Bookcraft (Bath) Ltd.,
Midsomer Norton, UK

The author has exerted every effort to ensure that drug selection and dosage set forth in this text are in accord with current recommendations and practice at the time of publication. However, in view of ongoing research, changes in government regulations, and the constant flow of information relating to drug therapy and drug reactions, the reader is urged to check the package insert for each drug for any change in indications and dosage and for added warnings and precautions. This is particularly important when the recommended agent is a new or infrequently employed drug.

Contents

List of contributors   vii

Preface   ix

1.   Infectious disease emergencies   1

2.   Neonatal infections   25

3.   Immunizations   37

4.   Travel medicine   45

5.   Prophylactic antimicrobial therapy   55

6.   Common outpatient infections   69

7.   Procedures   85

8.   Laboratory diagnosis   91

9.   Respiratory infections   103

10. Gastrointestinal infections   117

11. Bone and joint infections   137

12. Urinary tract infections   149

13. Skin and soft tissue infections   161

14. Central nervous system infections   167

15. Surgical infections   177

16. Sexually transmitted diseases and genital tract infections   189

17. AIDS   201

18. The immunocompromised host   213

19. Infection control   223

20. Antimicrobial therapy   227

Index   255

List of contributors

Brian M. Barkemeyer, MD
Associate Professor of Pediatrics
Division Head of Neonatology
Louisiana State University School of Medicine
New Orleans, Louisiana
USA

Randall D. Craver, MD
Professor of Pathology and Pediatrics
Louisiana State University School of Medicine
and
Medical Director
Children's Hospital Laboratory
New Orleans, Louisiana
USA

Stephen R. Deputy, MD
Diplomate of the National Board of
    Neurology and Psychiatry
Clinical Assistant Professor of Neurology
Louisiana State University School of Medicine
and
Children's Hospital
New Orleans, Louisiana
USA

Bonnie C. Desselle, MD
Assistant Professor of Pediatrics
Louisiana State University School of Medicine
and
Critical Care Intensivist
Children's Hospital
New Orleans, Louisiana
USA

Jay K. Kolls, MD
Associate Professor of Medicine and
    Pediatrics
Division Head of LSU Health Science
    Center Gene Therapy Program
Louisiana State University School of Medicine
New Orleans, Louisiana
USA

Donald C. Liu, MD, PhD
Assistant Professor of Surgery
Division Chief Pediatric Surgery
Louisiana State University School of Medicine
New Orleans, Louisiana
USA

Joseph Ortenberg, MD
Associate Professor
Departments of Urology and Pediatrics
Louisiana State University School of Medicine
    and
Director of Urologic Education
Children's Hospital
New Orleans, Louisiana
USA

Harriette Scarpero, MD
Chief Resident
Louisiana State University/Ochsner Urology
    Program
New Orleans, Louisiana
USA

Russell W. Steele, MD
Professor and Vice Chairman of Pediatrics
Division Head of Infectious Diseases
Louisiana State University School of Medicine
    and
Children's Hospital
New Orleans, Louisiana
USA

John N. Udall, MD, PhD
Richard E.L. Fowler Professor of Pediatrics
Louisiana State University School of Medicine
    and
Chief of Gastroenterology
Children's Hospital
New Orleans, Louisiana
USA

Preface

Physicians are expected to maintain, at their command, an extensive fund of knowledge. It is, of course, not realistic to commit all important information to memory or even to retain what would be considered essential aspects of diagnosis and treatment. We all, therefore, rely on reference sources for optimal patient care. Our personal libraries not only assure against omissions in medical management but also allow the most efficient method for keeping abreast of new developments in each subspeciality.

In the care of pediatric patients, infectious diseases make up over half of diagnostic considerations. For this reason, the pediatrician or primary care physician who treats children, must particularly prepare him or herself with a basic understanding of infectious processes. In many cases, knowledge of the disease must be applied in the clinical setting with minimal delay. These situations might be handled best if the physician has at hand a reliable and concise manual that condenses essential information related to diagnosis and treatment. In many cases, this may simply offer a rapid check of already planned management. In other cases, it may give guidance in an area less familiar to the clinician.

This handbook was designed to provide quick reference in the broad area of pediatric infectious diseases. Most information is in tabular or protocol form. The major efforts deal with diagnosis and treatment rather than pathophysiology. The latter should be reviewed as time permits with other standard texts.

Where there is some difference of opinion, particularly for modalities of treatment, we have often elected to present just one approach. This was done to avoid confusion. Every effort has been made to establish a consensus by reviewing standard texts and current medical journals. Major sources have included the following reference books: *Pediatrics*, edited by A.M. Rudolph, and the *Red Book* (Report of the Committee on Infectious Diseases) published by the American Academy of Pediatrics.

Changes from the previous edition, published in 1994, include not only an update for all infectious diseases but also the addition of two new Chapters; one on travel medicine (Chapter 4) and the other reviewing current prophylactic antimicrobial therapy (Chapter 5). The Chapter on travel medicine is important today in a world that has become much smaller with expanded air transport and a desire among all people to visit remote areas of the world. The section on AIDS (Chapter 17) has undergone extensive revision as a consequence of our progress in managing this viral disease and the numerous opportunistic infections that are a consequence of altered immune reactivity. All new antimicrobial agents approved since the last edition have been included and all new recommendations for therapies of choice have been updated.

Infectious disease emergencies 1

INTRODUCTION

Some infectious disease presentations must be diagnosed and treated rapidly to prevent mortality and optimize the opportunity to reduce morbidity. In most cases therapy is instituted before a diagnosis can be confirmed. These are true emergencies and fortunately only a few such entities are commonly encountered in pediatric patients. Sepsis and meningitis are the two most common. In the majority of cases, culture specimens should be obtained before treatment is begun.

In some instances only supportive therapy is available, either because specific treatment has not been developed (enteroviral encephalitis and myocarditis), the clinical progression is the consequence of a post-infectious process (chickenpox encephalitis, Guillain–Barré syndrome) or because eradication of the invading pathogen is unnecessary (infant botulism, herpes simplex meningitis).

Most infectious disease emergencies should be managed in a well-equipped intensive care unit, at least during the acute phase of illness. Progression of disease may require advanced life support including endotracheal intubation or other specialized support procedures. For this reason, transport to tertiary care centers should be considered if local facilities do not have intensive care capabilities.

BACTERIAL TRACHEITIS

Also termed membranous croup, bacterial tracheitis represents a secondary complication of viral laryngotracheobronchitis (LTB) characterized by necrotizing inflammation of the trachea, abundant thick secretions and occasionally sudden airway obstruction. Except for its viral prodrome, the clinical presentation is quite similar to that of *Haemophilus influenzae* epiglottitis; bacterial tracheitis is therefore a more likely diagnosis in a fully immunized child with high fever and rapid onset upper airway obstruction. Presenting symptoms are itemized in Table 1.1.

A diagnosis of bacterial tracheitis is most likely to be confirmed with airway radiographs showing tracheal irregularities or a membrane. Additional findings include pulmonary infiltrates, atelectasis, hyperinflation, and pulmonary edema.

The viral etiologies of the prodromal LTB include parainfluenza, influenza and adenoviruses. Recovered bacteria have been quite variable (Table 1.2). Earlier reports indicated that *Staphylococcus aureus* was most common, accounting for one half of cases. Recent outbreaks of disease caused by *Moraxella catarrhalis* and *Corynebacterium pseudodiphtheriticum* have been reported associated with less severe illness and a markedly decreased requirement for tracheal intubation.

Table 1.1 Epidemiology and presenting symptoms of bacterial tracheitis

Epidemiology
Peak age 4 years
Early winter outbreaks
Clinical course
Prodromal URI
Cough, stridor
High fever, > 39°C
Toxic appearance

URI, upper respiratory infection

Table 1.2 Etiology of bacterial tracheitis

Staphylococcus aureus	35–75%
Haemophilus influenzae	6–40%
α-hemolytic streptococcus	0–40%
Moraxella catarrhalis	0–27%
group A streptococcus	0–25%

Management includes empiric broad spectrum antibiotics for coverage of *S. aureus* and beta-lactamase producing *M. catarrhalis* and *H. influenzae*. A third generation cephalosporin (ceftriaxone or cefotaxime) plus nafcillin, oxacillin, or clindamycin combination are most appropriate. Protection of the airway and prevention of endotracheal occlusion are the priority. Humidification, frequent suctioning of the airway, and intravenous hydration should be started early. Endoscopy to confirm the diagnosis and remove any potentially obstructive membrane or exudative material should be undertaken for patients with significant airway symptoms. Even after endotracheal intubation these patients may develop obstructive plugs or membranes below the tube.

BOTULISM

Botulism is caused by ingestion of the organism *Clostridium botulinum*, or its preformed neurotoxin. There are three forms of the disease: food-borne, wound and infant botulism. The only form commonly seen in pediatrics is infant botulism. Disease in infants is caused by the release of toxin from organisms that have gained entry to the gastrointestinal tract.

Onset of illness usually occurs at 8–11 weeks of age with a reported range of 1 week to 10 months. Constipation and poor feeding are the first indications of the disease, with more suggestive neurologic signs beginning a few days later (Table 1.3). Diagnosis is best confirmed by identification of botulinus toxin in the stool (Table 1.4). Culture of the stool for *C. botulinum* should also be attempted but, because the organism is ubiquitous, it is not unusual to find it as normal flora in an infant's intestinal tract. Botulinus toxin has rarely been observed in the serum of infantile cases although the presence of toxin is fairly consistent in cases of food poisoning and wound botulism.

The differential diagnosis is rather limited (Table 1.5). Lumbar puncture should be performed to rule out other infectious etiologies.

A negative response to edrophonium (Tensilon) (1 mg intravenous or 2 mg intramuscular) and electromyographic studies will differentiate myasthenia gravis.

Treatment for botulism is primarily supportive as antibiotics or antitoxin have not been shown to alter the clinical course (Table 1.6). Aminoglycosides should be avoided because these agents can potentiate the neuromuscular blockade.

Table 1.3 Clinical diagnosis of infant botulism

Early symptoms	Later clinical findings
Constipation	Floppiness
Generalized hypotonia	Drooping eyelids
Poor feeding	Respiratory distress
Weak cry	Absent deep tendon reflexes
Muscle weakness	Dilated reactive pupils
	Poor suck
	Decreased to absent gag reflex
	Ptosis

Table 1.4 Laboratory diagnosis of infant botulism

Toxin in stools is diagnostic
Stool culture for *Clostridium botulinum*
Electromyography with repetitive stimulation
Lumbar puncture to exclude other diagnoses

Table 1.5 Differential diagnosis of infant botulism

Sepsis
Guillain–Barré syndrome
Myasthenia gravis
Aseptic meningitis
Polio
Diphtheria
Tick paralysis

Table 1.6 Treatment of infant botulism

Supportive care
  Monitor cardiac and respiratory function
  Endotracheal intubation and assisted ventilation
Avoid aminoglycosides

Specific predisposing factors to infant botulism remain speculative. A practical approach to prevention, however, might best focus on methods of reducing exposure to spores (Table 1.7), which infants might ingest.

CARDIAC INFECTIONS

Infections of the heart in children generally present as life-threatening disease requiring management by a pediatric cardiologist (Tables 1.8, 1.9 and 1.10). Endocarditis and

Table 1.7 Prevention of infant botulism

Infants under 1 year of age
  Wash objects placed to infants' mouths (pacifiers, toys, etc.)
  Wash or peel skin of fruits and vegetables
  Avoid honey

Table 1.8 Pediatric endocarditis

Bacterial etiology
  Staphylococcus aureus
  Staphylococcus epidermidis (neonates)
  Streptococcus viridans
  Streptococcus pneumoniae
  Enterococcus
Other etiology
  Acute rheumatic fever (ARF)
  Systemic lupus erythematosus (SLE)
  Libman–Sacks syndrome
Clinical findings
  Underlying congenital or valvular heart defect (neonate-associated central hyperalimentation lines)
  Presents slowly over weeks/months with fever, malaise, fatigue (occasionally acute with febrile illness, toxicity, congestive heart failure (CHF))
  Associated findings of ARF or SLE
  Examination may reveal prominent murmur (may have new murmur, usually valve insufficiency, findings of CHF)
  Embolic findings include petechiae, Roth spots, Osler nodes, splinter hemorrhages, Janeway lesions, embolic pneumonias, splenomegaly
  Chest X-ray may show enlarged heart or embolic pneumonias
  ECG findings are nonspecific (ARF may have increased PR interval)
  Echocardiography shows vegetations on valves or chambers
Laboratory findings
  Bacterial endocarditis-positive blood culture
  Anemia
  Elevated white blood cell count
  Left shift
  Elevated sedimentation rate (may be lowered with CHF)
  Increased acute-phase reactants
  Hematuria
  ARF-Jones criteria
  Elevated acute phase reactants, white blood cell count, sedimentation rate
  Antistreptolysin-O (ASO) or streptozyme confirmation of streptococcal infection
Treatment course
  Specific antibiotic therapy for 2–6 weeks
  If cultures are negative, vancomycin and aminoglycoside are appropriate
  Acute aortic insufficiency with CHF usually requires surgery
  For ARF, 3–6 week aspirin therapy (anti-inflammatory levels) and Bicillin/prophylaxis
  For severe carditis or CHF, short-course steroids are necessary

Table 1.9   Pediatric myocarditis

Viral etiology
  Coxsackie
  ECHO
  Polio
  Influenza
  Adenovirus
  Mumps
  Rubella
Bacterial etiology
  Staphylococcus aureus
  Neisseria meningitidis
  Corynebacterium diphtheriae (toxin)
  Rickettsia rickettsii (Rocky Mountain spotted fever)
Other etiology
  Acute rheumatic fever (pancarditis)
  Kawasaki disease
  Toxemia
  Parasitic disease
Clinical findings
  Febrile illness with chest pain followed by shortness of breath, malaise, fatigue over several weeks to
    months, may present as an arrhythmia or with a sudden fulminating course (especially in young
    infants) or with sudden collapse (sudden death), often associated with pericarditis (myopericarditis)
  Bacterial and rickettsial etiologies develop fulminant illness with sepsis, shock, and congestive heart failure
  Acute rheumatic fever-associated findings (Jones criteria), valvulitis (pancarditis)
  Kawasaki disease etiology during the acute phase manifesting diffuse myocarditis and small vessel arteritis
  Clinical examination gives findings of congestive heart failure
Laboratory findings
  Chest X-ray shows enlarged heart (left atrium and ventricle) and pulmonary edema
  ECG shows diffuse ST-T changes, low voltage, arrhythmias, left ventricular hypertrophy with strain
    pattern (late)
  Acute-phase reactants helpful only early in illness
  Laboratory studies for rheumatic or Kawasaki disease helpful but nonspecific
  Viral cultures usually negative; acute and convalescent viral titers (> 4-fold increase)
  Echocardiography shows enlarged left atrium and left ventricular poor contractility
  Multi-gated acquisition scan shows increased uptake by the heart
  Endomyocardial biopsy is diagnostic
Course of disease
  Variable course: may show spontaneous improvement with time or progress to chronic cardiomyopathy
  Bacterial and rickettsial etiologies have a severe course with high mortality despite early diagnosis and
    appropriate antibiotic coverage
Treatment
  Supportive therapy
  Inotropes and diuretics
  Afterload-reducing agents
  Extracorporeal support (ECMO, LVAD)
  Failure to respond or deterioration, may consider steroids and/or immunosuppressive agents

Table 1.10 Pediatric pericarditis

Viral etiology
  Coxsackie
  ECHO
  Adenovirus
  Influenza
  Mumps
  Cytomegalovirus
  Epstein–Barr virus
Bacterial etiology
  Staphylococcus aureus
  Streptococcus pneumoniae
  Neisseria meningitidis
Other etiologies
  Uremia
  Postpericardiotomy
  Collagen vascular disease
  Systemic lupus erythematosus, acute rheumatic fever
  Mycoplasma
  Tuberculosis
  Parasitic disease
Clinical findings
  Chest pain (precordial) referred to back and shoulder, relieved by sitting upright
  Dyspnea
  Fever, malaise (bacterial etiology with increased toxicity)
  Presents as sepsis associated with meningitis and septic arthritis (young infant)
  Examination reveals tachycardia, decreased heart sounds, rub, Kussmaul's sign (distension of neck
    veins with inspiration), paradoxical pulse > 10 mmHg (early tamponade)
  Associated illnesses include renal failure, previous heart surgery, systemic lupus erythematosus, juvenile
    rheumatoid arthritis, acute rheumatic fever, meningitis, pneumonia
Laboratory findings
  Chest X-ray shows enlarged, water bottle-shaped heart (initially may show just a straightened left-heart
    border)
  ECG shows diffuse ST-T changes, low voltage
  Elevated white blood cell count
  Left shift
  Elevated sedimentation rate
  Abnormal renal and collagen vascular studies if autoimmune etiology
  Positive blood cultures with bacterial etiology
  Echocardiography is diagnostic
  Pericardial fluid exudate has protein > 3 g/100 ml, inflammatory cells (bacterial), polymorphonuclear
    leukocytes, low glucose, specific gravity > 1.015
  Pericardial fluid transudate has protein < 2g/100 ml, few cells (mesothelial), normal glucose, specific
    gravity <1.015
Course and treatment
  Bacterial etiology: requires adequate drainage (repeated pericardiocentesis, tube drainage, or
    pericardial windows); most patients have organisms recovered via blood or pericardial fluid;
    appropriate antibiotics (14–21 days)
  *Viral etiology: 2–6 weeks' course, pain usually controlled with aspirin or NSAIDs; viral cultures usually
    negative, can progress occasionally to constriction; tamponade requires pericardiocentesis
  Other etiologies: usually follows course of other illness unless tamponade occurs

pericarditis are more commonly caused by bacterial agents, whereas myocarditis is more likely to have a viral etiology.

DIPHTHERIA

Diphtheria, an acute illness caused by the organism *Corynebacterium diphtheriae*, is relatively rare in the United States but is still occasionally seen among the non-immunized population. The incubation period for diphtheria is 1 to 6 days and may present in a number of clinical forms. These various presentations indicate that numerous etiologies must be considered in the differential diagnosis.

Diagnosis is confirmed by culture of material from beneath the pharyngeal membrane. Treatment, however, must be instituted as early as possible, usually based on clinical suspicion rather than culture results. The treatment prescribed varies with the severity of the disease as well as duration of symptoms before starting treatment (Table 1.11). Prognosis depends on the patient's age, the location and extent of the diphtheritic membrane, and the promptness with which antitoxin is given. Consideration must also be given to other persons exposed to the index case; treatment varies with the immune status of these individuals (Table 1.12).

ENCEPHALITIS

Encephalitis is a disorder of cerebral function (an encephalopathy) caused by infection or an inflammatory reaction in the central nervous system (Table 1.13). The differential

Table 1.11   Treatment of diphtheria

Drug/support	Dosage/duration
Antitoxin	Dilute 1:20 in isotonic sodium chloride and infuse i.v. not exceeding 1 ml/min
Symptom duration <48 h with mild symptoms	40 000 U antitoxin
Symptom duration > 3 days or severe symptoms	80 000 U antitoxin
Extremely severe or malignant diphtheria	100–120 000 U antitoxin
Diphtheria toxoid	First dose at end of 1st week of illness
	Second dose 1 month later
	Third dose 1 month after second dose
Antibiotics	
Penicillin	100 000 U/kg per day i.v. div. q.6 h for 10 days
or	
Erythromycin	20–50 mg/kg per day i.v. div. q.6 h for 10 days
Supportive intensive care	Airway protection with endotracheal intubation as needed to assure patent airway and prevent aspiration
	Mechanical ventilation for respiratory failure associated with paralysis of muscles of respiration
	Support for failing circulation
	Bedrest (minimum 2–3 weeks) until risk of myocarditis passes
	Prednisone 1–1.5 mg/kg per day for 2 weeks for myocarditis
	Provision for nutrition and hydration (enteral or parenteral)
	Isolation after completion of antibiotic therapy until three cultures of nose and throat (taken 24 h apart) are negative for toxigenic diphtheria bacilli

diagnosis of encephalitis includes other causes of encephalitis (Table 1.14). In determining the cause of encephalitis, obtaining a detailed history may be helpful (Table 1.15).

Diagnosis of encephalitis requires examination of cerebrospinal fluid and culture of blood, feces, throat and cerebrospinal fluid, and possibly immunologic testing for specific virus identification (Table 1.16). Additional information may be gained from electroencephalography (EEG), computerized tomography (CT) or magnetic resonance imaging (MRI), and brain biopsy. With the exception of herpes simplex and varicella-zoster in the immunocompromised host, the treatment of encephalitis is supportive (Table 1.17). Acyclovir has been shown to offer significant benefit in the treatment of herpes simplex encephalitis and is probably efficacious as antiviral therapy for the rare case of culture positive varicella-zoster encephalitis, only seen in the immunosuppressed host.

EPIGLOTTITIS

Acute epiglottitis is a life-threatening acute inflammation of the supraglottic region predominantly caused by *Haemophilus influenzae*

Table 1.12 Management of contacts of index cases of diphtheria

Contact	Management
Immunized household contacts	Schick test, observation
Non-immunized household contacts	Benzathine penicillin 1.2×10^6 U i.m. or Erythromycin 40 mg/kg per day for 7 days Culture before and after treatment Begin diphtheria toxoid immunization Observation daily for 7 days

Table 1.13 Signs and symptoms of encephalitis

Fever
Headache
Irritability
Nausea and vomiting
Upper respiratory symptoms
Lethargy and stupor
Delirium
Convulsions
Meningismus
Focal neurologic signs
Enuresis
Encopresis

Table 1.14 Differential diagnosis of acute encephalopathy

Infectious
  Meningitis, encephalitis
  Brain abscess
Trauma
Vascular
  Hypertensive encephalopathy
  Stroke
  Vasculitis
  Aneurysm
  Arteriovenous malformation
Toxic ingestion
Hydrocephalus
Metabolic disorders
  Uremia
  Hepatic encephalopathy
  Inborn error of metabolism
  Reye syndrome
  Diabetic ketoacidosis (DKA)
  Hyponatremia, hypernatremia, hypoglycemia
Anoxic encephalopathy
Status epilepticus: post-ictal

Table 1.15 Historic details of importance in encephalitis

Exposure to illnesses in other humans
Exposure to vectors such as ticks or mosquitoes
Exposure to animals, especially sick animals, such as horses
Recent travel
Recent injections
Exposure to environmental toxins

Table 1.16   Diagnosis of encephalitis

Cerebrospinal fluid
   Smear and culture for bacteria
   Viral culture
   PCR for herpes simplex virus and enteroviruses
   Smear and culture for acid-fast bacteria
   Special preparations for fungi and protozoa
   Leukocyte count (up to several thousand cells,
      frequently polymorphonuclear leukocyte
      predominance in early stages)
   Normal or moderately elevated protein
   Normal glucose
Blood, feces, and throat
   Viral culture
   Immunologic methods
   Detection of viral antigen
   Detection of specific antibodies
Electroencephalogram
CT scan
MRI
Brain biopsy

Table 1.17   Diagnosis of encephalitis

Supportive intensive care
   Assess airway for adequate gas exchange and
      risk of aspiration (patients without
      purposeful response to pain, comatose)
   Endotracheal intubation for airway protection
      (as needed)
   Mechanical ventilator support to correct
      hypoventilation or hypoxemia (as needed)
   Anticonvulsants for seizure control (as needed)
   Careful observation for and treatment of fluid
      electrolyte imbalances, particularly
      syndrome of inappropriate antidiuretic
      hormone secretion
   Hourly monitoring of urine output via bladder
      catheter
Specific antiviral therapy
   Acyclovir: for herpes simplex encephalitis
      (diagnosed on brain biopsy or suggested by
      paroxysmal lateralizing eleptiform discharges
      (PLED) on EEG or PCR)

type b. Since the advent of *H. influenzae* type b (Hib) vaccine, the prevalence of disease caused by this pathogen has dramatically decreased. Mostly affecting children under 4 years of age, epiglottitis presents with a rapid onset of toxicity and respiratory distress (Table 1.18).

A diagnosis can be made from the characteristic presentation in most cases. In severe or classic cases, nothing is to be gained by obtaining a lateral neck radiograph to confirm the diagnosis. Hyperextending the neck to obtain a proper radiograph may actually induce laryngospasm. A patent airway must be established as rapidly as possible. However, radiographic examination may provide useful information in the patient with mild symptoms in whom the diagnosis of croup is more likely. With this diagnosis, X-rays demonstrate a subglottic 'steeple sign' which is representative of viral induced edema. If radiographic examination is elected, the physician should accompany the patient at all times. Acute epiglottitis must be differentiated from other disorders which produce supraglottic and subglottic upper airway obstruction (Table 1.19).

Table 1.18   Signs and symptoms of epiglottitis at time of hospital admission

Sign or symptom	Incidence (% of patients)
Respiratory distress	100
Stridor	92
Fever	92
Drooling	63
Delirium	58
Dysphagia	58
Pharyngitis	50
Hoarseness	33
Cough	29

Table 1.19   Differential diagnosis of epiglottitis

Croup
Bacterial tracheitis
Peritonsillar abscess
Retropharyngeal abscess
Severe tonsillitis
Foreign body aspiration
Angioedema
Infectious mononucleosis

Table 1.20   Treatment of epiglottitis

Secure airway
  Keep child calm
  Let child assume most comfortable position, preferably in parent's arms
  Administer oxygen by face mask without agitating the child
  Contact anesthesiologist, otolaryngologist, and operating room supervisor
  Transport child as soon as possible to operating room with parent (to calm child), physician, and all
    equipment needed to secure airway if distress increases
  Induce anesthesia by allowing child to breathe spontaneously from mask (halothane and 100% oxygen)
    while in sitting position; then establish intravenous line
  Epiglottis is visualized by direct examination
  Nasotracheal tube is inserted and taped securely (if not possible, orotracheal intubation is attempted,
    followed by bronchoscopic intubation, or tracheostomy as a last resort)
Antibiotics
  Ceftriaxone or cefotaxime
Supportive care
  Observe in intensive care unit
  Keep sedated and restrained
  Provide 2–4 cmH$_2$O continuous positive airway pressure and humidification through endotracheal tube
  Assure hydration (intravenous)
Extubation
  After approximately 48 h intubation, the epiglottis is again examined directly
  If edema and inflammation have subsided, and a leak is present around the tube, it may be removed
  If not, tube is left in place and epiglottis is re-examined in 24 h

Once a diagnosis of epiglottitis is seriously suspected preparations must begin immediately to secure the airway. When treated early and aggressively, the prognosis for epiglottitis is excellent (Table 1.20).

GUILLAIN–BARRÉ SYNDROME

Guillain–Barré syndrome (GBS), or acute idiopathic polyneuritis, is potentially one of the most serious pediatric neurologic disorders. Although the majority of cases of GBS are mild and self-limited, at times the disorder may progress to complete respiratory paralysis and severe autonomic dysfunction. The overall incidence is 1 or 2 cases per 100 000 population. Although GBS generally peaks during the winter and spring, it may occur at any time of year. Factors associated with onset of the disease are listed in Table 1.21.

The underlying pathology is a nearly symmetrical, segmental demyelination of the peripheral nervous system distal to the ventral and dorsal root ganglia. Lymphocytic and macrophagic infiltration is characteristic, but the inflammatory mechanism resulting in infiltration has not been determined.

The clinical presentation of GBS is notoriously variable, and diagnosis is complex (Table 1.22). The classic case includes an ascending paralysis with sensory symptoms such as muscle cramps but few sensory signs. However, GBS may present atypically with a descending paralysis, ophthalmoplegia, or a 'locked-in' state with complete motor paralysis in which the patient appears comatose.

The course of severe GBS may be influenced by early recognition and the availability of intensive care, in particular ventilatory support (Table 1.23). With such support, all children with GBS should survive with a favorable outcome. The most common pediatric complications of GBS are respiratory arrest, aspiration pneumonia, autonomic dysfunction and iatrogenic complications of prolonged ventilation. Intravenous immunoglobulin or plasmapheresis may prevent progression of disease and decrease the development of late-stage GBS.

Management of children with GBS (Table 1.24) requires physicians, nurses, respiratory therapists, and physical and occupational therapists who are acquainted with the course and evolution of the disorder. In general, any patient with suspected GBS should be admitted to a pediatric intensive care unit or ward in which meticulous observation and neurologic re-examination are possible. Guillain–Barré syndrome may evolve acutely from minimal motor weakness to complete respiratory paralysis in some cases. Pulmonary function testing should be included for the evaluation of prognosis and to identify candidates for intravenous immunoglobulin therapy.

Pharmacologic treatment of GBS remains questionable. Corticosteroid therapy has not proved to be efficacious in GBS nor has the use of immunosuppressants, such as azothioprine or cyclophosphamide.

HANTAVIRUS PULMONARY SYNDROME

Hantavirus pulmonary syndrome (HPS) defines an acute respiratory illness caused by Sin Nombre, a hantavirus endemic in the southwestern United States. Disease is characterized by a short prodrome of fever and myalgia followed by interstitial pneumonia with massive pulmonary capillary leak, noncardiogenic pulmonary edema, cardiovascular collapse, and death in almost 50% of infected individuals. Additional clinical characteristics are summarized in Table 1.25.

First recognized in the spring of 1993 during a cluster outbreak in New Mexico, an additional 200 cases were reported over the next 4 years predominantly in southwestern and southeastern states of the USA. Etiologic confirmation can now be achieved with a number of highly specific serologic assays for hantavirus serum antibody or antigen identification in respiratory secretions and tissue (Table 1.26), available through diagnostic services at the Centers for Disease Control and Prevention (CDC).

Table 1.21 Factors associated with onset of Guillain–Barré syndrome

Infectious or postinfectious factors (60%)
  Viral
    Nonspecific upper respiratory or gastro-intestinal infections
    Epstein–Barr virus
    Cytomegalovirus
    Rickettsia
    Mycoplasma
    Bacterial
Noninfectious factors (10%)
  Vaccinations
  Immune disorders
  Endocrine disturbances
  Pregnancy
  Neoplasms
  Toxic exposures
  Surgery

Table 1.22 Diagnostic criteria for Guillain–Barré syndrome

Criteria required for diagnosis
  Progressive motor weakness of more than one limb and/or truncal or bulbar weakness
  Areflexia
Criteria strongly suggestive of diagnosis
  Minimal sensory findings
  Relative symmetry of weakness
  Progressive motor involvement (2–4 weeks) followed by a plateau and gradual complete recovery
  Cranial nerve involvement, especially bifacial paralysis
  Autoimmune system involvement
  Absence of fever at onset
  Elevated cerebrospinal fluid protein at some point of illness
Factors inconsistent with diagnosis
  Marked asymmetry of weakness
  Persistent bladder dysfunction
  Sudden onset of bowel or bladder dysfunction
  Over 50 mononuclear cells/mm^3 cerebrospinal fluid (or presence of any polymorphonuclear leukocytes)
  Sharp sensory level
Factors that exclude diagnosis
  History of toxic hydrocarbon or lead exposure, acute intermittent porphyria, diphtheria, botulism, poliomyelitis, or other well-recognized causes of neuropathy
  Purely sensory symptoms
  Electromyographic findings

Table 1.23 The course of Guillain–Barré syndrome

Development	Incidence (%)
Requirement of ventilatory support	20
Relapse	5–10
Complete recovery	50
Residual neurologic or orthopedic sequelae	10
Fatal pulmonary or cardiac (adults) complications	5

Table 1.24 Management of Guillain–Barré syndrome

Chronic care
  Prevention of urinary tract infection
  Prevention of decubiti
  Prevention of immobilization hypercalcemia and renal/bladder calculi
  Prevention of contractures
  Recognition and treatment (in some cases) of autonomic dysfunction
Respiratory care
  Admission to intensive care unit setting
  Recognition of deteriorating respiratory ability through clinical observation, pulmonary function tests, and arterial blood gas analysis
  Endotracheal intubation and mechanical ventilation should be considered:
    Forced vital capacity <15–20 ml/kg
    Maximum negative inspiratory pressure < 20–30 cm H_2O
    p_aCO_2 > 50 torr
    Weakness of protective reflexes (cough and gag)
Potential pharmacologic management
  Intravenous immunoglobulin (IVIG) 400 mg/kg per day for 5 days or until improvement is significant
  Corticosteroids have no proven efficacy in acute cases
  Treatment of autonomic dysfunction (rarely indicated)
    Antihypertensives (diuretic agents)
    Fludrocortisone for marked orthostatic hypotension
    Plasmapheresis (controlled studies underway) appropriate for severe cases not responding to IVIG

Table 1.25 Common clinical characteristics of Hantavirus pulmonary syndrome (HPS)

Rodent exposure; appropriate geographic regions
Fever > 38.3°C
Interstitial pneumonia
Rapidly progressive respiratory failure
Intubation 1–14 days (median 4 days) after onset of symptoms
Hemoconcentration (elevated hemoglobin, hematocrit)
Thrombocytopenia

Table 1.26 Diagnosis of Hantavirus pulmonary syndrome (HPS)

Compatible clinical course
Hantavirus-specific serology
  IgG, IgM
Lower respiratory tissue or secretions
  PCR for hantavirus RNA
  Immunohistochemical identification of hantavirus antigen

Treatment of HPS is largely supportive, with careful attention to fluid balance and cardiopulmonary support (Table 1.27). Assisted ventilation is usually required. Inhaled nitric oxide has been shown to provide significant benefit to patients with a persistent oxygenation index above 20 and evidence of pulmonary hypertension. Extracorporeal membrane oxygenation has also been used successfully in patients who, it is believed, would otherwise have had a 100% mortality risk.

MENINGITIS

Bacterial meningitis is a common cause of admission to intensive care units. Diagnosis is usually made by examination of cerebrospinal fluid in the child who presents with clinical signs of sepsis, particularly with physical signs localizing that infection to the central nervous system (i.e. irritability, lethargy, meningismus). Absence of these physical findings, however, does not rule out meningitis, particularly in the young infant.

Table 1.27 Management of hantavirus-related acute respiratory distress syndrome (ARDS)

Symptoms
  Rapid onset ARDS
  Neurologic disturbance
  Hemoconcentration (elevated hemoglobin)
  Coagulopathy including disseminated
    intravascular coagulation
  Renal failure
  Hepatic failure
Definition of ARDS
  Antecedent event (e.g. infection with hantavirus)
  Hypoxemia ($p_aO_2/FIO_2 < 200$ mmHg)
  Exclusion of left heart failure
  Bilateral diffuse infiltrates
  Noncardiogenic pulmonary edema
Treatment of ARDS
  Aerosolized ribavirin may be of benefit
  Supportive treatment
  Extracorporeal life support

Table 1.28 Etiology of bacterial meningitis

Neonatal
  Group B streptococcus
  Escherichia coli
  Listeria monocytogenes
  Group D streptococcus
  Gram-negative coliforms
  Staphylococcus aureus
Older children
  Streptococcus pneumoniae
  Neisseria meningitidis
  Haemophilus influenzae type b (in the non-
    immunized child)

Meningitis should be suspected and tested for in infants with fever, lethargy, irritability, and/or poor feeding. The clinician's assessment of the degree of 'toxicity' has proven to be the most valuable tool in identifying the child with possible meningitis. The etiology for bacterial meningitis is given in Table 1.28.

Management of meningitis includes administration of antibiotics as well as observation and treatment for any secondary complications that may occur (Table 1.29). A variety of problems may complicate the course of meningitis in both the early phase of the disease and chronically (Table 1.30).

The secondary attack rate for household contacts of meningococcal meningitis or meningococcemid is 1 per 250 (0.4%). Prophylaxis of household and daycare nursery contacts of index cases of meningococcal meningitis is discussed further in Chapter 5. Rifampin prophylaxis of household contacts of *H. influenzae* meningitis cases is only recommended if there is a susceptible (non-immunized) child in the home. Rifampin is given at a dosage of 20 mg/kg/day div. q.i.d. for 4 days, 600 mg/day for adults and 10 mg/kg/day for neonates.

MENINGOCOCCEMIA

The organism *Neisseria meningitidis* causes illness in humans with a variety of clinical presentations, ranging from benign upper respiratory infection to acute endotoxemia and vasculitis. Chronic disease has also been described. The common signs and symptoms of acute and chronic meningococcemia may initially be subtle, but fever accompanied by a petechial rash should always suggest meningococcal infection. Diagnosis of meningococcemia is made by a characteristic clinical presentation and is usually confirmed by culture (Table 1.31).

Care must be taken to differentiate meningococcemia from other febrile illnesses with rashes. These include septicemia and disseminated intravascular coagulation (DIC) due to other bacteria, endocarditis, Rocky Mountain spotted fever, and enteroviral infections.

Treatment of meningococcemia includes antibiotics and intensive supportive care when shock is present (Table 1.32). In addition, prophylactic treatment of family members and other close contacts of the index case is indicated (Tables 1.33, 1.34).

Table 1.29   Management of meningitis

Initial evaluation
    Lumbar puncture
    Blood culture
    Complete blood and platelet count
    Electrolyte analysis with serum and urine osmolarity (SIADH)
    Blood urea nitrogen (dehydration/renal function)
    Creatinine (dehydration/renal function)
    Glucose (hypoglycemia, comparison with cerebrospinal fluid glucose)
    Arterial blood gases (for shock or severe illness)
Inpatient evaluation
    Chest X-ray
    Prothrombin/partial thromboplastin times
    Liver enzyme analysis
    Serum (to hold; when other diagnoses are considered)
    Urinalysis
Supportive care
    Monitor blood pressure, fluid balance, neurologic and cardiac signs
    Restrict fluids to 75% of maintenance
    Anticonvulsants for seizures
Antibiotics (for dosages see Table 20.11 to 20.16)
    Neonates (birth to 2 months): ampicillin plus cefotaxime, ceftriaxone, or gentamicin
    Infants and children (>2 months): ceftriaxone or cefotaxime plus vancomycin (for resistant *Streptococcus pneumoniae*)
Corticosteroids (particularly if *Haemophilus influenzae* suspected) to prevent deafness and neurologic sequelae. Infants over 2 months; 0.6 mg/kg per day div. q.6h for 4 days – attempt to begin before first dose of antibiotics
Laboratory monitoring
    Complete blood count daily (when disseminated intravascular coagulation (DIC) suspected)
    Electrolytes as indicated (SIADH)
    Renal and liver function as indicated
    Urine sodium and osmolality (SIADH)
    Antibiotic drug levels (aminoglycosides, vancomycin)
    Cerebrospinal fluid (24–48 h into therapy for pneumococcal meningitis in all ages and all neonates)
    Ultrasound prior to discharge
Outpatient follow-up
    2 weeks
        Auditory testing
        Head circumference
        Neurologic examination
    6 weeks, 1 month, 1 year (depending on clinical course)
        Neurologic examination

SIADH, syndrome of inappropriate antidiuretic hormone secretion

PERITONITIS

Acute bacterial peritonitis occurs in two distinct forms as determined by the source of infection (Tables 1.35 and 1.36). Peritonitis should be suspected from the clinical presentation (Table 1.37) and confirmed by laboratory evaluation (Table 1.38).

Table 1.30 Complications of bacterial meningitis

Early complications
  Deafness
  Cerebral edema
  Seizures
  Syndrome of inappropriate antidiuretic
    hormone secretion
  Cranial nerve palsies
  Shock
  Disseminated intravascular coagulation
  Myocarditis
  Pericarditis
  Endocarditis
  Subdural effusion
  Brain abscess

Table 1.31 Laboratory diagnosis of meningococcemia

Complete blood count characteristically shows
  leukocytosis and thrombocytopenia
Cultures (blood, cerebrospinal fluid (CSF), skin
  lesion, nasopharynx)
CSF analysis for evidence of meningitis
Latex agglutination of blood, CSF and urine
Clotting studies for evidence of disseminated intra-
  vascular coagulation (DIC): low prothrombin
  time, fibrinogen, and fibrin split products with
  DIC

Table 1.32 Treatment of meningococcemia

Ceftriaxone 80 mg/kg per day i.v. div. q.d. for
  5–7 days
Aggressive fluid resuscitation for patient in shock
  to replete intravascular volume (see Table 1.54
  for supportive care)
Platelet or clotting factor replacement therapy for
  patient with disseminated intravascular coagulation and hemorrhage
Steroids not shown to improve survival
Burn-type wound care for skin sloughs in areas of
  thrombosis
Hyperbaric oxygen may be useful in wound
  management

Table 1.33 High risk contacts of meningococcal disease

All household contacts
Nursery or day care center contacts
Hospital personnel and individual(s) who had
  intimate exposure to oral secretions from the
  index case

The treatment for bacterial peritonitis is nonoperative for primary peritonitis and operative for secondary peritonitis (Table 1.39). Common postoperative complications include formation of adhesions with subsequent intestinal obstruction and intra-abdominal abscess formation.

RABIES

Rabies is an acute encephalitis caused by a rhabdovirus. Transmitted via secretions, urine or saliva following the bite of an infected animal, the virus passes along peripheral nerves to the central nervous system where neuronal necrosis occurs, principally in the brainstem and medulla. Incubation varies from 10 days to as long as 2 years, with mean onset being within 2 months of the bite (Table 1.40). In the United States most human rabies cases are transmitted by bats as determined by viral strain analysis. There is rarely a known history of exposure to infected animals.

There are two basic presentations of rabies in humans, classic and paralytic. The classic symptom of hydrophobia (Table 1.41) is caused by inspiratory muscle spasms, a consequence of destruction of brainstem neurons inhibitory to neurons of the nucleus ambiguous, which control inspiration.

Diagnosis may be confirmed by demonstration of the antigen, antibody, or viral complexes (Table 1.42). The differential diagnosis of rabies includes other causes of encephalitis and ascending neuritis.

Prevention of rabies includes measures to control the virus reservoir in the animal population as well as vaccination of domestic animals (95% effective). Postexposure treatment of humans also includes human rabies immunoglobulin and human diploid cell vaccine (see Chapter 6). The only true protection, however, is immunity acquired from pre-exposure vaccination.

Once a victim is clinically symptomatic, the prognosis is grim; there have only been three reported survivors. Treatment centers around intensive supportive care so should be given

Table 1.34 Antibiotics for meningococcal prophylaxis

Antibiotic prophylaxis	Dosage	Comments
Rifampin	<1 month: 5 mg/kg twice daily p.o. for 2 days	Contraindicated for pregnant women
	>1 month: 10 mg/kg twice daily p.o. for 2 days (max. 600 mg/dose)	Orange-red urine Stains contact lenses
Ceftriaxone	<12 yr: 125 mg i.m. as single dose	Safe for pregnant women
	>12 yr: 250 mg i.m. as a single dose	Better compliance
Ciprofloxacin	Single adult p.o. dose 500 mg	Contraindicated for pregnant women and children younger than 18 years

Table 1.35 Characteristic forms of peritonitis

Primary form
  Focus of infection outside abdominal cavity
  Infection is blood- or lymph-borne
  Commonly seen in children with ascites
    secondary to nephrosis or cirrhosis
Secondary form
  Infection disseminated by extension from or
    rupture of an intra-abdominal viscus or
    abscess of an intra-abdominal organ

Table 1.36 Bacteriology of peritonitis

Primary peritonitis
  Streptococcus pneumoniae
  Streptococci
  Gram-negative rods
  Mycobacterium tuberculosis
  Haemophilus influenzae
Secondary peritonitis
  Aerobic bacteria
    Escherichia coli
    Streptococci
    Enterococci
    Staphylococcus aureus
    Enterobacteriaceae
    Klebsiella
    Proteus
    Pseudomonas
    Candida
  Anaerobic bacteria
    Bacteroides fragilis
    Eubacteria
    Clostridia
    Peptostreptococci
    Peptococci
    Propionibacteria
    Fusobacteria

Table 1.37 Signs and symptoms of generalized peritonitis

Abdominal pain and tenderness
Edema
Ascites
Fever
Anorexia, vomiting, constipation, or diarrhea
Ileus
Lethargic, toxic-appearing child
Abdominal wall cellulitis

Table 1.38 Laboratory diagnosis of peritonitis

Leukocytosis
Ultrasonographic examination of abdomen
Radiographic examination of abdomen
  Dilation of large and small intestines
  Edema of small intestinal wall
  Peritoneal fluid
  Obliteration of psoas shadow
  Free air within peritoneal cavity (secondary
    peritonitis)
Paracentesis (see Chapter 7)
  Elevated protein concentration
  Pleocytosis (> 800 leukocytes/mm^3, more than
    25% of which are polymorphonuclear leuko-
    cytes)
Positive Gram smear and culture of fluid

Table 1.39 Treatment of peritonitis

Primary peritonitis	
Systemic antibiotics	Ceftriaxone
	Cefotaxime
Secondary peritonitis	
Preoperative disturbances	Correct hypovolemia and stabilize electrolytes to re-establish adequate urine output
	Correct hypoxemia with supplemental oxygen and mechanical ventilation if necessary
	Decompress gastrointestinal tract using nasogastric suction or long intestinal tube
Antibiotic therapy	Ampicillin
	plus
	Clindamycin
	plus
	Ceftriaxone, cefotaxime or gentamicin (dosing increments vary for neonates)
Operative therapy	Close, exclude, or resect perforated viscus followed by either
	Complete exposure of peritoneal cavity with radical debridement of peritoneum, followed by massive irrigation with or without antibiotics or
	Placement of drains after repair of perforation without further exploration or irrigation
Postoperative management	Continued administration of systemic antibiotics
	Intraperitoneal lavage with antibiotic solution
	Attention to repletion of intravascular fluid volume
	Observation for autonomic hyper-reflexia when draining peritoneum
	Nutritional support to meet high metabolic demands
	Close observation for intra-abdominal abscess formation

Table 1.40 Factors affecting time to onset of symptoms in rabies

Distance of site of initial inoculum from central nervous system
Amount of inoculum
Virulence of virus
Resistance of host

in facilities able to provide optional intervention to control the airway and assure ventilation in the patient with hydrophobia or obtundation, as well as circulatory system support.

ROCKY MOUNTAIN SPOTTED FEVER

Rocky Mountain spotted fever is a disease caused by inoculation with *Rickettsia rickettsii*, transmitted via the bite of a tick. The organisms replicate within the endothelial lining and smooth muscle cells of blood vessels, causing generalized vasculitis. Vasculitic changes of various organ systems account for the observed clinical findings (Table 1.43).

The incubation period in children is 1 to 8 days. When early non-specific symptoms appear in a child with a history of a tick bite, Rocky Mountain spotted fever should be seriously considered and early treatment instituted. Most laboratory findings in Rocky

Table 1.41 Symptoms of the classic form of rabies

Prodrome (2 days to 2 weeks)	Malaise, anorexia, headache, fever, irritability, pain, numbness or tingling at site of bite spreading upward. Later symptoms; jerky movements, pupillary dilatation, increased tearing and salivation
Acute neurologic phase (2–7 days)	Dysphagia, hydrophobia, mania (alternating with lethargy), increased salivation, abnormal biting and chewing, excitement, fear, apathy, terror, convulsive movements, choking, distended bladder, constipation, penile pain
Final phase (7–10 days)	Coma, dysrhythmias, hypotension, heart block, bradycardia, respiratory muscle spasm, hypoventilation, disturbance in fluid balance, metabolic upsets, cardiorespiratory arrest

Table 1.42 Diagnosis of rabies

Identification of antigen on cell culture
    Electron microscopy
    Immunofluorescent rabies-antibody staining
Antibody titers
    Diagnostic in nonvaccinated persons
    Cerebrospinal fluid titers to diagnose
        postvaccination encephalomyelitis
Viral complexes
    Corneal touch preparations
    Fluorescent antibody staining of parafollicular
        neurons of neck skin biopsy

Table 1.43 Clinical findings in Rocky Mountain spotted fever

History of tick bite (70–80% of cases)
Fever
Headache
Anorexia
Chills
Sore throat
Nausea and vomiting
Abdominal pain
Mild diarrhea
Arthralgias and myalgias
Rash
    Petechial but may begin as macular or maculo-
        papular rash, blanching lesions, affects
        extremities first, spreads centripetally,
        occasionally appears later (or not at all)
Noncardiogenic pulmonary edema
Occasional manifestations
    Edema (periorbital early, generalized later),
        splenomegaly in one-third of cases,
        hepatomegaly, pneumonitis, myocardial
        involvement, conjunctivitis, photophobia,
        papilledema, transient deafness,
        meningismus, delirium, seizures, coma

Mountain spotted fever are nonspecific until positive convalescent titers appear (Table 1.44). The exception to this is the appearance of the organism on skin lesion stains or by use of immunofluorescent biopsy of skin for early specific diagnosis.

It is difficult to differentiate Rocky Mountain spotted fever from the myriad other causes of febrile exanthemas. Its diagnosis is also frequently overlooked in patients who do not present with the typical rash or in whom a history of tick bite cannot be elicited (Table 1.45).

Treatment of Rocky Mountain spotted fever should be instituted as soon as the diagnosis is suspected clinically (Table 1.46). In addition to antibiotic therapy, careful supportive intensive care is needed with aggressive intervention necessary to stabilize the most severely ill patients.

SEPTIC SHOCK

No other problem is encountered as commonly in pediatric intensive care as sepsis. The diagnosis of sepsis in the child, particularly without an obvious source of infection, requires a high degree of suspicion (Tables 1.47 and 1.48).

Progressing sepsis usually results in multiple organ system involvement and subsequent system failure (Table 1.49). Septic shock is encountered in a number of severe cases of sepsis, most commonly with Gram-negative infections (Table 1.50). The cause and progression of unchecked septic shock are outlined in Table 1.51.

Table 1.44   Laboratory studies in Rocky Mountain spotted fever

Type of study	Result
White blood cell count	Normal or slightly decreased with left shift in first week; leukocytosis in second week
Platelet count	Depressed
Fibrinogen	Depressed with disseminated intravascular coagulation
Electrolytes	Hyponatremia and hypochloremia
Liver function tests	Elevated AST (asparate aminotransferase), ALT (alanine aminotransferase) and bilirubin; depressed total protein and albumin
Creatinine	Increased
Lactate dehydrogenase	Increased
Urinalysis	Hematuria
Cerebrospinal fluid	White blood cell count <300/mm^3, predominantly lymphocytes in most cases; normal glucose; mildly elevated protein
Weil–Felix reaction	Proteus OX-19 and OX-2 single titer >1:160 or 4-fold rise in titer diagnostic
Rocky Mountain spotted fever complement fixation titers	Convalescent titers may increase after 14 days of illness
Giemsa stain of skin lesion	May demonstrate organism
Immunofluorescent biopsy of skin	Possible to make diagnosis using this technique

Table 1.45   Differential diagnosis of Rocky Mountain spotted fever

Ehrlichiosis
Meningococcemia
Measles
Enteroviral infections
Typhoid fever
Endemic murine typhus
Rickettsialpox
Colorado tick fever
Tularemia
Immune-complex vasculitis
Collagen vascular diseases
Thrombotic thrombocytopenic purpura
Idiopathic thrombocytopenic purpura

Table 1.46   Treatment of Rocky Mountain spotted fever

Tetracycline (25 mg/kg per day) or chloramphenicol (100 mg/kg per day) i.v. div. q.6h for 10 days

Fluid management with replacement (as needed) of intravascular volume, lost to third spacing, in order to restore circulation

Mechanical ventilation and positive end expiratory pressure may be needed to correct hypoxemia from noncardiogenic pulmonary edema

Replacement of platelets and clotting factors in cases with disseminated intravascular coagulation and associated hemorrhage

Present and future understanding of the role of nitric oxide and endothelial defects caused by Rocky Mountain spotted fever may lead to new treatment regimens

Table 1.47 Clinical findings in presumed septicemia

Fever and chills (or hypothermia)
Toxic appearance
Poor peripheral perfusion (cold extremities)
Shock
Disseminated intravascular coagulation
Multi-organ failure
Documented source of infection
Host predisposition

Table 1.48 Clinical syndromes commonly associated with sepsis in children

Primary bacteremia
  Newborns
  Compromised host Malignancy, immuno-deficiency syndrome, immunosuppressive drug therapy
  Normal children Meningococcemia, pneumococcemia, *Staphylococcus aureus* or ß-hemolytic streptococcal septicemia
Secondary bacteremia
  Secondary to remote infection Meningitis, osteomyelitis, septic arthritis, pneumonia, orbital cellulitis, wound infection, intestinal obstruction, pyelonephritis, burns, diarrhea
  Secondary to operation or instrumentation

Table 1.49 Effects of sepsis on organ systems

Organ/system	Effect of sepsis
Hematologic	Granulocytosis, thrombocytopenia, disseminated intravascular coagulation
Pulmonary	Acute respiratory distress syndrome
Renal	Oliguria, acute renal insufficiency
Cardiac	Hypotension, myocardial depression (late)
Hepatic	Elevation of serum glutamic oxalo-acetic transaminase, glutamic pyruvic transaminate and bilirubin
Brain	Altered level of consciousness or confusion (especially with hypotension)

Table 1.50 Incidence of shock with bacteremia

Organism causing bacteremia	Percentage with shock
Gram-negative bacilli	40–45
Staphylococcus aureus	25–35
Streptococcus pneumoniae	10–15

TETANUS

Tetanus is caused by inoculation with the organism *Clostridium tetani*, which exists in both vegetative and sporulated forms. Spores introduced into a wound may convert into the vegetative form that produce a potent exotoxin, tetanospasmin, which affects the nervous system in several ways. The incubation period for the development of tetanus varies from 3 days to 3 weeks. There are four forms of the disease with distinct presentations (Table 1.55). Generalized tetanus is the most common. Cephalic tetanus is unusual and is seen following otitis media or injuries to the head and face.

Management of septicemia in children and empiric antibiotic therapy for presumed septicemia of unknown etiology are summarized in Tables 1.52 and 1.53. A general outline for treatment of septic shock should follow the familiar ABCs of cardiopulmonary resuscitation (Table 1.54).

Table 1.51 Progression of septic shock

Early symptoms
  Fever
  Increased VO_2
  Increased cardiac output
  Normal A VdO_2
Followed by
  'Warm' shock
  Vasodilatation
  Decreased systemic vascular resistance
  Redistribution of blood volume
  Decreased ventricular preload
  Increased cardiac output
  Hypotension
  Wide pulse pressure
  Oliguria
  Hypoxemia
Progressing to
  Generalized capillary leak
  Further decreased ventricular preload
  Hypotension
  Edema
  Acute respiratory distress syndrome
  Multiple organ system dysfunction
Late symptoms
  Oxygen extraction failure
  Decreased VO_2 and A VdO_2
  Increased cardiac output
Progressing to
  'Cold' shock
  Vasoconstriction
  Increased systemic vascular resistance
  Release of myocardial depressant factor
  Poor coronary perfusion
  Decreased cardiac output
  Increased A VdO_2
  Lactic acidosis
Progressing to death

VO_2, oxygen consumption; A VdO_2, arterio-venous dissolved oxygen

Table 1.52 Management of septicemia in children

Attempt to identify source of infection
  Careful physical examination, cultures, and
    radiographs as needed
Antibiotics
Surgical exploration and/or drainage if indicated
Monitoring for development of multiple organ
    system failure
  Arterial blood pressure monitoring
  Accurate recording of fluid balance (hourly)
  Neurological checks to assess level of
    consciousness (hourly)
  Frequent arterial blood gas determination and
    observation for signs of respiratory distress
  Determination of white blood cell and platelet
    count, hematocrit, and liver and renal func-
    tion tests may be desirable daily during acute
    phase of illness

Table 1.53 Initial antibiotic therapy for presumed septicemia of unknown source

Patient	Therapy
Neonatal	Ampicillin plus Cefotaxime, ceftriaxone, or gentamicin
Pediatric	Ceftriaxone or cefotaxime plus Vancomycin plus Clindamycin* (when group A streptococcus suspected)
Immunocompromised host	Ticarillin plus Tobramycin plus Vancomycin

* See tables 20.11 to 20.16 for antibiotic dosages

Neonatal tetanus usually presents in the first week of life after a contaminated delivery.

The diagnosis of tetanus is essentially a clinical diagnosis with a history of injury, followed by development of the symptoms described in Table 1.55. Laboratory findings are non-specific in most cases of tetanus.

Treatment of tetanus focuses on removal of the source of the toxin, neutralization of the toxin, and supportive care until the toxin (which is fixed to neural tissue) is metabolized (Table 1.56). The average mortality of tetanus is 50%, with even greater mortality for neonates. Recovery from

Table 1.54   Treatment of septic shock

Airway oxygenation
    Endotracheal intubation
    Mechanical ventilation with supplemental oxygen
    Positive end expiratory pressure as needed to correct hypoxemia if adult
       respiratory distress syndrome is present
    Goal is maintenance of over 95% arterial oxyhemoglobin saturation

Cardiac output
    Transfusion of packed red blood cells as needed to assure optimal red cell mass for adequate tissue
       oxygen delivery
    Optimize ventricular preload using fluid resuscitation with isotonic crystalloid solution or colloid
       (20 ml/kg over 20 min) repeated as needed until circulation has stabilized or CVP>10 mmHg or
       PCWP>12 mmHg
    Correct acidosis with bicarbonate if pH<7.2 (0.3 × base deficit x weight (kg))
    Correct hypocalcemia if present
    Inotropic support indicated if ventricular preload has already been optimized and cardiac output is still
       insufficient to meet tissue oxygen demands
    Vasoactive agents as needed to maintain normal systemic vascular resistance

Steroids
    Efficacy in septic shock still not established in children

Access and monitoring lines
    Intravenous line
    Intra-arterial line
    CVP or PCWP lines
    Urinary catheter
    Nasogastric tube (to buffer gastric pH)

Developing treatments
    Monoclonal antibodies
    Antitumor necrosis antibody
    Nitric oxide scavengers/nitric oxidase inhibitors
    Pentoxyphylline
    Naloxone and other opiate antagonists

CVP, central venous pressure; PCWP, pulmonary capillary wedge pressure

tetanus does not confer immunity and prevention is best accomplished by active immunization.

TOXIC SHOCK SYNDROME

Group A, ß-hemolytic streptococci (GABHS) and *Staphylococcus aureus* are causative agents of this syndrome. Toxic shock syndrome (TSS) is an illness seen in all age groups, though it is more commonly found in the clinical settings of antecedent fasciitis (GABHS), chickenpox (GABHS) or in young menstruating women (*S. aureus*). Shock is the result of exotoxins produced by these organisms (Tables 1.57 to 1.62).

Table 1.55 Clinical manifestations of tetanus

Localized tetanus
  Pain, continuous rigidity and spasm of muscles
    in proximity to site of injury

Generalized tetanus
  Trismus
  Dysphagia
  Restlessness
  Irritability
  Headache
  Risus sardonicus
  Tonic contractions of somatic musculature
  Opisthotonus
  Tetanic seizures
  Spasm of laryngeal and respiratory muscles
    with airway obstruction
  Urinary retention
  Fever
  Hyperhydrosis
  Tachycardia
  Hypertension
  Cardiac arrhythmias

Cephalic tetanus
  Dysfunction of cranial nerves III, IV, VII, IX,
    X and XI

Tetanus neonatorum
  Difficulty in sucking
  Excessive crying
  Dysphagia
  Opisthotonus
  Spasms

Table 1.56 Treatment of tetanus

Antitoxin
  Tetanus immunoglobulin (3–6000 U i.m.);
    begin tetanus toxoid active immunization

Antibiotics
  Parenteral penicillin G (200 000 U/kg per day)
    or tetracycline (30–40 mg/kg per day) for
    10–14 days to eliminate vegetative forms of
    Clostridium tetani

Surgical wound care

Supportive measures
  Decrease external stimuli (noise, light)
  Endotracheal intubation or tracheostomy as
    needed to protect against laryngospasm and
    aspiration
  Sedation
  Barbiturates, muscle relaxants, or non-polarizing
    neuromuscular blocking agents to decrease
    severity of muscle spasms
  Assure adequate ventilation, using mechanical
    ventilator if needed
  Treatment of sympathetic nervous system
    overactivity (extreme hypertension and
    tachycardia) with cautious use of ß-and/or
    α-adrenergic blockers
  Nutritional support

Table 1.57 Incubation period for staphylococcal toxic shock syndrome

Clinical setting	Onset of symptoms
Menstruation	1–11 days after vaginal bleeding begins
Surgical wounds	2 days after surgery
Skin, subcutaneous soft tissue, wound, or osseous infection	1 day to 8 weeks after inoculation
Postpartum and postabortion	1 day to 8 weeks after delivery/abortion

Table 1.58 Clinical manifestations of toxic shock syndrome

Signs	Symptoms
Rash	Myalgia
Desquamation	Vomiting
Fever	Dizziness
Hypotension	Sore throat
Pharyngitis	Headache
Strawberry tongue	Diarrhea
Conjunctivitis	Arthralgia
Vaginitis	Cough
Edema	
Confusion	
Agitation	
Somnolence	
Polyarthritis	

Table 1.59 Criteria for diagnosis of toxic shock syndrome

Body temperature ≥ 38.9°C
Diffuse macular erythroderma or polymorphic maculopapular rash
Desquamation of palms or soles 1–2 weeks after onset of illness
Hypotension: systolic BP ≤ 90 mmHg (adults) or <5th percentile by age (children under 16 years), or orthostatic dizziness or syncope
Involvement of three or more of the following organ systems:
    Gastrointestinal
        Vomiting or diarrhea at onset of illness
    Hepatic
        Total bilirubin, SGOT, or SGPT over twice upper normal value
    Hematologic
        Platelet count ≤ 100 000/mm^3
    Mucous membrane
        Conjunctival, pharyngeal, or vaginal hyperemia
    Muscular
        Severe myalgia or creatine phosphokinase over twice upper normal value
    Renal
        ≥ 5 white blood cells per high power field, or blood urea nitrogen or creatinine over twice upper normal value
    Neurologic
        Disorientation or altered level of consciousness without focal neurologic signs when fever and hypotension absent
    Metabolic
        Decreased total serum protein, albumin, calcium, and/or phosphorus
Reasonable evidence for absence of other bacterial, viral, or rickettsial infections, drug reactions, or autoimmune disorders

SGOT, serum glutamic oxalo-acetic transaminase; SGPT, serum glutamic pyruvic transaminase

Table 1.60 Laboratory abnormalities in toxic shock syndrome

High serum creatinine
Elevated serum creatine phosphokinase
Low serum calcium
Low serum phosphorus
Low total serum protein
Hypoalbuminemia
Leukocytosis with left shift
Anemia
Thrombocytopenia
Elevation of liver function results (bilirubin, AST (aspartate aminotransferase), ALT (alanine aminotransferase), prothrombin time)
Pyuria

Table 1.61 Factors associated with increased risk for toxic shock syndrome

Staphylococcal
   Previous history of vaginal infection
   Similar illness during a previous menstrual period
   Use of tampons, particularly highly absorbent brands
Streptococcal
   Fasciitis
   Chickenpox
   Pharyngitis
   Pelvic infection

Table 1.62 Treatment for toxic shock syndrome

Supportive intensive care – see Septic Shock (Table 1.54)
Antibiotics (clindamycin plus penicillin for streptococcus; oxacillin, nafcillin or vancomycin for staphylcoccus)
Discontinue tampon use
Steroids (use remains controversial)

Neonatal infections

2

BACTERIAL INFECTIONS

Serious bacterial infections are more common in the neonatal period than at any other time in life, in large part as a consequence of immature host defense mechanisms. During the first 28 days of life, the incidence of sepsis is reported to be as high as 8 cases per thousand live births with 20–25% of these having associated meningitis. With advances in neonatal intensive care and antibiotic therapy, mortality rates for such infections have been lowered to 5–20%.

Neonatal sepsis can be divided into early-onset and late-onset, each having distinct features (Table 2.1). Late onset neonatal sepsis typically affects previously well infants who have been discharged from the hospital.

Early clinical manifestations of neonatal sepsis are frequently non-specific and subtle, often showing overlap with non-infectious diseases. Perinatal factors (Table 2.2) can be helpful in identifying which infants are at greatest risk for infection. Prematurity markedly increases risk.

Clinical manifestations of neonatal sepsis (Table 2.3) are variable in their occurrence and involve many different organ systems.

Laboratory studies can be helpful during initial clinical evaluation. Despite many attempts to develop more sensitive and specific rapid laboratory tests for infection, the white blood cell (WBC) count and differential remain the most frequently used screening studies. Neutropenia, especially an absolute neutrophil count below 1800/mm³, or an immature to total neutrophil ratio above 0.2 in the first 24 h of life are suggestive of infection. Leukocytosis with WBC count above 25 000/mm³ may also result from infection, but is more often associated with non-infectious causes. Other hematologic

Table 2.1 Common features of early-onset vs. late-onset neonatal sepsis

Feature	Early onset	Late onset
Time	0–7 days	Beyond 7 days
Perinatal risk factors	High	Possible
Source of organism	Maternal genital tract	Environment
Progress of infection	Fulminant	Insidious
Meningitis present	Moderate	High

Table 2.2 Perinatal risk factors for bacterial infection

Prematurity
Low birthweight
Prolonged rupture of membranes
Maternal fever
Maternal urinary tract infection
Chorioamnionitis
Maternal group B streptococcal colonization
Fetal distress
Perinatal asphyxia
Male gender
Low socioeconomic status

Table 2.3 Clinical manifestations of neonatal sepsis

Temperature instability
  Hypothermia
  Hyperthermia
Respiratory distress
  Tachypnea
  Retractions
  Grunting
  Nasal flaring
  Apnea
Feeding disturbances
  Poor suck
  Vomiting
  Gastric residuals
  Abdominal distention
  Diarrhea
CNS dysfunction
  Lethargy
  Irritability
  Seizures
Cardiovascular
  Tachycardia
  Bradycardia
  Cyanosis
  Pallor
  Hypotension
Hematologic
  Bruising
  Petechiae
  Bleeding
  Jaundice

findings include thrombocytopenia, WBC vacuolization and toxic granulations.

An elevation in the C-reactive protein has gained increasing clinical utilization as a predictor for infection. Rapid antigen tests, such as latex-particle agglutination or countercurrent immunoelectrophoresis, can be helpful as supporting evidence for infection, but false positive results have limited their use. Cultures of blood and cerebrospinal fluid should be obtained from all neonates with suspected sepsis, although clinical judgement must be used in determining the safety of lumbar puncture in infants at risk for respiratory compromise or preterm infants at risk for intraventricular hemorrhage. Tracheal aspirate cultures are useful when available in infants with respiratory symptoms, although endotracheal tube colonization is inevitable with prolonged intubation. Urine culture is of limited use in the evaluation of early-onset infection, but is very useful in late-onset infection. Urine for culture should be obtained by suprapubic aspiration of the bladder when possible. Cultures of the gastric aspirate and skin may reflect the infant's bacterial colonization at birth, but do not always correlate with systemic infection. Chest X-ray is indicated in infants with respiratory distress as a screen for both pneumonia and non-infectious causes.

Normal values for cerebrospinal fluid in neonates differ from those in older infants. Cerebrospinal fluid WBC counts as high as $30/mm^3$, protein values as high as 170 mg/dl, and glucose values as low as 24 mg/dl may be normal in the neonatal period.

Etiology

Early-onset neonatal infections are typically transmitted vertically from the mother to the infant. Organisms can be acquired transplacentally, via infected amniotic fluid, or by direct contact in passage through the birth canal. Group B streptococci and *Escherichia coli* cause most infections, but a number of other organisms may be involved (Table 2.4). Late-onset infection typically involves group B streptococci, although Gram-negative organisms and *Listeria* sp. may also be involved.

Prevention of group B streptococcal disease

Group B streptococcus is the most common cause of neonatal sepsis, with an incidence of up to 4 per 1000 live births, which is increased to one per 50 preterm infants weighing less than 2000 g. While there is ongoing debate over the optimal method for prevention of early onset group B streptococcal disease, the American Academy of Pediatrics in conjunction with the American College of Obstetrics and Gynecology and others put forth a consensus statement on the use of intrapartum chemoprophylaxis in 1997 (Table 2.5).

Table 2.4 Bacterial etiology of neonatal infection

Organism	Incidence (%)
Group B streptococci	35–40
Other Gram-positive cocci	20–25
Staphylococcus sp.	
Enterococcus sp.	
Other streptococci	
Escherichia coli	20
Other Gram-negative enterics	10–15
Klebsiella sp.	
Haemophilus sp.	
Pseudomonas sp.	
Listeria monocytogenes	1–2

Intravenous penicillin G (5 million units initially, then 2.5 million units every 4 h) is the preferred method for intrapartum prophylaxis. Ampicillin or other broader spectrum drugs may be used based on additional maternal indications (urinary tract infection or chorioamnionitis). Intravenous clindamycin or erythromycin may be used for mothers allergic to penicillin. Management of the infant whose mother has received intrapartum prophylaxis for group B streptococcal infection should be individualized, but the algorithm in Table 2.6 has been suggested.

Management of neonatal sepsis

Because of the high morbidity associated with delayed therapy for neonatal sepsis, empiric antibiotic therapy should be initiated for any neonate with suspected sepsis after appropriate cultures have been obtained;

Table 2.5 Two prevention strategies for early onset Group B streptococcal (GBS) infection

(1) Screening method	
Risk factors present?	If yes to any, intrapartum penicillin
Prior infant with GBS disease	
GBS bacteruria this pregnancy	
Delivery < 37 weeks' gestation	
Maternal GBS screen at 35–37 weeks (rectal & vaginal swab)	If yes, intrapartum penicillin
GBS screen results unavailable and maternal risk factors present (Temp ≥ 38°C or membranes ruptured ≥ 18 h)	If yes, intrapartum penicillin
GBS screen negative	No prophylaxis
(2) Risk factor method	
Risk factor present?	If yes to any, intrapartum penicillin
Prior infant with GBS disease GBS bacteruria this pregnancy Delivery < 37 weeks' gestation Membranes ruptured ≥ 18 h Maternal temp ≥ 38°C	If no to all, no prophylaxis

Table 2.6 Management of an infant born to a mother who received intrapartum antimicrobial prophylaxis

Signs and symptoms of sepsis	Full diagnostic evaluation: complete blood count, differential, blood culture, consider chest X-ray and lumbar puncture
	Empiric antibiotic therapy
Gestational age < 35 weeks or Less than 2 doses antibiotics given to mother	Limited evaluation (complete blood count, differential, blood culture) Observe for 48 h If sepsis suspected, full evaluation and therapy
2 or more doses of antibiotics given to mother	No evaluation No therapy
< 32 weeks' gestation	Full diagnostic evaluation and therapy pending results of cultures

Table 2.7 Management of suspected neonatal sepsis

Suspected sepsis based on clinical signs and perinatal risk factors	Complete blood count, chest X-ray Blood and cerebrospinal fluid (CSF) cultures Tracheal and urine cultures (if appropriate) Empiric antibiotic therapy
Positive CSF cultures	Antibiotics for 21 days
Positive blood/urine cultures	Antibiotics for 10–14 days
Pneumonia	Antibiotics for 10–14 days
Negative cultures	
High suspicion remains	Antibiotics for 7–10 days
Low suspicion	Discontinue antibiotics at 48–72 h

however, antibiotic administration should not be delayed owing to difficulty or inability to obtain the appropriate specimens for culture. Because of the relatively low incidence of neonatal sepsis coupled with the uncertainties in making a definite diagnosis, a majority of infants who are treated for suspected sepsis will not have this condition. Empiric antibiotics are chosen to treat the most common pathologic organisms. Typical antibiotic choices are ampicillin to provide therapy against Gram-positive organisms (group B streptococci, *Listeria* sp., and enterococcus) coupled with an aminoglycoside (gentamicin most commonly) or a third generation cephalosporin (cefotaxime or ceftriaxone) to provide therapy against Gram-negative organisms. Aminoglycoside concentrations must be monitored to prevent toxicity. Third generation cephalosporins have less toxicity, but present greater problems with alteration of normal flora and selection of resistant organisms. Ceftriaxone should be avoided in infants with significant hyperbilirubinemia as it may displace bilirubin from albumin binding sites. When culture and sensitivity results are available, antibiotic choices should be adjusted to provide more specific therapy (Table 2.7).

In addition to antibiotic therapy, supportive care of the infected neonate is essential. Close attention to respiratory, cardiovascular, fluid and electrolyte, and hematologic support are essential to optimize outcome. Adjunctive immunologic therapies continue to be investigated. WBC transfusions have been beneficial in some infants with severe neutropenia, but are often not readily accomplished. Therapy with granulocyte colony stimulating factor (G-CSF, Filgrastim) in neonatal sepsis with associated neutropenia has resulted in increased neutrophil counts, but its effect on outcome requires further study. Similarly, the efficacy of intravenous immunoglobulin therapy to treat or prevent neonatal sepsis remains undetermined.

CONGENITAL INFECTIONS

Congenital infections with non-bacterial pathogens can result in significant morbidity and mortality. TORCH has been used as an acronym for what were once the more common pathogens involved in congenital infections – *Toxoplasma* sp., rubella virus, cytomegalovirus (CMV), and herpes simplex virus (actually a perinatal infection). Changing incidence of the common pathogens involved in congenital infections, however, have made the TORCH acronym less useful. CMV is the most common agent involved in congenital infection, estimated to infect 1 to 2% of all newborns in the United States. Increased prevalence of sexually transmitted diseases

such as syphilis and human immunodeficiency virus (HIV) has resulted in increasing numbers of newborns infected with these pathogens, while screening and immunization for rubella have all but eliminated this pathogen as a cause of congenital infection. Herpes can occasionally manifest as a congenital infection with growth retardation and deep dermal scars, but it occurs more frequently as a perinatally acquired infection.

Clinical manifestations of congenital infection are variable, but there is considerable overlap between different pathogens (Table 2.8). Clinical manifestations which should arouse suspicion for congenital infection include intrauterine growth restriction, microcephaly, hepatosplenomegaly, anemia, and thrombocytopenia. It should be noted, however, that most cases of intrauterine growth restriction and microcephaly are not caused by infection.

When a congenital infection is suspected, appropriate laboratory studies should be performed (Table 2.9). Because of the limited blood volume in a neonate, judicious use of the available laboratory studies is required. Before initiating such tests on the infant, a close review of available maternal history is essential.

Table 2.8   Clinical manifestations of congenital infections

	CMV	Syphilis	Toxoplasmosis	Rubella
IUGR	+ +	+	+	+ +
Microcephaly	+ +	–	+	+
Hydrocephaly	+	+	+	+
Intracranial calcifications	+ +	–	+ +	–
Hepatosplenomegaly	+ +	+ +	+ +	+ +
Jaundice	+ +	+ +	+ +	+
Anemia	+	+ +	+ +	+
Thrombocytopenia	+ +	+ +	+	+ +
Petechiae/purpura	+ +	+ +	+	+ +
Cataracts	+	–	–	+ +
Chorioretinitis	+	+	+ +	+
Deafness	+ +	+	+	+ +
Cardiac defects	–	–	–	+ +
Bone lesions	–	+	–	+ +

CMV, cytomegalovirus; IUGR, intrauterine growth restriction;
+ +, prominent manifestation; +, occasionally seen; –, not a manifestation

Toxoplasmosis

Congenital toxoplasmosis occurs in approximately 1 in 1000 deliveries in the United States as a result of transplacental acquisition of *Toxoplasma gondii* during maternal primary infection. Most infected infants are asymptomatic at birth but may develop symptoms later in infancy. Chorioretinitis occurs in over 80% of infected infants. Other common clinical manifestations are listed in Table 2.8. Diagnosis can be confirmed by testing for IgM to toxoplasma; isolation of this protozoan is difficult. Major sequelae of infection are neurologic problems including seizures, mental retardation, and deafness. Treatment of the infant (Table 2.10) may limit adverse sequelae.

Hepatitis B virus

Hepatitis B virus can be spread transplacentally, but the majority of affected infants are exposed at the time of birth. In the United States, almost 1% of pregnant women test positive for hepatitis B surface antigen (HBsAg). Hepatitis B infection in the neonate may result in acute hepatitis, but more worrisome is the very high likelihood of infected infants becoming chronic carriers with increased risks for cirrhosis and hepatocellular carcinoma.

Because of the high prevalence and chance for adverse outcome in infected neonates, universal screening of all pregnant women is recommended. All infants should receive the hepatitis B vaccine, and infants born to HBsAg positive mothers should also be passively immunized with hepatitis B immune globulin. After such passive and active immunization, breastfeeding for infants born to HBsAg positive mothers poses no additional risk of infection. Management of hepatitis B is shown in Table 2.11.

Hepatitis C virus

Hepatitis C virus is transmitted in similar fashion to hepatitis B virus. Seroprevalence of hepatitis C in pregnant women in the United States is 1–2%, with maternal–fetal

Table 2.9 Laboratory evaluation of suspected congenital infection

Initial studies on neonate
  Blood: complete blood count, IgM, VDRL, toxoplasmosis and rubella serologies (IgG and IgM), extra serum to 'hold'
  Urine: CMV culture
  CSF: cell count, protein, glucose, VDRL, Gram stain, bacterial and viral cultures
  X-ray: long bones, skull series

Studies on mother
  Blood: VDRL and rubella serology (if not done), toxoplasmosis serology, extra serum to 'hold'
  Cervix: consider culture for herpes simplex and CMV

Additional studies when organism highly suspected
  CMV: culture of pharynx, biopsy and culture of involved organ (liver, lung), acute and convalescent sera for antibody
  Syphilis: MHA-TP, FTA-ABS, convalescent serum for VDRL
  Toxoplasmosis: special serologic studies on neonate and mother
  Rubella: culture of placenta, pharynx, urine and stool
  Herpes simplex: cytologic exam (Giemsa, fluorescence or Tzanck smear) and viral culture of skin or mucosal lesions
  HIV: HIV antibody on mother and infant, blood for PCR antigen or HIV culture on infant (See Chapter 17)

CMV, cytomegalovirus

Table 2.10 Treatment of congenital toxoplasmosis

Pyrimethamine 1 mg/kg/day p.o.
plus
Sulfadiazine 100 mg/kg/day p.o. divided q.6h for 28 days or longer (up to 6 months)
Folinic acid (Leucovorin calcium) 5 mg every 3 days during pyrimethamine therapy to prevent hematologic problems
Corticosteroids may be helpful during the inflammatory stages of this illness (elevated CSF protein, chorioretinitis)
No special isolation is required

transmission rates ranging from zero to 25%. Routine screening for hepatitis C in pregnancy is not recommended, but if a mother has risk factors (blood transfusion, intravenous

Table 2.11 Management of hepatitis B in neonates

Hepatitis B vaccine to all infants at 0–2, 1–4, and
  6–12 months
Hepatitis B immune globulin 0.5 ml i.m. and
  vaccine within 12 h of birth to infants born to
  HBsAg positive mothers and premature
  neonates < 2000 g whose mother's HBsAg
  status is unknown

HBsAg, hepatitis B surface antigen

drug abuse, or other repeated exposure to percutaneous or mucosal blood), screening should be performed. The risk of maternal–fetal transmission is increased for mothers with HIV infection. Infants born to mothers with hepatitis C virus should be screened for infection postnatally. Antibody tests may give false positive results for up to 12 months as a result of transplacentally derived antibodies, and accurate antigen tests for hepatitis C are in development. Transmission of hepatitis C by breastfeeding is possible, although such transmission has not been documented.

Human immunodeficiency virus

Human immunodeficiency virus (HIV) is the etiologic agent of acquired immunodeficiency syndrome and can be spread from an infected mother to her neonate. Transmission may occur by transplacental spread or by exposure to maternal blood and secretions at the time of delivery. Earlier estimates were higher but it now appears that infection occurs in less than 25% of infants born to infected mothers. Transplacentally acquired antibody to HIV results in all infants born to seropositive mothers testing positive for HIV antibody at birth. Uninfected infants should be seronegative in follow-up testing by 15 months of age. More sensitive early diagnostic methods such as polymerase chain reaction (PCR), viral culture, and p24 antigen are currently recommended as methods for identifying infected infants (see Chapter 17).

Most infected newborns are normal at birth, with symptoms developing in the first year of life. The efficacy of pre- and postnatal antiviral therapy has now been well documented. Cesarean section delivery may result in an additive reduction to the risk of vertical transmission. Since HIV can be transmitted via breast milk, infants of infected mothers should be formula fed.

Syphilis

Congenital syphilis infections have had a resurgence in recent years owing to the illicit drug epidemic. Transplacental passage of this spirochete may result in fetal wastage, non-immune hydrops, or postnatal manifestations such as snuffles, rash, hepatitis and osteochondritis/periostitis. If untreated, late manifestations include neurosyphilis, deafness, and dental and bone abnormalities.

Infants may be infected with syphilis at birth and be asymptomatic, thus evaluation of maternal serology and therapy is essential to identify such infants and prevent subsequent complications. An infant should be evaluated for congenital syphilis if he or she is symptomatic or with active disease as determined by radiographic studies or the mother has a positive nontreponemal test confirmed by a treponemal test and one or more of the following:

  not treated;
  penicillin dose inadequate or unknown;
  treated with any antibiotic other than
    penicillin; treated during the last month
    of pregnancy;
  less than four-fold decrease in serologic
    screening assay following treatment.

Serology may involve a nontreponemal test (e.g. VDRL, ART, RPR) and a subsequent confirmatory treponemal test (e.g. MHA-TP, FTA-ABS). Nontreponemal tests provide quantitative titers to correlate with disease activity; treponemal tests provide confirmation of positive nontreponemal results, but remain reactive for life despite adequate therapy (see Chapter 16).

Evaluation of infants at risk should include physical examination, nontreponemal screening assay, MHA-TP or FTA-ABS, lumbar puncture, long bone X-rays, and chest roentgenogram (see Chapter 16). Cerebrospinal fluid findings suggestive of neurosyphilis include leukocytosis, elevated protein, or positive VDRL. Treatment should follow Table 2.12.

Treated infants and seropositive untreated infants of treated mothers should be followed closely with repeat nontreponemal serology at 3, 6 and 12 months of age for evidence of declining nontreponemal titers. Most infants who have been effectively treated will have negative nontreponemal serology by 6 months of age. If titers fail to decline, the infant should be re-evaluated and treated. Infants with abnormal cerebrospinal fluid (CSF) findings should have repeat CSF evaluations every 6 months until normal, with repeat treatment indicated for persistent evidence of neurosyphilis.

Varicella-zoster virus

Varicella-zoster virus can result in congenital infection with variable expression depending on the timing of maternal infection. Maternal

Table 2.12 Treatment for congenital syphilis

Neonates with	
physical examination or X-ray evidence of active disease, or abnormal cerebrospinal fluid (CSF) findings, or nontreponemal titers four-fold or greater than mother's, or maternal treatment absent, unknown, undocumented, non-penicillin, or within 1 month of delivery, or undocumented fall in maternal nontreponemal titers, or negative work-up but uncertain follow-up after discharge	
Age < 4 weeks, normal CSF	Aqueous crystalline penicillin G 100–150 000 U/kg/day i.v. or i.m. div. b.i.d. (< 7 days of age) or t.i.d. (> 7 days) for 10 days or Procaine penicillin 50 000 U/kg/day i.m. div. q.d. for 10 days
Age < 4 weeks, abnormal CSF	Aqueous crystalline penicillin G 100–150 000 U/kg/day i.v. div. b.i.d. (< 7 days) or t.i.d. (> 7 days) for 10 days
Age > 4 wk to 1 yr, normal CSF	Aqueous crystalline penicillin G 200 000 U/kg/day i.v. div. q.i.d. for 10 days
Age > 4 wk to 1 yr, abnormal CSF	Aqueous crystalline penicillin G 200 000 U/kg/day i.v. div. q.i.d. for 10 days followed by benzathine penicillin G 50 000 U/kg i.m. weekly x 3
Age > 1 yr normal CSF	Benzathine penicillin G 50 000 U/kg i.m. weekly x 3
Age > 1 yr abnormal CSF	Aqueous crystalline penicillin G 200–300 000 U/kg/day i.v. or i.m. div. q.i.d. for 10 days followed by benzathine penicillin G 50 000 U/kg i.m. weekly x 3

varicella infection in the first 20 weeks of pregnancy can sometimes result in fetal varicella syndrome manifested by growth retardation, cicatricial skin lesions, limb hypoplasia and neurologic insults. Maternal chickenpox in the final 21 days of gestation can result in congenital chickenpox, with infants born to mothers with onset of rash from 5 days before to 2 days after delivery at highest risk for severe infection. Varicella-zoster immune globulin (VZIG) 125 U i.m. should be given to these high-risk infants (Table 2.13). Infants born to mothers with chickenpox in the perinatal period should be isolated from susceptible infants until 21 days postnatally (28 days if VZIG given).

Infants who are exposed to chickenpox postnatally generally have a benign course, but preterm and other immunocompromised infants are at high risk for more severe infection.

Rubella

Rubella virus, transplacentally acquired during the course of primary maternal infection, may result in growth retardation, heart defects, hepatosplenomegaly, thrombocytopenia, cataracts and deafness. The incidence and severity of malformations increase with infection early in gestation. Diagnosis can be made by viral isolation or by testing for IgM to rubella. Treatment is supportive and

Table 2.13 Management of postnatal varicella exposure

Varicella-zoster immune globulin (VZIG) 125 U i.m. should be given to the following high-risk infants exposed postnatally to chickenpox:
    infants born prior to 28 weeks gestation or with birthweight less than 1000 g
    preterm infants with negative maternal history of varicella
    immunocompromised infants

Isolation of exposed infants from other susceptible infants should be undertaken from 10 to 21 days post-exposure (28 days if VZIG given)

infected infants require isolation because virus excretion may be prolonged.

Cytomegalovirus

Cytomegalovirus (CMV) may be vertically transmitted to the fetus in primary or recurrent maternal infection. Approximately 10% of infected infants are symptomatic at birth with the classic manifestations; these infants have a mortality rate of 25% and almost all survivors have long-term morbidity. Of the 90% of infected infants who are asymptomatic at birth, up to 15% will develop significant late neurologic morbidity, sensorineural hearing loss being most common. Diagnosis is confirmed by urine culture for CMV.

Acquired CMV infection may be severe in premature and other immunocompromised infants. CMV is transmitted by blood products or by breast milk. Infected infants may develop pulmonary, hepatic, hematologic and neurologic manifestations. Ganciclovir is active *in vitro* against CMV infection, but its effectiveness in congenital infection with established disease is still under investigation. Prevention is best accomplished by the use of CMV-negative or frozen deglycerolyzed blood for transfusion to infants at risk.

Herpes simplex virus

Herpes simplex virus (HSV) types 1 (15%) and 2 (85%) cause maternal herpes genitalis and can result in congenital infection. The more common presentation of neonatal herpes infection, though, is perinatally acquired infection. Neonatal disease may result from ascending infection prior to birth, acquisition from the birth canal during delivery, or post-natal acquisition from an infected carer. The incidence remains low at 0.2 to 0.5 cases per 1000 births. Infection is most likely with maternal primary HSV infection, but can also occur with recurrent infection. Most infected infants are born to mothers who are asymptomatic but actively shedding virus from a genital infection at the time of delivery. Cesarean delivery should be performed within 4 hours of rupture of membranes for women with active lesions. Prenatal screening with serial cervical cultures for HSV to predict status at delivery is not effective and no longer recommended. Infants at high risk for infection should be isolated initially until the results of viral cultures from the mother and infant are known. These infants should be closely observed in the hospital for evidence of infection, with cultures obtained from the eyes, mouth and any suspicious skin lesions. Use of acyclovir during this observation period should be individualized. Infants at lower risk for infection should also be isolated while hospitalized, and carers should be educated about the early signs of infection.

Neonatal herpes infection presents in the first 42 days of life as a rapidly evolving disease with clinical symptoms similar to those of bacterial sepsis. Disease may subsequently be categorized into one of three classifications: localized infection of the skin, eyes, or mouth; central nervous system infection with or without skin, eye, or mouth involvement; and disseminated infection. Mortality is highest for infants with disseminated infection, while morbidity is high for infants with disseminated or central nervous system infection. Diagnosis can be confirmed by culture of the virus from skin vesicles, mucosal lesions, blood, or CSF. Cytologic examination with fluorescent or Tzanck smears of lesion scrapings may be helpful in early diagnosis. Early therapy with acyclovir 30 mg/kg/day i.v. div. t.i.d. for 10–14 days has resulted in improved outcome in many cases. Many experts recommend starting acyclovir in neonates and infants younger than 42 days with CSF findings suggestive of aseptic meningitis.

COMMON FOCAL INFECTIONS

Conjunctivitis

Conjunctivitis in the newborn is common, with chemical irritation from prophylactic silver nitrate the most common cause. Chemical conjunctivitis occurs in the first 48 h of life and is self-limited. Conjunctivitis beginning after 48 h of life is usually of infectious origin and of greater clinical significance. Gram stain and appropriate cultures are required to identify the pathogen involved (Table 2.14).

Omphalitis

Omphalitis is characterized by purulent discharge from the umbilical stump with erythema and induration of the periumbilical area. Etiologic bacteria include *Staphylococcus aureus*, group A and B streptococci, diphtheroids, and Gram-negative enteric bacilli. Complications include sepsis, umbilical arteritis or phlebitis, peritonitis, and necrotizing fasciitis. Recommended initial therapy is intravenous methicillin plus an aminoglycoside or third generation cephalosporin.

Table 2.14 Common neonatal eye infections

Infecting organism	Age at onset	Clinical features	Therapy
Staphylococcus aureus	2–5 days	Unilateral, crusted, purulent discharge	Topical sulfacetamide, neomycin erythromycin, or tetracycline
Neisseria gonorrhoeae	3 days to 3 wks	Bilateral hyperemia and chemosis; copious thick white discharge	Ceftriaxone i.v. or i.m., 50 mg/kg (max 125 mg) as a single dose; saline irrigation; contact isolation
Chlamydia trachomatis	2–20 wks	Unilateral or bilateral mild conjunctivitis, copious purulent discharge	Oral erythromycin 50 mg/kg/day div. q.i.d. for 14 days

Scalp abscess

Fetal monitoring with internal scalp electrodes may result in a break in skin continuity with subsequent abscess formation. Treatment consists of local antiseptic care, incision, and drainage. Culture and sensitivity of the abscess drainage should be performed. If there is evidence of extension or systemic illness, intravenous methicillin plus an aminoglycoside or third generation cephalosporin should be administered. Consideration should be given for scalp electrode site infection with herpes simplex virus or *Neisseria gonorrhoeae* when the mother is infected with these organisms.

NOSOCOMIAL INFECTIONS

Nosocomial infection in the newborn is defined as an infection that was neither present nor incubating at birth, generally occurring after 48 h of life. The incidence of nosocomial infections in normal newborn nurseries is around 1% while in neonatal intensive care units (NICU) the incidence may be as high as 20%, especially in very low birthweight infants. Factors that contribute to higher rates of nosocomial infection include immature host-defense mechanisms, prolonged hospitalization, invasive supportive measures, and crowding.

Organisms responsible for nosocomial infections in the NICU include coagulase-negative staphylococci, *Staphylococcus aureus*, Gram-negative enteric bacilli, and *Candida* sp. Nosocomial infection should be considered in any hospitalized infant who exhibits unexplained clinical deterioration. As with early-onset neonatal infections, clinical manifestations of nosocomial infections are frequently subtle and non-specific.

Empiric antibiotic therapy for nosocomial infections should be based on the pathogens most prevalent in that nursery and the hospital organism susceptibility profile. Vancomycin in combination with a third generation cephalosporin offers broad-spectrum coverage of the most frequent pathogens. Empiric therapy should be changed to more specific therapy when culture and sensitivity results are available. Antifungal therapy is usually not begun empirically owing to the toxicity of such therapy, but this choice should be individualized.

Nosocomial viral infections are also of clinical significance. Respiratory syncytial virus (RSV) infections are associated with high morbidity and mortality in preterm infants and infants with underlying cardiorespiratory disease. Spread is by direct contact and droplet contamination. Nosocomial outbreaks are common during community epidemics which may occur from late fall to early spring. Therapy with ribavirin may be beneficial for high-risk infants. Infected infants should be isolated. Passive immunization with Palivizumab, a monoclonal antibody product against RSV, may help reduce the frequency and severity of infection in high-risk groups such as infants with severe prematurity and those with bronchopulmonary dysplasia (see Chapter 3). The incidence of nosocomial infections can be reduced by paying close attention to infection control measures, with special emphasis on strict handwashing practices.

Coagulase-negative staphylococci

Coagulase-negative staphylococci, typically *Staphylococcus epidermidis*, have become the most common cause of nosocomial bacterial infection in the NICU. These organisms are present on skin and mucosal surfaces, and are especially prone to cause infection in infants with foreign bodies in place such as umbilical catheters, central venous lines and shunts. *S. epidermidis* produces a slime layer on the foreign body that serves to isolate the bacteria from both host defenses and antibiotics. While some strains may be susceptible to penicillinase-resistant penicillins such as methicillin or oxacillin, most infections require treatment with vancomycin. Rifampin or gentamicin may offer synergy with vancomycin, but serious infections often require the removal of the colonized foreign body.

Candida species

Candida species, typically *Candida albicans*, are a ubiquitous group of fungal organisms that colonize the skin and mucous membranes. In the absence of competing bacterial flora – as may occur with broad-spectrum antibiotic use or in immunocompromised patients – infections with *Candida* may occur. Superficial infections such as thrush or diaper dermatitis may be treated with oral or topical nystatin preparations.

Candida invasive disease is a more serious infection that is more difficult to diagnose and treat. Infants with such invasive infections may present with features similar to bacterial sepsis. Diagnosis requires isolation of *Candida* from a normally sterile body site, such as the blood, CSF or tissue. Urine culture positive for *Candida* may represent contamination, depending on the method by which the specimen was obtained. Ophthalmologic examination to assess for candidal endophthalmitis may be useful.

Amphotericin B therapy is the most proven therapy for *Candida* invasive disease, although its toxicity has resulted in an ongoing search for alternative therapies. Flucytosine may be synergistic with amphotericin B for very severe infections. Alternative therapies that show promise include fluconazole and liposomal forms of amphotericin B. The duration of therapy can be individualized, but more severe infections in high-risk newborns may require treatment for 4 to 6 weeks. With less severe infections associated with an indwelling catheter, prompt therapy and catheter removal may allow for shorter courses of therapy. Judicious use of antibiotics and indwelling catheters is important in the prevention of nosocomial infections with both coagulase-negative *Staphylococcus* and *Candida* species.

Immutizations

3

ACTIVE IMMUNIZATION

Routine vaccination

The ultimate goal in medicine is not treatment but prevention of disease and vaccine administration represents the most efficacious and cost-effective measure for accomplishing this goal. Success is best indicated by the worldwide eradication of smallpox, elimination of polio in the western hemisphere and control of previously common severe infectious diseases such as measles, diphtheria, tetanus and pertussis. Twelve vaccines should be routinely administered to all children before they begin school. They comprise hepatitis B, *Haemophilus influenzae*, pneumococcus, diphtheria, tetanus toxoid, pertussis, trivalent polio, rotavirus, measles, mumps, rubella and varicella-zoster. The current recommendations from the Committee on Infectious Diseases, American Academy of Pediatrics (Report of the Committee on Infectious Diseases, 25th ed., 2000) for immunization in children are outlined in Table 3.1. Additional vaccines and vaccine combinations available in the United States are itemized in Table 3.2.

Methods for providing these vaccines are simple, essentially requiring only a concerned attitude on the part of parents and physicians. It is, therefore, unfortunate that many children in the United States are inadequately immunized against these infectious agents. Recent surveys of private pediatric practices have indicated that, even under optimal circumstances, 30–40% of pre-school children were not appropriately vaccinated. In addition, screening for tuberculosis with intradermal skin testing is necessary for children in high prevalence regions and/or for children with increased risk factors. The general compliance with this recommended screening procedure is even lower.

Other recommendations for vaccine use

If the immunization program for a young child is begun but not completed, the physician can simply continue where the program was interrupted. Original doses do not have to be repeated. There are, however, a few caveats. Rotavirus vaccine is not recommended if immunization cannot be completed before one year of age. If the child is past the seventh birthday, pertussis vaccine should be eliminated and the adult form of diphtheria vaccine (Td) should be substituted; Td vaccine contains approximately 15% of material included in childhood diphtheria. Otherwise, diphtheria–tetanus–acellular pertussis (DTaP) or adult tetanus diphtheria (Td) are given at 2-month intervals with measles–mumps–rubella (MMR) administered as soon as is practical.

Tetanus prophylaxis in wound management is simple if patients have received their

Table 3.1 Routine immunization schedule

Vaccine	Age for administration; months except where stated
Hepatitis B	0–2, 1–4, 6–18
H. influenzae	2, 4, (6), 12–15
Pneumococcus	2, 4, 6, 12–18 (pending licensure)
DTaP	2, 4, 6, 15–18
Polio	2 (IPV), 4 (IPV), 6–18 (IPV or OPV), 4–6 yr (IPV or OPV)
Rotavirus	2, 4, 6
MMR	12–15, 4–6 yr
Varicella	12–18

Table 3.2 Vaccines available in the United States

Vaccine	Type	Route
Adenovirus	Live virus	Oral
Anthrax	Inactivated bacteria	Subcutaneous
BCG (Bacillus of Calmette and Guérin)	Live bacteria	Intradermal or subcutaneous
Cholera	Inactivated bacteria	Subcutaneous
Diphtheria–Tetanus–Pertussis (DTP) or	Toxoids and inactivated bacteria	Intramuscular
–Acellular–Pertussis (DTaP)	Bacterial component	Intramuscular
Hepatitis A	Recombinant viral antigen	Intramuscular
Hepatitis B	Inactive viral antigen	Intramuscular
Hib conjugates	Polysaccharide–protein conjugate	Intramuscular
Hib conjugate–DTP (HbOC-DTP and PRP-T reconstituted with DTP)	Polysaccharide–protein conjugate with toxoids and inactivated bacteria	Intramuscular
Hib conjugate–DTaP (PRP-T reconstituted with DTaP)	Polysaccharide–protein conjugate with toxoids and inactivated bacterial components	Intramuscular
Hib conjugate (PRP-OMP) hepatitis B	Polysaccharide–protein conjugate with inactivated virus	Intramuscular
Influenza	Inactivated virus (whole-virus), viral components	Intramuscular
Japanese encephalitis	Inactivated virus	Subcutaneous
Measles	Live virus	Subcutaneous
Meningococcal	Polysaccharide	Subcutaneous
MMR	Live viruses	Subcutaneous
Measles-rubella	Live viruses	Subcutaneous
Mumps	Live virus	Subcutaneous
Pertussis	Inactivated bacteria	Intramuscular
Plague	Inactivated bacteria	Intramuscular
Pneumococcal	Polysaccharide	Intramuscular or subcutaneous
Pneumococcal conjugate	Polysaccharide–protein conjugate	Intramuscular
Poliovirus		
OPV	Live virus	Oral
IPV	Inactivated virus	Subcutaneous
Rabies	Inactivated virus	Intramuscular or intradermal
Rubella	Live virus	Subcutaneous
Tetanus	Inactivated toxin (toxoid)	Intramuscular
Tetanus–diphtheria (Td, DT)	Inactivated toxins	Intramuscular
Typhoid		
Parenteral	Inactivated bacteria	Subcutaneous
Parenteral	Capsular polysaccharide	Subcutaneous (boosters may be intradermal)
Oral	Live bacteria	Oral
Varicella-zoster	Live virus	Subcutaneous
Yellow fever	Live virus	Subcutaneous

primary immunization doses. Under these circumstances, tetanus toxoid, usually along with diphtheria, is given for a tetanus-prone wound if the patient has not received tetanus toxoid within 5 years of the accident. If the individual has received three doses of tetanus toxoid during his or her lifetime, this is considered adequate and tetanus immunoglobulin need not be given. Fewer than three doses of tetanus toxoid is considered inadequate for protection and, under these circumstances, for a tetanus-prone wound 250 U of tetanus immunoglobulin should be given along with tetanus toxoid, and the immunization procedure should be completed during long-term management with the next dose of DTaP or Td given 4 weeks later.

The simultaneous administration of vaccines, particularly when 'catching-up' on immunization programs, is a common practice. A great deal of clinical data now support the efficacy of vaccines administered on the same day if circumstances make this the only practical approach. The one drawback is that simultaneously administered vaccines are more likely to cause local or systemic side-effects and, if any reaction is severe, the clinician would not know which agent was responsible.

Additional vaccines are generally administered only to individuals traveling to foreign countries where other infectious agents are endemic. This is discussed in Chapter 4. Additional information for these travelers is available in the periodic publication of a supplement to *Morbidity and Mortality Weekly Report* entitled 'Health Information for International Travel,' which can be obtained from the Superintendent of Documents, US Government Printing Office, Washington, DC 20402, or from state health departments.

Local side-effects, such as erythema and induration with tenderness, are common after the administration of all vaccines, but particularly with pertussis. Reactions are self-limited and do not require specific therapy, although most physicians routinely administer acetaminophen before offering immunizations. A nodule may appear at the injection site and persist for several weeks but this should not be considered a significant reaction. Rarely, systemic reactions occur and these necessitate the alteration of immunization programs (Table 3.3).

If reactions occur with DTaP injections, the physician can usually assume that the pertussis antigen is the causative agent and immunizations should then be completed with DT or Td. The only contraindication to tetanus and diphtheria toxoids is the history of a neurologic or a severe hypersensitivity reaction following a previous dose when pertussis had been excluded. When the causative agent cannot be determined, skin testing (prick and intradermal) may be useful with tetanus and diphtheria toxoids to document immediate hypersensitivity. Tetanus toxoid should not be routinely given more frequently than every 10 years since with more frequent injections a percentage of recipients will develop major local reactions. These are essentially Arthus reactions, resulting from very high serum tetanus antitoxin levels.

Other contraindications to pertussis vaccine

Hypersensitivity to vaccine components, presence of an evolving neurologic disorder, or a history of a severe reaction (usually within 48 h) following a previous dose are definitive contraindications to the receipt of pertussis

Table 3.3 Contraindications to immunizations

Reaction to previous dose
Neurologic
Allergic
Live vaccines
Immunodeficiency
Malignancy
Immunosuppressive therapy
Plasma or blood transfusion within 2 months or immunoglobulin within 2–10 months, depending on dosage (for measles only)
Pregnancy

vaccine. Some authorities recommend discontinuing pertussis vaccine for other severe reactions (Table 3.4).

Premature infants

Premature infants are generally immunized at the usual chronologic age using routine vaccine dosages. At 2 months DTaP, *H. influenzae* type B (Hib) and inactivated polio vaccines can be given, even if the infant weighs < 1500 g at birth. Rotavirus vaccine has not been fully evaluated in prematurely born infants but should be safe and effective in those who weigh > 2000 g when immunization is begun.

Preterm neonates born to HBsAg-positive mothers should be managed identically to full-term neonates (Table 3.5), receiving hepatitis B immunoglobulin (HBIG) and the first dose of hepatitis B vaccine (at a different site) within 12 h of birth.

In premature neonates with birthweight less than 2000 g whose mothers are HBsAg-negative, hepatitis B vaccine should be delayed until the weight is more than 2000 g or until 2 months of age, whichever comes first. There is no urgency in administering this vaccine early in life, so the first dose can be given at hospital discharge if the weight is adequate. If the birthweight is less than 2000 g and the mother's hepatitis B status cannot be determined within the initial 12 h of life, both HBIG and hepatitis B vaccine should be given at birth (Table 3.6).

Immunosuppressed patients

Immunization of immuncompromised patients may not elicit a protective immune response, and in the case of live vaccines may cause severe disease. Risks must therefore be carefully balanced against potential benefits. However, it should be emphasized that data are quite limited concerning adverse reactions of live vaccine products in immunosuppressed individuals. Inadvertent immunization of HIV-infected infants with live vaccines have rarely resulted in disease, offering reassurance that even these vaccines are relatively

safe. Children with congenital disorders of immune function appear most vulnerable to dissemination of bacterial and virus vaccine micro-organisms, particularly BCG, polio and measles, so these should not be given when host immune responses are severely compromised.

Only live oral polio vaccine needs to be withheld from normal children in households with a family member who is immune deficient. IPV should be substituted for all doses. On the other hand, MMR, varicella, and

Table 3.4 Consider discontinuation of whole cell or acellular pertussis vaccine

Hypotonic/hyporesponsive episode
Excessive somnolence of 3 h duration
Persistent crying or screaming of 3 h duration
Temperature higher than 40.5°C (104.9°F)

Table 3.5 Hepatitis B prevention for premature and full-term infants of HBsAG-positive mothers

Birth	Hepatitis B immunoglobulin (HBIG) 0.5 ml i.m. within 12 h of birth Hepatitis B vaccine 0.5 ml i.m. within 12 h of birth
1 months	Hepatitis B vaccine
6 months	Hepatitis B vaccine

Table 3.6 Hepatitis B virus vaccine and hepatitis B immunoglobulin (HBIG) in neonates

Mother HBsAg-Positive (as Table 3.5)
Mother HBsAg-negative
Full-term and premature > 2000 g:
vaccine begun birth to 2 months
Premature < 2000 g: delay vaccine until
> 2000 g or 2 months of age
Mother HBsAg status unknown
Full-term and premature > 2000 g:
vaccine at birth (< 12 h)
determine mother's HBsAg status
HBIG within 7 days if mother positive
Premature < 2000 g:
HBIG and vaccine within 12 h of birth

rotavirus vaccines can be given to children in these households and the former two vaccine products are even more important under these circumstances since wild measles and varicella have caused significant disease in immunosuppressed children and adults (Table 3.7).

Influenza vaccine

Annual vaccination is recommended for all with medical problems that would result in more extensive infection if they developed influenza and for all individuals with increased exposure to potential outbreaks (Table 3.8). The type of vaccine and dosage recommended for various age groups vary with the vaccine prepared each year. Therefore, the physician should consult the package insert or the state health department for specific information.

Field trials of influenza vaccines in the past have usually shown vaccine efficacy in the range of 70% to 80%. The greatest success is achieved when the antigenic drift of viral strains is anticipated so that the vaccines would include appropriate components. Vaccines now provide protection for both influenza A and influenza B. If an individual receives vaccine each year, only one dose is needed. If vaccine is given for the first time, however, often two doses are required for adequate immunization.

Outbreaks of influenza occur between October and the end of February in the USA. Therefore, the vaccine should be administered before or during the month of October and discontinued by March 1. Often, an outbreak that occurs in December or January is not documented until February when it receives national attention. This is too late to begin an immunization program since, historically, cases rarely appear after March 1 in the USA. The best and most efficient system is for the primary care physician to maintain a list of patients who should receive vaccine and, during the month of September, notify these patients so that they may plan for a brief office appointment. The most important aspect in assuring success for vaccination practices is a compulsive and methodical attitude on the part of primary care physicians. The individual patient cannot be expected to remember this aspect of health care.

Rabies vaccine

Rabies vaccine is currently recommended for animal handlers and anyone traveling to regions of the world where rabies is endemic in domestic animals. It is also used for post-

Table 3.7 Vaccines for immunodeficient and immunosuppressed children

Definition of immunosuppression
immunosuppressive chemotherapeutic agents for malignancy or management of transplant rejection
congenital or acquired (AIDS) immunodeficiency conditions
corticosteroids
2 mg/kg/day of prednisone or equivalent or 20 mg/day total dose
given > 14 days
Avoid live vaccines
IPV rather than OPV
MMR may be given to AIDS patients who are not severely immunosuppressed
Varicella vaccine can be given to children when there is an immunosuppressed individual in the household

Table 3.8 Indications for influenza vaccine

Chronic diseases
Pulmonary
Cardiac
Renal
Diabetes mellitus
Metabolic disorders
Anemia
Malignancies
Immunosuppressive therapy
Age > 65 years
Hospital personnel
School teachers

exposure prophylaxis in conjunction with rabies immunoglobulin (RIG). For pre-exposure prevention a three-dose regimen, which can be given intradermally, is required. This is preferred for ease of administration and markedly reduced cost. If pre-immunized individuals are bitten by potentially rabid animals they will still require two post-exposure doses of rabies vaccine, but rabies immunoglobulin will not be required. For post-exposure treatment five doses of vaccine along with RIG should be administered. The Centers for Disease Control (CDC) now recommend that the full dose of RIG be infiltrated in the area around and into the wound if possible. If the volume is too large, any remaining volume should be injected by the intramuscular route at a site distant from administration of the rabies vaccine (Table 3.9).

PASSIVE IMMUNIZATION

Immunoglobulin

Passive immunization may be accomplished by administering immunoglobulin (previously called immune serum globulin) to individuals exposed to infectious hepatitis or those traveling into endemic regions of the world where probability of exposure is significant, and to non-immune children exposed to measles. The other indication for immuno-globulin is hypogammaglobulinemia. However, this product has been in greatly limited supply for quite a few years and has been

largely replaced by newer vaccines (such as hepatitis A) and intravenous immunoglob-ulin preparations.

Hyperimmune human immunoglobulin

Gammaglobulin prepared from selected hyperimmune donors is particularly useful as passive immunotherapy in modifying or preventing clinical illness from a number of infectious agents (Table 3.10).

The need for consultation concerning the indications for varicella-zoster hyperimmune globulin (VZIG) is more frequent than for any of the other globulin products. This is the result of both the ubiquitous nature of the virus and the large number of patients who benefit from its administration. The most common circumstance is a child with malignancy, usually leukemia, who is exposed to chickenpox. Table 3.11 outlines the guidelines for using VZIG. It is now more readily available through regional distribution centers around the country, which can be located through a central service at one of the following addresses:-

American Red Cross
Blood Services
Northeast region
(617) 449-0773
or
American Red Cross
Blood Services
(800) GIVELIFE

Table 3.9 FDA approved rabies vaccines

Vaccine	Manufacturer	Cell culture	Method of administration
Human diploid cell vaccine (HDCV) (Imovax)	Pasteur-Mérieux Connaught	Human diploid cells	i.m. or i.d.
Rabies vaccine adsorbed (RVA)	Michigan Biologics Products Institute*	Fetal rhesus diploid lung cells	i.m.
Purified chick embryo cell (PCEC) (RabAvert)	Chiron Behring GmbH & Co	Chick embryo	i.m.

*Distributed by Smith Kline Beecham Pharmaceutics; i.m., intramuscular; i.d., intradermal

Hyperimmune animal immunoglobulin

In addition to human hyperimmune globulin preparations, antisera of animal origin are also available for clinical use. These products carry with them a high probability of serum reactions, particularly if the recipient has been exposed to similar animal products previously. Information for these and other products can be obtained through the Centers for Disease Control, telephone: (404) 329-3311 or 329-3644. Materials include: black widow spider equine antivenin, equine western equine encephalitis, botulism ABE polyvalent equine antitoxin, diphtheria equine antitoxin, antirabies serum, polyvalent gas gangrene equine antitoxin, coral snake equine antivenin, and crotalid polyvalent antivenin.

Table 3.10 Hyperimmune human immunoglobulin

Immune globulin	Trade name	Manufacturer
Cytomegalovirus	Cytogam	Connaught Laboratories
Hepatitis B	HBIG	Cutter Biological, Abbott, Merck Sharp and Dohme
Rabies	R.I.G.	Cutter Biological
Respiratory syncytial virus	Synagis	Medimmune
Tetanus	T.I.G.	Cutter Biological, Savage, Hyland, Parke-Davis, Wyeth, Elkins-Sinn, Merck Sharp and Dohme, Hyland Therapeutics
Varicella-zoster	VZIG	Massachusetts Public Health

Table 3.11 Guidelines for the use of varicella-zoster hyperimmune globulin (VZIG)

1. One of the following underlying illnesses or conditions:
    Leukemia or lymphoma
    Congenital or acquired immunodeficiency
    Under immunosuppressive treatment
    Newborn of mother who had onset of chickenpox < 5 days before delivery or within 48 h after delivery
2. One of the following types of exposure to chickenpox or zoster patient(s):
    Household contact
    Playmate contact (> 1 h play indoors)
    Hospital contact (in same 2- to 4-bed room or adjacent beds in a large ward)
    Newborn contact (newborn of mother who had onset of chickenpox < 5 days before delivery or within 48 h after delivery)
3. Negative or unknown prior history of chickenpox
4. Age < 15 years, with administration to older patients on an individual basis
5. Time elapsed after exposure is such that VZIG can be administered within 96 h

Travel medicine

INTRODUCTION

Immigrants and naturalized citizens residing in the USA constitute the population most likely to travel with young children to developing countries. These periodic trips are often the only way relatives can maintain family relationships. Clinicians' assessment of priorities and approaches to counseling are therefore very different from those for adults who are simply planning business or exotic leisure travel. The usual conservative approach must be tempered by consideration of more personal issues, otherwise parents would be strongly encouraged to delay exposing young children to serious health problems more prevalent in their (or their parents') native countries.

RESTRICTIONS FOR FAMILY TRAVEL

As a general recommendation, families should be advised to avoid traveling with infants younger than 6 months old because in this age group diarrheal diseases are more severe, and insect-borne illnesses are extremely difficult to prevent and treat. In fact, very few medications for diseases such as malaria, leishmaniasis, or filariasis have been adequately studied in young infants. Perhaps more importantly, immunizations for polio, rotavirus, hepatitis B, *Haemophilus influenzae* type b, tetanus, diphtheria and pertussis are not completed until 6 months and measles, mumps, rubella (MMR) and varicella not routinely before 12 months. As discussed later consideration can be given to administering MMR and perhaps varicella vaccines as early as 6 months of age.

It is obvious that most children born in developing countries do well without any unique medical intervention. They do not routinely receive special vaccines nor malaria

prophylaxis. Also, any infant being breast fed is afforded maximal protection from most infectious agents and is unlikely to develop difficulty following exposure to gastrointestinal pathogens such as *Salmonella* and *Shigella* sp. However, because special steps can reduce disease in infants and young children, potential preventive measures should be carefully explained to parents. For infants not being breast fed, bottled water and canned fruits and vegetables must be provided, or at the very least, meticulously boiled water and freshly cooked food should be prepared. These same recommendations pertain to older children and adults as well, but there is greater emphasis on this advice for infants because food-borne disease is more serious in this age group.

MISSIONARY FAMILIES

Missionaries and their families represent a unique, high-risk group for tropical diseases, a consequence of long duration exposure in rural communities much different from the usual vacation or business travel destination. Recommendations for preventive medical interventions are quite varied since there is disagreement as to whether these individuals should be managed like all other residents of the host country or whether they should receive special care similar to that offered to transient travelers. There is not a single publication in the medical literature which specifically addresses their needs, yet missionaries routinely seek medical advice from their physicians. A survey of the missionary offices of various religious denominations also failed to identify consistent guidelines for medical management of these families.

Anticipated length of stay in a particular region often plays a major role in decisions made by travel medicine clinics. This variable particularly pertains to chemoprophylaxis for malaria. Clinicians' assessment of priorities and approaches to counseling are therefore very different from those for adults who are simply planning business or exotic leisure travel. The usual conservative approach must be tempered by consideration of more personal issues, otherwise missionaries would be strongly encouraged to delay exposing young children to serious health problems more prevalent in developing countries.

ROUTINE IMMUNIZATIONS

All family members should complete the recommended basic series of immunizations that prevent common childhood diseases (Table 4.1). In the case of *H. influenzae* type b conjugate vaccine, adequate protection is actually achieved after 2 doses in the primary series. A minimum of 3 immunizations is necessary for hepatitis B, pneumococcus, DTP, polio and rotavirus. Booster doses of some vaccines may be given earlier than generally recommended to maximize protection before travel. Measles, mumps and rubella (MMR) combined vaccine and varicella may be given as early as 6 months of

age rather than the usual 12 months, if the family will be traveling to or residing in any region where these diseases are highly endemic.

TRAVEL VACCINES

Limitations for young children

There are major limitations in making recommendations for children traveling to foreign countries. For example, many vaccines and prophylactic chemotherapeutic agents used against pathogens that are relatively rare in the USA have simply not been thoroughly studied in this population (e.g. mefloquine for malaria prophylaxis) or have been shown to be inadequate (e.g. some components of the meningococcal vaccine in children younger than 2 years of age). Yellow fever vaccine is associated with a higher incidence of vaccine-related encephalitis in young infants as compared with adults, so it should only be given if the benefits clearly outweigh the risks. The yellow fever vaccine is never recommended for infants less than 4 months of age.

There is, in fact, considerable unpublished information concerning the use of most vaccines and medications in young children because this age group has received many of these agents for years in developing countries in spite of non-approval. In most cases,

Table 4.1 Routine immunizations and the age when protection is provided

Disease	Recommended vaccine schedule	Age when protection adequate for travel
Hepatitis B	0, 1, 6 months	6 months
Diphtheria	2, 4, 6, 15 months, 5 yr	6 months
Tetanus	2, 4, 6, 15 months, 5 yr	6 months
Pertussis	2, 4, 6, 15 months, 5 yr	6 months
Polio	2, 4, 6 months, 5 yr	6 months
Rotavirus	2, 4, 6 months	6 months
H. influenzae b	2, 4, 6, 12 months	4 months
Measles	12 months	12 months
Mumps	12 months	12 months
Rubella	12 months	12 months
Varicella	12 months	12 months

Table 4.2 Age limitations for vaccines and chemoprophylaxis

Agent	Limitation and reason
Meningococcal vaccine	< 2 years
	Poor antibody response to groups C, Y, and W-135
Oral typhoid vaccine	Not approved < 6 years
	Limited data and no suspension formulation but safe and effective
Yellow fever vaccine	Contraindicated < 4 months
	Vaccine-associated encephalitis
Mefloquine	< 15 kg (approx. 30 months of age)
	Limited pharmacologic data but safe and effective
Loperamide	≤ 2 years
	Not approved as data are limited
Bismuth subsalicylate	≤ 3 years
	Not approved as data are limited
Fluoroquinolones	≤ 18 years
	Not approved, potential damage to developing cartilage

few adverse reactions have been reported. Table 4.2 includes information currently available from suppliers concerning reported side-effects as well as identified limitations.

Reviews of travel medicine issues have been remarkably conservative in recommendations for infants and young children. Conclusions probably reflect gaps in published management data, as discussed.

Active immunizations for other infectious diseases vary according to the country of residence. The necessity for active immunization in children is no different from that in adults and schedules are generally identical (Table 4.3).

Hyperimmune human immunoglobulin for rabies and hepatitis B are necessary for unimmunized individuals of all ages immediately following direct exposure to these diseases. This would have to be given in the host country and may not be readily available. Families should be apprised of this limitation, which further supports routine vaccination for rabies and hepatitis B.

Hepatitis A

One of the greatest risks during residence in developing countries is exposure to hepatitis A from contaminated food and water. Because the disease is usually anicteric and quite mild in young children, many experts do not recommend preventive measures for this age group. However, these young family members could subsequently become the contact source of infection for their parents and adult relatives, in whom disease can be more severe. Reported mortality among the older age groups is 3 per 1000 cases.

Hepatitis A vaccine has been licensed and recommended for children as young as 2 years of age who travel to or reside in regions of the world where disease is endemic. Limited data indicate good antibody conversion in infants younger than one year of age. For this reason it seems prudent to immunize children who are as young as 6 months old. One dose is required with a booster administration 6 to 12 months later. Another dose might be considered for infants immunized before they are two years old, given some time after the second birthday.

Typhoid fever

A common infection in developing countries is typhoid fever, accounting for significant morbidity and mortality in residents of all ages. Although two killed vaccines are available, the live oral vaccine is as efficacious as

Table 4.3 Recommended preventive measures for travel to countries where specific diseases are endemic

Vaccine	Schedule

Hepatitis A vaccine
  Vaqta
  (Merck)
	2 weeks prior to travel
	  and 6–18 months later
	
	2–17 years of age, 0.5 ml (25U) i.m.
	> 18 years, 1.0 ml (50U) i.m.

Typhoid vaccine, live oral Ty21a
  Vivotif Berna
  (Berna Products Corp)
  or
	1 capsule q.o.d. x 4

Typhoid Vi polysaccharide vaccine
  Typhim Vi
  (Pasteur-Mérieux Connaught)
	0.5 ml i.m.
	  repeat q. 2 years if high risk

Meningococcal polysaccharide vaccine
  Menomune – A/C/Y/W-135
  (Connaught)
	0.5 ml subcutaneous (SQ)
	single dose q. 2 years if less than 10 years of age

Yellow Fever, 17D	Single dose SQ recommended for age > 9 months
	  4–9 months: individualized based on estimates of risk
	    < 4 months: contraindicated
	  booster every 10 years

Rabies
  Rabies vaccine adsorbed (RVA)
  (Smith Kline Beecham)
  Imovax Rabies
  Imovax Rabies i.d.
	1 ml i.m. 0, 7, and 21 or 28 days
	
	1 ml i.m. 0, 7, and 21 or 28 days
	0.1 ml i.d. 0, 7, and 21 or 28 days

Japanese Encephalitis	SQ doses, 0, 7, 30 days or 0, 7, 14 days
	  > 3 years of age: 1.0 ml
	  6 months to 3 years: 0.5 ml
	  < 6 months: no data but 0.5 ml
	  appropriate

Cholera vaccine, USP vaccine
  (Wyeth-Ayerst)
	No country currently requires
	  for entry
	SQ or i.m. doses, 2 doses at least 1 week apart
	  > 10 years of age: 0.5 ml
	  5–10 years: 0.3 ml
	  6 months to 4 years: 0.2 ml
	  < 6 months: not recommended

the killed vaccines and preferred for all ages. However, at this time it is not approved in the USA for children younger than 6 years of age. The primary reason for this limitation is that these children are usually unwilling to swallow capsules. Vaccine trials using a suspension formulation actually demonstrated higher efficacy and safety in children than that observed for the capsule when employed in adult studies. Unfortunately, this oral suspension is not commercially available.

A parenteral vaccine, Typhoid Vi, the capsular polysaccharide (ViCPS) of *Salmonella typhi*, is approved for administration to children 2 years of age and older. It requires only a single injection for immunization, but local reactions occur in 7% of recipients. Protective efficacy for the oral vaccine lasts for 5 to 6 years, compared with the ViCPS vaccine which requires a booster every two years. Of the three typhoid vaccines currently licensed in the USA, only the older parenteral heat-phenol-inactivated product is licensed for children as young as 6 months of age.

A reasonable approach for young children is to give the capsule with a gelatin dessert, banana or other preferred food of infants using the same schedule recommended for older children. It is important to keep in mind that this is a live bacterial vaccine, quite safe, but not recommended for patients who are immunosuppressed or for young children in a household where any adult is immunosuppressed. For reasons not completely understood, mefloquine may reduce the immunogenicity of typhoid vaccine, so this drug should be given more than 24 h before or after a vaccine dose.

Meningococcus

Meningococcal vaccine contains polysaccharide antigens that elicit a T-cell independent immune response markedly limited in infants. It is therefore not generally recommended until two years of age. However, the group A component is immunogenic as early as 3 months of age, and this is the serogroup most likely to cause outbreaks in developing countries. Immunization is therefore appropriate for any infant older than 90 days. The risk of invasive meningococcal disease from other serogroups, even in countries which report a high incidence of Group A infection, is low enough that immunization for Groups C, W135, and Y is rarely essential. However, the current quadrivalent vaccine contains these serogroups so protection is routinely afforded following immunization for Group A. Parents can also be counseled to prevent their children from having close contact with adults during reported outbreaks of meningococcal disease in local communities; early rifampin prophylaxis is advised following

potential exposure. Direct household exposure to infected patients still represents the only well documented risk factor for secondary cases.

Yellow fever

Prevention of yellow fever in infants is problematic because immunization is associated with a relatively high incidence of vaccine-induced encephalitis. This reaction can be severe in children younger than 4 months of age. Most authorities believe that yellow fever vaccine should never be given to young infants, but this contraindication must be balanced against disease prevalence and the likelihood of exposure for children older than 4 months. The vaccine is considered safe in children over 9 months of age. Yellow fever is endemic in tropical South America, sub-Saharan Africa, and periodically in Central America.

Rabies

Few Americans realize that rabies is endemic among domestic animals in most developing countries. It is therefore prudent to consider immunization if living circumstances are likely to create unpreventable exposure. This is usually defined as residence in rural regions for more than 6 months. Because they are less cautious, children are more likely to be bitten by potentially rabid animals and thus are higher priority candidates for vaccine. Two vaccines may be administered by the intramuscular (i.m.) and one by the intradermal route. Both methods have been shown to be equally efficacious. Most patients prefer the intradermal route because of reduced cost of the 0.1 ml dose used. Only the human diploid cell vaccine (HDCV) is approved for intradermal injection, while both HDCV and rabies absorbed (RVA) may be administered i.m. using a 1.0 ml dose. A special syringe must be used for the intradermal injection. Both routes require 3 doses given at 0, 7, and 21 or 28 days. Immunization does not mean that additional treatment is unnecessary following an animal bite, but it does offer adequate protection so that only two intramuscular booster doses of vaccine at 0 and 3 days following exposure would be required; rabies immunoglobulin does not have to be given to immunized individuals bitten by potentially rabid animals.

Japanese encephalitis

Japanese encephalitis is an arthropod-borne disease seen in rural regions of Japan, China, Southeast Asia, and India, primarily during wet summer months. Risk for disease in urban areas is low, and even in endemic regions few cases are reported during the fall, winter and spring. If risk of exposure is considered high, vaccine (JE-VAX; Connaught, Swiftwater, PA) may be administered to children at any age. Specific information pertaining to reported infection and availability of vaccine may be obtained from the Division of Vector-Borne Infectious Diseases, Centers for Disease Control and Prevention (970/221-6400).

Infant cribs should be covered with mosquito nets, and aerosol insecticidal sprays should be applied to exposed skin during daytime activity when there is increased risk of exposure to biting mosquitoes. Incidence of disease is highest in children 2 to 7 years of age. The relatively lower rates in infants may be the consequence of protective maternal antibody or reduced exposure to mosquitoes, which are more likely to bite in outside environments. Reported mortality is between 5% and 35%, a difference largely reflecting availability of intensive medical care for various study locations. These high figures support routine immunization for any missionary families at risk. The preferred dosing schedule is 0, 7, and 30 days, if time allows. The 0, 7, and 14 day schedule is also highly protective, but final antibody titers are somewhat lower.

Cholera

Cholera immunization is mentioned only to emphasize that the World Health Organization no longer recommends vaccination for travel to or from cholera-endemic regions, and currently no country requires immunization for entry or re-entry. Although quite safe, this vaccine offers only 50% protective efficacy of very short duration, 3 to 6 months, for selected epidemic serotypes. Risk remains minimal for families residing in homes where proper hygienic precautions are employed.

Tuberculosis screening and BCG

All long-term emigrants to virtually any country outside of the US should have a Mantoux skin test for tuberculosis. This test serves as important baseline information if exposure occurs during residence. Some countries require documentation of tuberculin skin test responses before entry. For US children younger than 12 months of age, such testing is probably unnecessary because the likelihood of prior exposure in the USA is so low. On the other hand, if the infant has received Bacille Calmette-Guerin (BCG) vaccine, recording of the Mantoux response is very useful for interpretation of later skin testing. Tuberculin skin testing can be done simultaneously with measles vaccination, but testing should be delayed for 4 to 6 weeks if MMR was previously given.

BCG should be given prior to residence in almost all developing countries, concordant with local recommendations for universal immunization. Methods for BCG administration using a scarification technique are well understood in travel medicine clinics so vaccination is best accomplished in this setting. The Tice strain of BCG is administered percutaneously; 0.3 ml of the reconstituted vaccine is usually placed on the skin in the lower deltoid area (i.e. the upper arm) and delivered through a multiple-puncture disc. Infants < 30 days of age should receive one half the usual dose, prepared by increasing the amount of diluent added to the lyophilized vaccine. If the indications for vaccination persist, these children should receive a full dose of the vaccine after they are one year old if they have an induration of

< 5 mm when tested with 5 TU of PPD tuberculin. If time allows, a tuberculosis skin test (IPPD) should be placed and read to document adequacy of BCG vaccination.

TRAVELER'S DIARRHEA

Traveler's diarrhea usually occurs during the first week of travel and is generally a mild self-limited disease. The incidence is highest among persons visiting Latin America, Africa, Asia, and the Middle East. Numerous organisms are responsible, with the vast majority being due to enterotoxigenic *E. coli* in Americans who travel to Mexico or South America.

If meticulous attention is paid to avoiding potentially contaminated food and water, the incidence of infection is extremely low. Prophylactic antibiotics are no longer routinely recommended because their use leads to the rapid development of bacterial resistance. Antimicrobial therapy should be reserved for symptomatic cases or for individuals entering an extremely high-risk area (poor sanitation) and who will be remaining there for more than 5 days. Recommended antibiotics are trimethoprim/sulfamethoxazole (TMP/SMX), trimethoprim alone, and the quinolones: ciprofloxacin or norfloxacin (for patients older than 18 years) (Table 4.4). It is most practical to allow travelers to bring appropriate medication with them if they are staying for more than 5 days, but with instructions to begin therapy only if symptoms occur. Loperamide (Imodium®), an antimotility medication is safe, available over-the-counter, and can be combined with antibiotics for more effective symptomatic care. Bismuth subsalicylate has also been shown to be a useful adjunct to antimicrobial therapy in adults.

For infants and children less than 2 years of age, prophylaxis is not recommended. Once symptomatic, these young patients should be given fluids with a higher electrolyte content such as that contained in oral rehydration solutions.

Table 4.4 Traveler's diarrhea

Prophylaxis not recommended
Early treatment for 5 days if symptomatic
TMP/SMX
8–12 mg TMP/40–60 mg SMX/kg
div. q. 12 h
Doxycycline
5 mg/kg div. q.12 h
Ciprofloxacin
20–30 mg/kg div. q. 12 h

PREVENTIVE INTERVENTIONS FOR DEVELOPING COUNTRIES

Malaria

Primary prevention of malaria relies on a combination of personal protective measures and antimicrobial prophylaxis. International travelers visiting areas where malaria is endemic should be encouraged to avoid exposure to mosquitoes, use insect repellents and pesticides and wear long pants and long-sleeved shirts. For most malarious areas, oral chloroquine is the drug of choice for primary prophylaxis. For travel to regions reporting chloroquine-resistant *Plasmodium falciparum*, mefloquine alone or chloroquine plus pyrimethamine/sulfadoxine or doxycycline should be used (Table 4.5).

All individuals residing in malaria-endemic regions for short periods of time (< 6 months) should receive chemoprophylaxis (weekly chloroquine or mefloquine) beginning one week before arrival and continued for four weeks after returning to a developed country. This recommendation applies to family members of all ages, although data concerning the safety and efficacy of appropriate chemoprophylactic regimens are limited in very young children. For regions where chloroquine-resistant *Plasmodium falciparum* has not been identified, chloroquine remains the drug of choice. Such regions include Haiti, the Dominican Republic, Central America west of the Panama Canal, and the Middle East,

Table 4.5   Recommended antibiotic regimens and dosage for malaria prevention

Category	Antibiotic regimen
Non-chloroquine-resistant malaria strains (*Plasmodium vivax, P. ovale, P. malariae*, and chloroquine-sensitive *P. falciparum*)	Chloroquine phosphate, 5 mg/kg (max. 300 mg) base (equivalent to 8.3 mg/kg; max. 500 mg salt) once/week starting 2 weeks before travel to a malarious area and continuing during travel until 4 weeks after leaving the area or Hydroxychloroquine sulfate, 5 mg/kg (max. 310 mg) base (equivalent to 6.5 mg/kg; max. 400 mg salt) once/week before travel to a malarious area and continuing during travel until 4 weeks after leaving the area
P. vivax and *P. ovale* endemic areas (relapse prevention)	Chloroquine phosphate or hydroxychloroquine sulfate, same dose and regimen as above plus Primaquine, 0.3 mg/kg/day (max. 15 mg/day) for 14 days after leaving the malarious area

Chloroquine-resistant malaria strain (chloroquine-resistant *P. falciparum*)	Mefloquine hydrochloride (tablet, 250 mg)
	  < 15 kg: not recommended
	  15–19 kg: ¼ tablet/week
	  20–30 kg: ½ tablet/week
	  31–45 kg: ¾ tablet/week
	  > 45 kg: 1 tablet/week
	Starting 1 week before travel and continuing during travel until 4 weeks after leaving the malarious area
	or
	Chloroquine phosphate, same dose and regimen as above
	plus
	Pyrimethamine/sulfaxine (tablet, 25 mg/500 mg)
	  < 1 yr: ¼ tablet
	  1–3 yr: ½ tablet
	  4–8 yr: 1 tablet
	  9–14 yr: 2 tablets
	  > 14 yr: 3 tablets
	Given as a single dose for self-treatment for febrile disease when medical facility unavailable
	or
	Doxycycline (alone)
	  < 8 yr: contraindicated
	  > 8 yr: 2 mg/kg (max. 100 mg/day) once/day
	starting 1–2 days before travel and continuing during travel until 4 weeks after leaving the malarious area

including Egypt. Mefloquine is the drug of choice for travel into chloroquine-resistant malaria regions. Although mefloquine is not approved for use in children weighing less than 15 kg, a great deal of experience using this drug for prophylaxis – and even more for treatment – indicates that it is safe and effective using dosages outlined in Table 4.6.

Doxycycline can be used as prophylaxis for short-term travelers, but at the daily dosages recommended is likely to stain teeth in children younger than 9 years of age. The only other alternative is to bring medication appropriate for treatment of

Table 4.6 Malaria chemoprophylaxis

Chloroquine phosphate	5 mg/kg base (8.3 mg/kg/salt) once weekly, maximum dose 300 mg base beginning one week before entering endemic regions and continuing for 4 weeks after leaving
Mefloquine	> 45 kg: 1 tablet/week 31–45 kg: ¾ tablet/week 20–30 kg: ½ tablet/week 10–20 kg: ¼ tablet/week < 10 kg: ⅛ tablet/week

Table 4.7 Schedule for immunization and chemoprophylaxis

Time before travel	Vaccine or chemoprophylaxis
6 months	Hepatitis B
5 months	Hepatitis B
1 month	Measles, Mumps, Rubella (MMR) TB Mantoux Skin Test Hepatitis A Typhoid oral or i.m. Japanese encephalitis Rabies
1 week to 1 month	DTP Polio Meningococcal Rabies x 2 Yellow fever Japanese encephalitis
1 week	Hepatitis B Chloroquine or mefloquine Japanese encephalitis

young infants and begin therapy once a physician diagnoses malaria. Although anti-malaria agents should be available locally, there may be exceptions in medically under-served areas.

SCHEDULING

Table 4.7 summarizes required vaccines, chemoprophylaxis and other recommended intervention prior to travel. Planning should begin far in advance, which in many cases will necessitate multiple visits. A calendar should be prepared for each traveler, and printed sheets that detail medical problems unique to specific host countries should be provided. This latter information is available from the Centers for Disease Control and Prevention, Information Service and Traveler's Health Hotline (404) 639-2572.

Travel supplies

The usual protective measures should be strictly applied to family members. These include providing insecticide-impregnated mosquito nets for cribs and beds, protective clothing and mosquito repellents. Infants should also spend the majority of time in well-screened areas, and have repellents applied every two hours. Only products containing low concentrations of DEET should be used and applied to exposed skin (excluding the face, hands, or abraded areas). DEET should be removed by washing after the infant returns to indoor screened environments. Families should also consider bringing with them some other materials which may be helpful in preventing or treating tropical diseases. Suggestions are provided in the following list.

Recommended
    Routine medications
    Aspirin or acetaminophen
    Disinfectant for skin cuts and wounds
    Bandages, gauze, Band-aids, tweezers
    Antibiotic ointment
    Sunblock
    Sunhat
    DEET-based insect repellent
    Heating coil (to boil water)
    Iodine tablets or hand-filter (to treat water if no electricity)
    Antihistamine
    Plastic water bottle or flask
Necessary if applicable
    Over-supply of regular prescription drugs
    Copy of important prescriptions using generic names
    Nasal decongestant spray

Oil of wintergreen (for toothache) ± emergency dental kit

Antifungal skin cream and foot powder

Oral rehydration packets (for travel to remote areas)

Antimotion sickness pills

Cough syrup

Thermometer

Sunburn cream

Insect sting kit (Epi-pen)

Ipecac (if traveling with small children)

Items of practical importance that may be necessary or helpful

Mosquito bed net

Permethrin insect spray to impregnate clothes

AIDS-free certificate (for long-term visitors, students, or workers)

Swiss army knife

Sunglasses, spare eyeglasses, copy of eye prescription

Sewing kit

Small flashlight

Knockdown insect spray

Tissues and toilet paper

Commercial AIDS prevention kit (needles, syringes, i.v. infusion tubing)

Copies of passport front page, airline ticket, important phone numbers (e.g. US embassy, personal physician), credit card date

Supplementary health insurance

Trip disruption insurance (should include medical evacuation coverage)

Pretravel dental checkup

Presigned consent form for medical treatment to minor children left at home

Prophylactic antimicrobial therapy 5

The concept of chemoprophylaxis was introduced with the assumption that an antibiotic that eradicates an infection should also be able to prevent disease. Although data have confirmed the efficacy of prophylaxis for many well-defined indications (Table 5.1), some applications have actually led to an increase in infection, e.g., penicillin prophylaxis for meningococcal disease has been associated with a higher incidence of secondary disease. Therefore, any recommendation must be supported by well-designed clinical studies.

In general, prophylaxis works best when directed at a single specific pathogen to either prevent the progression of infection or eradicate colonization before disease becomes clinically established. Benefit is also most likely when the antibiotics used for prophylaxis have the following additional attributes: safety, low propensity for generating antibiotic resistance, and achievement of adequate serum concentrations at a tolerable and cost-effective dosage. Patient compliance is also a critical issue.

OTITIS MEDIA

It is estimated that 30% of a pediatrician's time is spent in managing various aspects of otitis media. Even more important than treatment of acute episodes is recognition of those children with persistent middle ear effusions since this may result in delay of psychomotor and language development or permanent conductive hearing loss. It should be appreciated that recurrent acute otitis media (RAOM) is a common source of discomfort in children, parental anxiety, and cost for acute medical care. With the high incidence of RAOM and frequent sequelae, a variety of strategies have been examined for prevention that employ various combinations of

Table 5.1 Infections or diseases for which antimicrobial chemoprophylaxis has been established

Bacterial diseases (various pathogens)
   Bacterial endocarditis
   Otitis media
   Recurrent urinary tract infection
   Respiratory pathogens in cystic fibrosis
     (Chapter 9)
   Sexually transmitted diseases (Chapter 16)
   Surgical procedures (Chapter 15)
   Traveler's diarrhea
Specific bacteria
   Atypical mycobacteria (MAC)
   Group A streptococcus (rheumatic fever)
   Haemophilus influenzae type b
   Infections in pediatric AIDS (Chapter 17)
   Meningococcus
   Neonatal group B streptococcal infection
     (Chapter 2)
   Pertussis
   Pneumococcus
   Tuberculosis
Viral
   Cytomegalovirus
   Herpes simplex
   HIV (Chapter 17)
   Influenza A
Others
   Malaria (Chapter 4)
   Pneumocystis carinii (Chapter 17)
   Scrub typhus

prophylactic antibiotics, ventilation tubes, steroids, and nonsteroidal anti-inflammatory agents. Vaccines and immunoglobulin have also been investigated. Of all approaches, a regimen of prophylactic antibiotics alone followed by ventilation tubes only for the more recalcitrant cases appears most rational. A 7-day course of steroids (0.5 to 1.0 mg/kg/day divided every 12 h) with antibiotics – after antibiotics alone have failed – has also been shown to be of benefit before beginning a longer course of prophylactic treatment.

Recurrent acute otitis media is defined as three episodes of infection within a 6-month period or four within 12 months. Data now exist that support the efficacy of amoxicillin and sulfisoxazole in reducing acute attacks of otitis media and in clearing middle ear effusions for children who are otitis media prone (Table 5.2). Additional studies have suggested that ventilation tubes in combination with prophylactic antibiotics may be necessary for some patients. However, most investigators agree that a trial of chemoprophylaxis is warranted before any decision for ventilation tube placement is made.

Trimethoprim–sulfamethoxazole (TMP/SMX) is equally effective as other regimens and is associated with a very low incidence of adverse reactions. However, the pharmaceutical companies that manufacture TMP/SMX have not requested approval from the Food and Drug Administration for this prophylactic indication, and a disclaimer

Table 5.2 Antibiotic prophylaxis for recurrent otitis media (OM)

Candidates for therapy
  3 episodes of acute OM within 6 months
  4 episodes of acute OM within 12 months
  1 episode before 6 months of age
    plus an otitis media-prone sibling
  2 episodes in the first year of life
  Down syndrome
  Turner syndrome
Chemoprophylaxis
  Sulfisoxazole, 35 mg/kg/day once or twice daily
  or
  Amoxicillin, 20 mg/kg/day divided or once daily
Duration of therapy
  90 days following the last episode of OM
  or
  During the winter months
  or
  For the duration of each new upper respiratory
    infection
Consider ventilating tubes
  Failure of chemoprophylaxis alone
  Poor compliance

---

emphasizing this restriction appears in the current *Physicians' Desk Reference*. The only theoretical adverse consequence of long-term prophylaxis is selection of antibiotic-resistant pathogens in the respiratory tract. This has been observed in some studies but not in others. Additional strategies for the prevention of RAOM do not appear to be effective. These include immunoglobulin, antihistamines, and decongestants.

URINARY TRACT INFECTIONS

Recurrent urinary tract infections (UTIs) are observed in 30% to 50% of children following acute pyelonephritis or cystitis, with approximately 90% of these occurring within 3 months after the initial episode. Eighty per cent of recurrences are new infections by different fecal-colonic bacterial species that have become resistant to recently administered antibiotics. The recurrence rate is not altered by extending the duration of treatment. Failure to eradicate an organism from the urine suggests an anatomic or physiologic defect. These patients require suppressive antibiotics until the underlying abnormality resolves or is surgically corrected. Recurrent UTI, if unrecognized, may lead to serious renal injury, hypertension, or end-stage renal disease.

The anatomic status of the upper urinary tract and the presence or absence or vesico-ureteral reflux (VUR) can have an important bearing on the long-term treatment chosen (Chapter 12). Vesicoureteral reflux has been reported in up to 50% of children with UTI, and chemoprophylaxis is an integral part of the management of these patients. Posterior urethral valves also predispose to infection and renal damage, but the value of antimicrobial prophylaxis is not as clear for this anatomic defect.

Children who have three or more UTIs in a 12-month period may need chronic suppressive antibiotic therapy for 3 to 6 months to allow repair of intrinsic bladder defense mechanisms. Girls with frequent UTIs tend to have asymptomatic recurrences. Children with recurrent UTI and anatomic defects or reflux may need suppressive antibiotics for as long as the defect exists. Resistance to antibiotics commonly develops, however, because of resistance (R) factors in fecal-colonic bacteria in patients receiving long-term suppressive therapy.

Other methods for decreasing reinfections of the lower urinary tract include avoiding bubble bath and detergents in the bath water, wiping the perineal area from front to back after voiding or defecation, increasing water intake, emptying the bladder every 3 to 4 hours during the day, and wearing cotton panties that have no permanent or aniline dyes. Agents that have been shown to be efficacious for chronic suppressive therapy include the sulfonamides, TMP/SMX, nitrofurantoin, fluoroquinolones, nalidixic acid, and oxolinic acid (Table 5.3). Previously, sulfonamides were the preferred agents, but with the recognition of increased resistance among coliform bacteria, the combination of TMP/SMX appears superior. A unique advantage of the trimethoprim component is its ability at relatively low dosages to reduce colonization of Enterobacteriaceae in the urethral orifice, thus diminishing the incidence of ascending reinfection.

Nitrofurantoin has been effectively used as prophylaxis for recurrent UTI in infants and children. Although it is active against most strains of *Escherichia coli*, it is inactive against many isolates of *Proteus*, *Pseudomonas*, *Klebsiella*, and *Enterobacter*. Resistance rarely develops with this agent. Pulmonary, neurologic, and hepatic adverse effects have been reported, but these are rare. The fluoroquinolones (ciprofloxacin and norfloxacin) are effective chronic therapy for recurrent UTI but should not be used in pregnant women or prepubertal children because of potential cartilage damage. Nalidixic acid and oxolinic acid are both bactericidal for most of the common Gram-negative uropathogens. Oxolinic acid has been associated with central nervous system (CNS) toxicity. Moreover, rapid and frequent development of bacterial resistance has been reported in many series of trials.

RHEUMATIC FEVER

Although the incidence of rheumatic fever has markedly declined in the United States during the last two decades, periodic outbreaks have recently been reported in widespread regions, thus suggesting a change in epidemiologic patterns. During the same time period, rheumatic fever and rheumatic heart disease have remained relatively more common in developing countries.

The strategy for prevention of rheumatic fever, which has remained consistent since the 1950s, is directed at reducing both the initial attacks of streptococcal infection (primary prevention) and recurrent attacks of acute rheumatic fever (secondary prevention). Primary prevention is best achieved with immediate and appropriate antimicrobial therapy against group A, β-hemolytic streptococcal (GABHS) upper respiratory tract infections. Recommended therapy consists of intramuscular benzathine penicillin G, 600 000 units for children who weigh less

Table 5.3 Antibiotic prophylaxis for recurrent urinary tract infection

Antibiotic	Daily dosage
Trimethoprim/sulfamethoxazole (TMP/SMX)	2 mg of TMP/10 mg of SMX/kg as a single bedtime dose
	or
	5 mg TMP/25 mg SMX twice per week
Nitrofurantoin	1–2 mg/kg divided q.24h
Sulfisoxazole	10–20 mg/kg divided q.12h
Nalidixic acid	30 mg/kg divided q.12h
Methenamine mandelate	75 mg/kg divided q.12h

than 27 kg and 1.2 million units for those over 27 kg. Phenoxymethyl penicillin (penicillin V), 250 mg two or three times daily for 10 days orally, is considered equivalent. For patients allergic to penicillin, erythromycin, 20 to 40 mg/kg/day orally divided twice daily is recommended. Oral cephalosporins are acceptable alternatives for penicillin-allergic patients, except those who have had true anaphylactic reactions to penicillin. Sulfonamides and TMP/SMX are not effective for primary prevention; they do, however, have a role in secondary prevention.

Failure of primary prevention has been observed in asymptomatic patients and in mild cases of streptococcal tonsilopharyngitis, as well as in patients with poor compliance or those less likely to seek medical attention for minor illnesses.

After the initial attack of acute rheumatic fever, patients are highly susceptible to recurrent episodes following GABHS infection. Continuous antimicrobial prophylaxis has been shown to prevent or at least significantly reduce the recurrence of rheumatic fever and rheumatic heart disease. The risk of recurrence is increased in economically disadvantaged populations and decreases as the time interval since the most recent attack lengthens. Risk is also higher with a history of multiple previous episodes, carditis, or increased exposure to GABHS infection as seen among school teachers, health workers, military recruits, and parents of young children.

The best regimen for secondary antimicrobial prophylaxis is intramuscular benzathine penicillin G 1.2 million units (for those over 27 kg) or 600 000 units (for those less than 27 kg) at 3-to-4-week intervals. For high-risk patients this antibiotic should be given every 3 weeks. Oral amoxicillin, 250 mg twice daily, and oral sulfadiazine, 500 mg (for patients less than 27 kg) or 1.0 g (for patients over 27 kg) daily, are also recommended, but the risk of recurrence is somewhat higher with these oral regimens as compared with injectable penicillin, even with optimal compliance. For patients allergic to penicillin and sulfa, oral erythromycin, 250 mg twice daily, is an effective alternative (Table 5.4).

At present there is no consensus as to when antimicrobial prophylaxis can be safely discontinued. In general, secondary prevention should be continued for at least five years after the last episode of rheumatic fever and until the patient has reached early adulthood. At this time, some authorities recommend changing from parenteral to oral prophylaxis. Recent data have also supported discontinuation of prophylaxis in low-risk young adults as long as they are maintained under adequate medical follow-up (Table 5.5).

The continuous, long-term use of penicillin theoretically increases the risk of penicillin allergy. However, data reported from the International Rheumatic Fever Study Group indicated similar rates of serious penicillin allergy in rheumatic patients receiving long-term prophylaxis as compared with

Table 5.4 Chemoprophylaxis of recurrences of rheumatic fever

Drug	Dose	Route
Benzathine penicillin G or	1 200 000 U every 4 weeks	Intramuscular
Penicillin V or	250 mg twice a day	Oral
Sulfadiazine or sulfisoxazole	0.5 g once a day for patients ≤ 27 kg (60 lb) 1.0 g once a day for patients > 27 kg (60 lb)	Oral
For individuals allergic to penicillin and sulfonamide drugs:		
Erythromycin	250 mg twice a day	Oral

Table 5.5 Duration of prophylaxis for persons who have had rheumatic fever: recommendations of the American Heart Association

Category	Duration
Rheumatic fever without carditis	5 years or until age 21, whichever is longer
Rheumatic fever with carditis but no residual heart disease (no valvar disease)	10 years or well into adulthood, whichever is longer
Rheumatic fever with carditis and residual heart disease (persistent valvar disease)	At least 10 years since last episode and at least until age 40; sometimes lifelong prophylaxis

children without rheumatic fever who received short-term parenteral penicillin. Patients with rheumatic heart disease also require subacute bacterial endocarditis prophylaxis before dental and surgical procedures as outlined in the following sections.

BACTERIAL ENDOCARDITIS

Infective endocarditis is a potentially life-threatening disease that has decreased in incidence as a consequence of chemoprophylactic intervention. Early diagnosis and therapeutic intervention have also contributed to a decline in mortality by 80% over the past 50 years. Patients with congenital or acquired heart disease are at an increased risk for endocarditis following well-defined medical, dental and surgical procedures. Antimicrobial prophylaxis is recommended by both the American Heart Association and the Committee on Infectious Diseases of the American Academy of Pediatrics for use preoperatively at times when the risk of bacteremia from defined procedures is high. Table 5.6 lists those congenital or acquired cardiac conditions for which endocarditis prophylaxis is or is not recommended.

Mitral valve prolapse is a common disorder but is a relatively low risk factor for endocarditis, but definitive data to provide guidance and management are particularly limited. Patients with this condition associated with mitral regurgitation or thickened and/or redundant mitral valve leaflets are at a higher risk for bacterial endocarditis. The current consensus is that these patients should receive antimicrobial prophylaxis.

Procedures requiring endocarditis prophylaxis

Table 5.7 summarizes the recommendations for dental procedures and Table 5.8 the recommendations for other interventions for which endocarditis prophylaxis generally is or is not indicated. Decisions should be individualized according to the risk introduced by the procedure and the predisposition to infection for the specific cardiac defect. Because α-hemolytic (viridans) streptococci are most commonly implicated in endocarditis following dental procedures, prophylaxis should be specifically directed against these organisms. Certain upper respiratory tract procedures may also cause bacteremia with organisms having similar antibiotic susceptibilities to those producing bacteremia following dental procedures. Therefore the same regimens are recommended.

Table 5.9 contains suggested regimens of prophylaxis for dental procedures and instrumentation of the upper respiratory tract and esophagus. In those patients at particularly high risk for endocarditis (e.g. those with prosthetic heart valves or surgically constructed systemic pulmonary shunts), parenteral prophylactic antibiotics are favored.

Table 5.6   Endocarditis prophylaxis related to cardiac conditions

Endocarditis prophylaxis recommended
   High-risk category
      Prosthetic cardiac valves, including biosynthetic and homograft valves
      Previous bacterial endocarditis
      Complex cyanotic congenital heart disease (e.g. single ventricle states, transposition of the great
         arteries, tetralogy of Fallot)
      Surgically constructed systemic pulmonary shunts or conduits
   Moderate-risk category
      Most other congenital cardiac malformations (other than above and below)
      Acquired valvar dysfunction (e.g. rheumatic heart disease)
      Hypertrophic cardiomyopathy
      Mitral valve prolapse with valvar regurgitation and/or thickened leaflets

Endocarditis prophylaxis not recommended
   Negligible-risk category (no greater risk than the general population)
      Isolated secundum atrial septal defect
      Surgical repair of atrial septal defect, ventricular septal defect, or patent ductus arteriosus (without
         residua beyond 6 months)
      Previous coronary artery bypass graft surgery
      Mitral valve prolapse without valvar regurgitation
      Physiologic, functional, or innocent heart murmurs
      Previous Kawasaki disease without valvar dysfunction
      Previous rheumatic fever without valvar dysfunction
      Cardiac pacemakers (intravascular and epicardial) and implanted defibrillators

Table 5.7   Endocarditis prophylaxis for specific dental procedures

Endocarditis prophylaxis recommended
   Dental extractions
   Periodontal procedures including surgery, scaling and root planing, probing and recall maintenance
   Dental implant placement and reimplantation of avulsed teeth
   Endodontic (root canal) instrumentation or surgery only beyond the apex
   Subgingival placement of antibiotic fibers or strips
   Initial placement of orthodontic bands but not brackets
   Intraligamentary local anesthetic injections
   Prophylactic cleaning of teeth or implants where bleeding is anticipated

Endocarditis prophylaxis not recommended
   Restorative dentistry (operative and prosthodontic) with or without retraction cord
   Local anesthetic injections (nonintraligamentary)
   Intracanal endodontic treatment; post placement and buildup
   Placement of rubber dams
   Postoperative suture removal
   Placement of removable prosthodontic or orthodontic appliances
   Taking of oral impressions
   Fluoride treatments
   Taking of oral radiographs
   Orthodontic appliance adjustment
   Shedding of primary teeth

Table 5.8 Endocarditis prophylaxis for respiratory, gastrointestinal, genitourinary tract and other procedures

Endocarditis prophylaxis recommended
    Respiratory tract
        Tonsillectomy and/or adenoidectomy
        Surgical operations that involve respiratory mucosa
        Bronchoscopy with a rigid bronchoscope
    Gastrointestinal tract
        Sclerotherapy for esophageal varices
        Esophageal stricture dilation
        Endoscopic retrograde cholangiography with biliary obstruction
        Biliary tract surgery
        Surgical operations that involve intestinal mucosa
    Genitourinary tract
        Prostatic surgery
        Cystoscopy
        Urethral dilation

Endocarditis prophylaxis not recommended
    Respiratory tract
        Endotracheal intubation
        Bronchoscopy with a flexible bronchoscope, with or without biopsy
        Tympanostomy tube insertion
    Gastrointestinal tract
        Transesophageal echocardiography
        Endoscopy with or without gastrointestinal biopsy
    Genitourinary tract
        Vaginal hysterectomy
        Vaginal delivery
        Cesarean section
        In uninfected tissue:
            Urethral catheterization
            Uterine dilatation and curettage
            Therapeutic abortion
            Sterilization procedures
            Insertion or removal of intrauterine devices
    Other
        Cardiac catheterization, including balloon angioplasty
        Implanted cardiac pacemakers, implanted defibrillators, and coronary stents
        Incision or biopsy of surgically scrubbed skin
        Circumcision

Genitourinary and gastrointestinal tract surgery and instrumentation

Data are inadequate to support specific recommendations to cover the entire range of invasive diagnostic and therapeutic procedures. Table 5.10 contains suggested regimens of prophylaxis for genitourinary and gastrointestinal procedures for both standard and special-risk patients as adapted from the current American Heart Association recommendations. Bacteremia less often accompanies other genitourinary and gastrointestinal tract procedures, and endocarditis has rarely if ever developed subsequent to these procedures. These include percutaneous liver biopsy, upper gastrointestinal endoscopy or proctosigmoidoscopy without

Table 5.9 Recommended prophylactic antibiotic regimens for dental, respiratory tract and esophageal procedures

Situation	Agent	Regimen
Standard general prophylaxis	Amoxicillin	Adults: 2.0 g; children: 50 mg/kg orally 1 h before procedure
Unable to take oral medications	Ampicillin	Adults: 2.0 g i.m. or i.v.; children: 50 mg/kg i.m. or i.v. within 30 min before procedure
Allergic to penicillin	Clindamycin or	Adults: 600 mg; children: 20 mg/kg orally 1 h before procedure
	Cephalexin or cefadroxil or	Adults: 2.0 g; children: 50 mg/kg orally 1 h before procedure
	Azithromycin or clarithromycin	Adults: 500 mg; children: 15 mg/kg orally 1 h before procedure
Allergic to penicillin and unable to take oral medications	Clindamycin or	Adults: 600 mg; children: 20 mg/kg i.v. within 30 min before procedure
	Cefazolin	Adults: 1.0 g; children: 25 mg/kg i.m. or i.v. within 30 min before procedure

Table 5.10 Recommended prophylactic antibiotic regimens for genitourinary or gastrointestinal procedures

Situation	Agent	Regimen
High-risk patients	Ampicillin plus gentamicin	Adults: ampicillin 2.0 g i.m. or i.v. plus gentamicin 1.5 mg/kg (not to exceed 120 mg) within 30 min of starting the procedure; 6 h later, ampicillin 1 g i.m. or i.v. or amoxicillin 1 g orally Children: ampicillin 50 mg/kg i.m. or i.v. (not to exceed 2.0 g) plus gentamicin 1.5 mg/kg within 30 min of starting the procedure; 6 h later, ampicillin 25 mg/kg i.m. or i.v. or amoxicillin 25 mg/kg orally
High-risk patients allergic to ampicillin/amoxicillin	Vancomycin plus gentamicin	Adults: vancomycin 1.0 g i.v. over 1–2 h plus gentamicin 1.5 mg/kg i.v. or i.m. (not to exceed 120 mg); complete injection/infusion within 30 min of starting the procedure Children: vancomycin 20 mg/kg i.v. over 1–2 h plus gentamicin 1.5 mg/kg i.v. or i.m.; complete injection/infusion within 30 min of starting the procedure
Moderate-risk patients	Amoxicillin or ampicillin	Adults: amoxicillin 2.0 g orally 1 h before procedure, or ampicillin 2.0 g i.m. or i.v. within 30 min of starting the procedure Children: amoxicillin 50 mg/kg orally 1 h before procedure, or ampicillin 50 mg/kg i.m. or i.v within 30 min of starting the procedure
Moderate-risk patients allergic to ampicillin/ amoxicillin	Vancomycin	Adults: vancomycin 1.0 g i.v. over 1–2 h; complete infusion within 30 min of starting the procedure Children: vancomycin 20 mg/kg i.v. over 1–2 h; complete infusion within 30 min of starting the procedure

biopsy, barium enema, uncomplicated vaginal delivery, and brief (in and out) bladder catheterization with sterile urine.

Enterococci (e.g. *Streptococcus faecalis*) are most frequently responsible for endocarditis following genitourinary and gastrointestinal tract surgery or instrumentation. Although Gram-negative bacillary bacteremia may follow such procedures, these organisms are only rarely responsible for endocarditis.

SPECIFIC BACTERIAL PATHOGENS

Meningococcus

The secondary attack rate for household contacts of meningococcal meningitis or meningococcemia is 1 per 250 (0.4%). Rifampin prophylaxis at a dose of 20 mg/kg/day (maximum, 1200 mg) divided every 12 hours for 2 days effectively eliminates this risk. Half this dose (10 mg/kg/day) may be used in neonates. Soft contact lenses should be removed because rifampin causes permanent staining. Prophylaxis is also recommended for other groups that have had intimate contact with these patients.

Pregnancy is a contraindication to rifampin, but ceftriaxone, 250 mg intramuscularly as a single dose, may be substituted.

High-risk contacts for meningococcal disease include all household contacts, nursery or day care center contacts and hospital personnel and individuals who have had intimate exposure to oral secretions from the index case.

Table 5.11 lists the available alternative treatments for chemoprophylaxis of meningococcal disease. The fluoroquinolones are effective as prophylaxis for contacts with meningococcal disease; however, they are not licensed for prepubertal children and pregnant women. Penicillin G and chloramphenicol, despite their efficacy for treatment of meningococcal meningitis, are not effective in eradicating oropharyngeal carriage of *Neisseria meningitidis*.

Haemophilus influenzae type b (Hib)

The risk to un-immunized household contacts of a child with invasive *H. influenzae* disease is 600 times higher than that in the

Table 5.11 Antibiotics for meningococcal prophylaxis

Antibiotic prophylaxis	Dosage	Comments
Rifampin	< 1 month: 5 mg/kg twice daily p.o. for 2 days > 1 month: 10 mg/kg twice daily p.o. for 2 days (max. 600 mg/dose)	Contraindicated for pregnant women Orange-red urine Stains contact lenses
Sulfisoxazole	2 months to 1 yr: 500 mg daily p.o. for 2 days 1 yr–12 yr: 500 mg twice daily p.o. for 2 days > 12 yr: 1 g twice daily p.o. for 2 days	Contraindicated for pregnant women during the third trimester and infants younger than 2 months
Ceftriaxone	< 12 yr: 125 mg i.m. as single dose > 12 yr: 250 mg i.m. as single dose	Safe for pregnant women Better compliance
Fluoroquinolones	Single adult p.o. dose	Contraindicated for pregnant women and children younger than 18 years
Minocycline	100 mg twice daily p.o. for 5 days	Contraindicated for pregnant women and children younger than 8 years

general population and is age dependent; the secondary attack rate for young infants less than 1 year old is 6%, 1 to 4 years of age, 2.1% and 4 to 6 years of age, 0.5%. The risk to un-immunized contacts in day care centers has not been fully determined, but appears to be great enough to warrant prophylaxis for susceptible children attending these centers and for adult personnel once there have been two cases of *H. influenzae* systemic disease within 60 days. Rifampin treatment of culture positive individuals has been shown to reduce the oropharyngeal carriage of *H. influenzae* by 97%. Rifampin at a dose of 20 mg/kg (maximum, 600 mg) once daily for 4 days eradicates the oro- and nasopharyngeal carriage of Hib in the majority of contacts. For infants younger than 1 month of age, the dose should be reduced to 10 mg/kg once daily for 4 days.

Pneumococcus

Asplenia may be congenital, postsurgical, or functional, the latter primarily resulting from sickle cell disease or other hemoglobinopathies. Regardless of the cause, patients are susceptible to invasive infection caused by encapsulated bacteria, particularly *Streptococcus pneumoniae* but occasionally Hib and *N. meningitidis*. Continuous antibody prophylaxis in addition to vaccination for pneumococci and *H. influenzae* has been an effective strategy for reducing the incidence of fatal postsplenectomy infections. However, postsplenectomy pneumococcal sepsis in patients who had received pneumococcal vaccine and were currently receiving appropriate antimicrobial prophylaxis regimens has been reported. Adequate levels of penicillin for pneumococci can be achieved with oral penicillin V at doses of 125 mg three times daily for children younger than 5 years old and 250 mg three times daily for children 5 years of age or older. Although somewhat more expensive, amoxicillin has certain advantages over the penicillin regimen when given at a dose of 20 mg/kg/day. Because of more consistent absorption from the gastrointestinal tract, higher serum concentrations are achieved, and in addition, amoxicillin has excellent activity against most strains of *H. influenzae*. The more pleasant taste of amoxicillin suspension also increases compliance. Some authorities suggest that various antibiotics should be rotated for long-term prophylaxis to prevent the emergence of resistant organisms. Consideration may also be given to the use of TMP/SMX in a dose of 4 mg TMP/ kg/day for children younger than 5 years of age since this antibiotic offers enhanced coverage for *H. influenzae*. The required duration of antimicrobial prophylaxis in asplenic patients has not yet been defined. Some recommend continuation during the patient's entire lifetime, whereas others have suggested long-term prophylaxis during the adult years only if there are additional high-risk factors. Asplenic patients and patients with sickle cell disease who are 2 years of age or older should receive pneumococcal vaccine (23-valent polysaccharide vaccine), and a second dose should be given 3 to 5 years later to children who would be younger than 10 years old at revaccination. The polysaccharide conjugate *Haemophilus* and meningococcal vaccines should also be given routinely. For effective splenectomy prophylaxis, pneumococcal vaccination should preferably be given 2 weeks before surgery because this will result in a more vigorous immune response, probably resulting from the contribution of immunologically reactive splenic lymphocytes.

Tuberculosis

Tuberculosis (TB) remains the most common serious infectious disease worldwide and accounts for 10 to 12 million new infections and 3 million deaths per year. As a consequence of the AIDS epidemic, TB has undergone a change in epidemiology that necessitates a more defined and effective strategy for chemoprophylaxis and vaccination. Multiple randomized placebo-controlled trials of isoniazid chemoprophylaxis have been completed and published during the past four decades, and all have shown a protective effect. Skin testing and a history of exposure were the most critical determinants for intitiation of prophylaxis. More recently, recommendations for treatment have included tuberculin skin test-negative individuals at high risk of infection (Table 5.12). Table 5.13 summarizes recent changes in interpretation of the Mantoux skin test that are based on the risk of disease in relation to different clinical and historical circumstances.

Patients who receive BCG vaccine may react to Mantoux test antigen, but an induration of 15 mm or greater should usually be considered to have resulted from TB exposure for these individuals.

Isoniazid remains the drug of choice for TB chemoprophylaxis following skin test conversion and is given at a dose of 10 mg/kg/day (maximum 300 mg) once daily. When compliance cannot be ensured, a regimen consisting of 20 mg/kg (maximum, 900 mg) twice weekly under the direct observation of a health care worker is recommended. For infants and children, therapy should be continued for 6–9 months. For HIV-infected patients a minimum of 12 months of therapy is recommended. Compliance remains a significant problem in TB-preventive therapy, and for noncompliant individuals who have received less than 80% of the recommended medication, a new full course of chemoprophylaxis should be implemented.

The recommended chemoprophylactic therapy for contacts of patients with isoniazid-resistant *Mycobacterium tuberculosis* infection is rifampin at an oral dose of 10 mg/kg (maximum, 600 mg) once daily. For isoniazid and rifampin-resistant *M. tuberculosis*, pyrazinamide with ethambutol or pyfazinamide with ciprofloxacin (for postpubertal contacts only) is suggested.

Pertussis

Prophylactic erythromycin is effective in preventing symptomatic disease as well as eradicating colonization in contacts of pertussis cases. Although immunization affords protection in 70 to 80% of recipients, prophylaxis should be offered to immunized as well as un-immunized family members, day care center, or hospital contacts during outbreaks of pertussis. Erythromycin is given orally at 50 mg/kg/day (maximum, 1.5 g) divided three times daily for 14 days.

SPECIFIC VIRAL PATHOGENS

Influenza A

Prophylaxis is recommended for all with medical problems that would result in more extensive infection once influenza developed and for all individuals with increased exposure to potential outbreaks. Influenza vaccine remains the primary means for prevention of influenza infection in such high-risk individuals. However, during influenza outbreaks, rimantadine or amantadine is indicated for those who have not been immunized but have been exposed to active disease. Once vaccine is given, antiviral therapy need only be continued for 14 days. In extremely high-

Table 5.12   Children who should receive isoniazid for tuberculosis prophylaxis

Children	Duration of treatment
Asymptomatic skin test reactor with a normal chest X-ray	6 months
Skin test–negative household contact of an active case	3 months (then repeat skin test)
Previously skin test-positive children who are immune suppressed (malignancy, corticosteroid, or immunosuppressive therapy)	For the duration of immune suppression

Table 5.13 Definition of a positive Mantoux skin test (5 tuberculin units of purified protein derivative) in children

Reaction size of ≥ 5 mm
  Children in close contact with known or suspected infectious cases of tuberculosis
  Households with active cases
  Households with previously active cases if
    Treatment cannot be verified as adequate before the exposure
    Treatment was initiated after a period of contact with the child
    Reactivation is suspected
  Children suspected to have tuberculous disease
    Chest roentgenogram consistent with active or previously active tuberculosis
    Clinical evidence of tuberculosis
  Children with underlying conditions that put them at high risk of acquiring severe tuberculosis
    Immunocompromised conditions
    HIV infection
Reaction size of ≥ 10 mm
  Children at increased risk of dissemination
  Young (age < 4 years old)
  Other medical risk factors: Hodgkin's disease, lymphoma, diabetes mellitus, chronic renal failure, malnutrition
  Increased environmental exposure
    Those from or whose parent have emigrated from high-prevalence regions of the world
  Children frequently exposed to the following adults
    HIV infected
    Homeless persons
    Users of intravenous and other street drugs
    Poor and medically indigent city dwellers
    Residents of nursing homes
    Migrant farm workers
Reaction size of ≥ 15 mm
  Children ≥ 4 yr old without any risk factors

risk individuals, the combination of vaccine plus rimantadine offers maximum protection, 90% vs 70% for either alone. The dosage for both antiviral agents is 5 to 8 mg/kg/day (maximum, 200 mg/day) given orally once daily or divided into two doses.

Herpes simplex virus (HSV)

Oral acyclovir is effective in reducing recurrences of genital HSV in adolescents and adults who have experienced frequent episodes of reactivation. The usual recommended dosage is 800–1000 mg/day in 2 to 5 divided doses, continued for as long as 12 months. Some experts recommend acyclovir for prophylaxis in immunocompromised HSV-positive patients although the drug is not currently licensed for this indication. During low-risk periods it is given orally, 600–1000 mg/day in 3 to 5 divided doses. In children the total daily dosage should not exceed 80 mg/kg. With high-risk circumstances (increased immunosuppressive chemotherapy) it can be given intravenously, 750 mg/m^2/day in 3 divided doses.

Cytomegalovirus (CMV)

Acyclovir, valacyclovir and ganciclovir have been shown to offer some limited benefit for the prophylaxis of CMV infection in transplant recipients and other immunocompromised hosts, although these antiviral agents are not currently licensed for this clinical application. They are considered for high-risk patients who are CMV antibody positive or who are negative but have received organs from CMV positive donors. The dose of oral acyclovir is 800–3200 mg/day (not to exceed 80 mg/kg/day) in 1 to 4 divided doses or 1500 mg/m^2/day in 3 divided doses i.v. during the risk period. The i.v. dosage of ganciclovir is 10 mg/kg/day in 2 divided doses for 1 week, followed by 5 mg/kg/day in a daily dose. Valacyclovir has only been studied in adult renal transplant patients, using an oral dose of 2 g 4 times daily for 90 days after transplantation with the dosage adjusted for renal function; this treatment reduced the incidence of CMV disease after renal transplantation in CMV-negative recipients of a kidney from a seropositive donor and in CMV-positive recipients. Ganciclovir is also used for chronic suppressive or maintenance therapy in HIV-infected patients who have been treated for CMV retinitis and other types of CMV organ involvement (e.g. renal). The dosage is as listed above, continued for 3 months or longer.

Common outpatient infections

6

INTRODUCTION

Most infections can be managed on an out-patient basis and these compose, by most estimates, 60 to 80% of unscheduled pediatric office or emergency room visits. Approximately 90% of febrile episodes in children are caused by viruses rather than bacteria and are usually accompanied by upper respiratory signs and symptoms. Reassurance and medication for fever or congestion are the only interventions warranted. Distinguishing more severe infectious processes remains the most important aspect of outpatient evaluation.

ABSCESSES (CUTANEOUS)

The organisms most frequently recovered from skin and soft tissue abscesses are *Staphylococcus aureus* and group A ß-hemolytic streptococci (Table 6.1). Among these infections, cutaneous abscesses should be distinguished from impetigo, cellulitis and wound infections, where treatment is somewhat different. All abscesses should be incised and drained. When there is a question as to whether a lesion is fluctuant, EMLA cream can be applied to the skin and an 18-gauge needle and syringe used to aspirate material or probe the abscess. An incision can then be made and a wick placed to ensure continued drainage. This is all that is necessary for *S. aureus* and most other organisms. Group A streptococci require penicillin or an appropriate alternative oral antibiotic to penetrate the larger areas of cellulitis. Bacteremia from cutaneous abscesses is extremely rare but should be considered with extensive involvement, high fever, or in the immunocompromised host.

Abscesses in the perirectal region are almost always associated with mixed

Table 6.1 Organisms recovered from cutaneous abscesses in children

Aerobes (50%)
Staphylococcus aureus (25%)
Group A ß-hemolytic streptococci; a- and nonhemolytic streptococci
Enterobacteriaceae
Escherichia coli
Anaerobes (25%)
Bacteroides melaninogenicus
Bacteroides fragilis
Fusobacterium
Mixed aerobes and anaerobes (25%)

infection, including anaerobic bacteria and aerobic pathogens, mainly *S. aureus* and *Escherichia coli*, though streptococci and other aerobes each account for approximately 10% of infections. As with other cutaneous abscesses, incision with drainage is the most important aspect of therapy. In contrast to infection in other anatomic areas, simple drainage may be inadequate. Fistulae must be identified, opened, and excised. Perirectal abscesses therefore require surgical consultation. Suggested antibiotics are clindamycin and a third-generation cephalosporin (or as directed by Gram stain and culture). They should only be used for extensive involvement, systemic symptoms and compromised hosts.

ADENITIS

Adenitis (Table 6.2) should be distinguished from adenopathy (see Chapter 13) although considerable clinical overlap exists. Adenitis is usually painful, hot, and occurs more frequently (75%) in the 1- to 4-year-old age group. Untreated, these nodes will suppurate and occasionally progress to cellulitis and bacteremia. When there is no primary focus – such as pharyngitis or tonsillitis – fever and other systemic symptoms imply such progression. Pitting edema strongly suggests the presence of a suppurative node that requires drainage. Ultrasonography is a useful tool in determining the consistency of the node and in helping identify localized exudate. This test should be most strongly considered for the child who is toxic or has significant pain since he is more likely to benefit from early drainage. Cervical adenitis with minimal tenderness or persistence following 10 days of antimicrobial therapy increases the likelihood of atypical mycobacterial and *Mycobacterium tuberculosis* infection. This should be evaluated by intradermal testing with intermediate PPD (5 tuberculin units). Adenitis in all locations is caused most commonly by either *S. aureus* or group A streptococci and therapy is directed against these two pathogens (Table 6.3).

ANIMAL AND HUMAN BITES

Animal bites account for 1% of emergency room visits, with approximately 90% caused by dogs, 10% by cats, and 1% by rodents (rabbits, squirrels, hamsters and gerbils). Approximately 90% are pets owned by the family or neighbors, which suggests that better education of children (and parents) might reduce these all too common injuries. Human bites require similar management and are therefore included in this discussion.

A major focus of treatment concerns prevention of wound infection. Human bites most commonly become infected (more than 50%), followed by cat (30%), whereas dog and rodent bites are associated with a 5% incidence of cellulitis or abscess formation. Organisms recovered from infected animal bites include *Pasteurella multocida*, *Staphylococcus intermedius*, *Streptococcus* sp. and anaerobic bacteria. Such infection is usually clinically apparent within 24 h after the injury. Upper extremity injuries become infected more commonly than those to the face, scalp or lower extremities, because debridement and irrigation of the compartments of the hand

Table 6.2 Bacterial etiology of adenitis

All locations
  S. aureus 40–50%
  Group A streptococci 30–40%

Other organisms by location:
Cervical
  Atypical mycobacteria
  M. tuberculosis
  Gram-negative enterics
  H. influenzae
  Anaerobes
  Actinomyces israelii
  Tularemia

Preauricular
  Tularemia

Occipital
  Tinea capitis

Axillary
  Cat scratch disease
  Sporotrichosis

Inguinal
  Anaerobes
  Gram-negative enterics
  Tularemia

Generalized
  Infectious mononucleosis
  Toxoplasmosis
  Cytomegalovirus
  Other viruses
  Kawasaki disease
  Syphilis
  Hepatitis
  Brucellosis
  Sarcoidosis

Table 6.3 Treatment of adenitis

Prescribe any of the following:
  Dicloxacillin or cloxacillin
  Erythromycin
  Cephalexin, cephradine, cefadroxil, or
    cefuroxime axetil
  Amoxicillin/clavulanate
Incision and drainage when fluctuant

are more difficult. In contrast to animal attacks, human inflicted bites are commonly associated with infection caused by *Eikenella corrodens*.

Gram stains or cultures immediately following the injury are not predictive of organisms subsequently associated with infection. Therefore, these laboratory studies should only be obtained once cellulitis or abscess formation occurs. Every effort should be made primarily to close lacerations, both for cosmetic reasons and to reduce local bacterial colonization. Large wounds, those associated with extensive tissue destruction, or ones requiring optimal cosmetic repair may best be managed under general anesthesia in the operating room (Table 6.4).

BACTEREMIA

Reported studies have demonstrated that bacteremia occurs in fewer than 2% of febrile infants who do not appear toxic. The most common predisposing infections are otitis media and pneumonia. The majority of patients, however, have no obvious focus. In children who have received at least 2 doses of *Haemophilus influenzae* type b vaccine, more than 90% of positive cultures are pneumococcus (Table 6.5). Unique are children with sickle cell disease who exhibit a high incidence of pneumococcal bacteremia. These children, when febrile, require close observation.

Table 6.4 Treatment of animal and human bites

Cleansing and debridement
Extensive wound irrigation
Suturing for closure
Antibiotics: amoxicillin/clavulanate
Tetanus prophylaxis when indicated
Rabies prophylaxis when indicated
Re-examine in 24 hr

Table 6.5 Bacteremia in infants

S. pneumoniae (92%)
Salmonella sp. (6%)
N. meningitidis (1%)
Group A streptococci (1%)
S. aureus (< 1%)

Febrile neonates less than 28 days of age should usually be hospitalized and evaluated for sepsis. This includes blood culture, lumbar puncture, and urine for culture obtained by catheterization or bladder tap. Older infants are managed on an individual basis with decision for hospitalization based on physical assessment rather than any laboratory parameters. The decision to obtain a blood culture should usually be accompanied by one for observation in the hospital setting. If pneumococcal bacteremia is documented from an outpatient culture, the patient must be re-examined. If improved but showing no focus of infection, penicillin or an alternative antibiotic for penicillin-resistant strains should be given for ten days. Specific infections seen on follow-up, such as otitis media or pneumonia, are managed in the usual fashion. Salmonella bacteremia is usually associated with gastroenteritis. Although there is no direct evidence that bacteremic cases should be managed differently from those with simple intestinal infection, most experts recommend antimicrobial therapy, either parenteral or oral, depending on the severity of illness.

CELLULITIS

Infection of the skin and subcutaneous tissue is most commonly the result of local trauma or the extension of an underlying abscess. Periorbital cellulitis is most likely to arise following conjunctival colonization with pneumococcus or other potential pathogens, whereas orbital cellulitis is a consequence of ethmoid sinusitis with penetration into the retrobulbar space. Buccal cellulitis is frequently associated with ipsilateral otitis media. There are some features that help differentiate more probable etiologic agents and these should be used as guides to therapy (Table 6.6).

Selection of antibiotics is guided by an understanding of the pathogens most likely to cause cellulitis. Any abscess should first be incised and drained. In most cases, a penicillinase-resistant penicillin is used to

Table 6.6 Cellulitis: clinical features associated with specific bacteria

Clinical feature	Organism
Neonatal cellulitis	
Facial	Group B streptococci
Funicitis (periumbilical)	Group A streptococci
Predisposing trauma	S. aureus, Group A streptococci
Foot (puncture wound)	Pseudomonas sp.
Burn	Group A streptococci
Chickenpox	Group A streptococci, S. aureus
Infant cellulitis	
Facial, periorbital	S. pneumoniae
Ascending lymphangitis	Group A streptococci
Erysipelas (distinct borders)	Group A streptococci

Table 6.7 Treatment of cellulitis

Patient/condition	Treatment
Neonate	Nafcillin or oxacillin + ceftriaxone or cefotaxime
1 month to 5 years	Ceftriaxone or cefotaxime
Predisposing trauma	Nafcillin or oxacillin
Ascending lymphangitis	Penicillin

Table 6.8 Etiology and treatment of conjunctivitis

Age	Etiology	Treatment
< 3 days	Silver nitrate	None
3 days–3 weeks	N. gonorrhoeae	Ceftriaxone, one dose
3 weeks–20 weeks	C. trachomatis	Sulfonamide eye drops plus erythromycin p.o. for 14 days
> 12 weeks	H. aegypticus ('pink eye')	Sulfonamide eye drops for 5–10 days
	S. aureus	Topical bacitracin
	H. influenzae	Sulfonamide eye drops
	S. pneumoniae	Sulfonamide eye drops
	Moraxella lacunata	Sulfonamide eye drops
	Streptococci	Sulfonamide eye drops
	Adenoviruses	Cold soaks
	Enterovirus 70	Cold soaks
	Herpes simplex	Vidarabine ointment or trifluridine eye drops

cover staphylococci and group A streptococci (Table 6.7). When *Streptococcus pneumoniae* is a probable agent, such as with facial cellulitis, a third generation cephalosporin is most appropriate. Blood and, when practical, an aspirate of the advancing margin of the cellulitis should be cultured.

CONJUNCTIVITIS

Causes of conjunctivitis are largely age dependent and include sensitivity to environmental agents (allergic conjunctivitis) as well as viral and bacterial pathogens. Microscopic examination of exudate with Gram stain (*Neisseria gonorrhoeae*) and Giemsa stain (*Chlamydia trachomatis*) when appropriate will help differentiate the varied etiologies. Cultures should be obtained prior to treatment (Table 6.8).

DERMATOPHYTOSES AND CANDIDIASIS

Dermatophytes have the unique ability to colonize skin, hair and nails, but almost never invade deeper tissues. Diagnosis is made clinically by noting characteristic patterns such as a ring with central clearing or kerion formation. Confirmation is best achieved with a KOH preparation. Wood light examination will occasionally demonstrate the characteristic apple green fluorescence of *Microsporum* and some other organisms. Up to the present, 37 species of dermatophytes have been identified, hence it is more practical to approach diagnosis and selection of antifungal agents according to clinical presentation (Table 6.9). Cultures are most useful for infections that do not respond to initial therapy.

FEVER AND OCCULT BACTEREMIA

Although children 3 to 36 months of age with fever ≥ 39.0°C, white blood cell count (WBC) > 15 000/mm^3 and no focus of infection are at increased risk for having pneumococcal occult bacteremia, antimicrobial treatment is only warranted for those who appear toxic. The preferred antibiotic for outpatient treatment is ceftriaxone 50–75 mg/kg (maximum 1 g) as a single dose. The vast majority resolve their fever without subsequent focal or systemic infection. If the child's condition worsens, he/she should be admitted to the hospital for a sepsis work-up and begun on parenteral antibiotics (Table 6.10). Much more important than fever *per se* is its underlying cause. Once this has been determined, antipyretics (Table 6.11) may be used for the child's comfort and to help prevent febrile convulsions in the susceptible age group. Newer pharmacokinetic data offer better guidelines for administration of acetaminophen or aspirin.

Table 6.10 Laboratory studies for children 1 month to 3 years of age with fever and no apparent source

Urinalysis – all children
Urine culture – Uncircumcised males Females < 2 years
Optional
Complete blood count
Chest roentgenogram (with respiratory   symptoms)
Stool culture (with GI symptoms)
Blood culture (temp ≥ 39.0°C)

Table 6.9 Treatment of dermatophytoses

Clinical disease	Therapy
Tinea capitis	
Kerion	Griseofulvin 20–25 mg/kg/day p.o. div. q.24h for 4–8 weeks
Black-dot ringworm	
Gray-patch ringworm	
Tinea corporis	Topical clotrimazole, miconazole or tolnaftate b.i.d. for 4 weeks
Tinea cruris	Topical (as above) for 4–6 weeks
Tinea pedis	Topical (as above) for 6–12 weeks; oral griseofulvin for *Trichophyton rubrum*
Onychomycosis	Oral griseofulvin for 3–4 months
Candidiasis	
Thrush	Nystatin p.o. 200 000 U q.i.d. for 10–14 days or fluconazole 6 mg/kg on the first day followed by 3 mg/kg daily for 14 days
Diaper rash	Nystatin cream q.i.d.

Table 6.11 Antipyretic therapy

Acetaminophen
　　Loading dose: 22 mg/kg
　　Maintenance: 13 mg/kg q.6h
Aspirin
　　Loading dose: 18 mg/kg
　　Maintenance: 8.5 mg/kg q.6h

FEVER OF UNKNOWN ORIGIN (FUO)

Fever of unknown origin (FUO) is a convenient term used to classify patients who warrant a particular systematic approach to diagnostic evaluation and management. Criteria first proposed for adult patients by Petersdorf and Beeson in 1961 have been used for over three decades for all ages but may not be applicable today. In contrast to adults, prognosis for children who fulfill criteria for FUO is much better since they are less likely to have malignancies or autoimmune processes as the cause of prolonged fever. Definition is generally the following: an immunologically normal host with oral or rectal temperature ≥ 38.0°C (100.4°F) at least twice a week for more than 3 weeks, a noncontributory history and physical examination, and one week of outpatient investigation. Early diagnostic studies would normally include a complete blood cell count, lactic dehydrogenase (LDH), uric acid, urinalysis and culture, chest roentgenogram, tuberculin skin test, erythrocyte sedimentation rate (ESR) and, in the older child, an antinuclear antibody titer. Certain medical circumstances would greatly influence both diagnostic and management approaches. These include patients with acquired or congenital immunodeficiency, neutropenic patients, and those whose fevers have occurred during prolonged hospital stays.

The greatest clinical concern in evaluating FUO is identifying patients whose fever has a serious or life-threatening etiology for whom a delay in diagnosis could jeopardize successful intervention. Cancer and severe bacterial infections are the causes most frequently discussed and likely to influence diagnostic and management approaches. However, it should be emphasized that a vast majority of children with prolonged FUO resolve their illnesses without a diagnosis and do not exhibit long-lasting effects. Therefore it appears appropriate for most children to delay extensive diagnostic evaluation until the child has remained febrile for at least six weeks. Diagnostic evaluation should begin with basic studies done during outpatient observation as summarized in Table 6.12.

The initial outpatient evaluation generally requires 1 week to complete laboratory testing and to obtain final results. After this time the physician must decide whether simple continued observation or progressive laboratory investigation is more appropriate. Decisions are based primarily on the clinical status of the child and results of initial evaluation. For most patients, observation is most prudent since the majority will become afebrile by 6 weeks. A practical approach to continued evaluation once this appears necessary is summarized in Table 6.13.

OROPHARYNGEAL INFECTION

Almost all 'upper respiratory infections' are caused by viral agents and require only symptomatic therapy. Pharyngitis or tonsillitis without nasal involvement is more commonly associated with group A streptococci and a

Table 6.12 Initial evaluation of children with fever of unknown origin (FUO) and rationale for screen

History and physical (all causes)
Complete blood cell count (leukemia and
　infections)
Lactic dehydrogenase (LDH) , uric acid
　(leukemia and lymphomas)
Urinalysis and culture (infection)
Chest roentgenogram (infections and
　malignancies)
Tuberculin skin test (tuberculosis)
Antinuclear antibody titer – older child
　(autoimmune)
ESR or CRP (all causes)

Table 6.13 Protocol for continued evaluation of children with FUO

Phase 1 Outpatient (after 3–6 weeks of fever)
   Complete blood cell count (repeat)
   Erythrocyte sedimentation rate
   Urinalysis and culture (repeat)
   EBV serology
   Chest roentgenogram (review if already
     obtained)
   Blood culture
   Anti-streptolysin O
   Human immunodeficiency virus antibody (if
     there are risk factors)
   Twice daily temperature recordings (by
     parents at home)

Phase 2 Inpatient (after 6 weeks of fever)
   Hospitalize for observation
   Lumbar puncture (partial treatment or any
     toxicity in a young infant)
   Repeat blood cultures
   Sinus radiographs
   Ophthalmologic examination for iridocyclitis
   Liver enzymes
   Serologic tests
     Cytomegalovirus
     Toxoplasmosis
     Hepatitis A, B, and C
     Tularemia (in endemic regions)
     Brucellosis (with risk factors)
     Leptospirosis
     Salmonellosis

Phase 3 Inpatient (after 6 weeks of fever if
  condition worsens)
   Abdominal ultrasonography
   Abdominal CT scanning
   Gallium or indium scanning
   Upper gastrointestinal tract X-ray series with
     follow-through
     (older child with any abdominal symptoms)
   Bone marrow (if any abnormalities in
     complete blood cell count)
   Technetium bone scanning

throat culture or test for streptococcal antigen is essential for determining this bacterial etiology. Often, documentation of an outbreak of oropharyngeal infection caused by a particular viral pathogen offers guidance to management of subsequent cases. Rare but important bacterial pathogens causing pharyngitis are *Arcanobacterium hemolyticum*, *Neisseria gonorrhoeae*, *Corynebacterium diphtheriae*, and *Francisella tularensis* with other groups of streptococci, particularly C and G, accounting for isolated outbreaks of disease (Table 6.14).

OTITIS EXTERNA (SWIMMER'S EAR)

Otitis externa is caused by retention of water in the external canal with resulting bacterial replication and inflammation. Recovered bacterial pathogens are those which commonly colonize skin and thrive in moist environments, that is *S. aureus*, *Pseudomonas aeruginosa*, *Proteus vulgaris*, *Streptococcus pyogenes*, Enterobacteriaceae and *Aspergillus* sp.

Therapy is directed at eradication of probable organisms with broad spectrum topical antibiotics which can be accomplished with a 10-day course (Table 6.15). Children who swim frequently or have had repeated bouts of otitis externa should instill an acidified alcohol solution into the external canals after swimming or showering.

OTITIS MEDIA

It has been estimated that pediatricians spend as much as 30% of their time in the management of otitis media, second only to well child care in clinical responsibilities. Early and aggressive intervention is essential for the child's comfort as well as prevention of severe suppurative complications such as mastoiditis and meningitis. As important is prevention of the persistent conductive hearing loss, which has been shown to delay speech development and cognitive function.

Definitions

A diagnosis of acute otitis media (AOM) requires the presence of middle ear effusion along with the rapid onset of clinical signs and symptoms, specifically fever, pain, irritability, anorexia, or vomiting. This definition separates AOM from otitis media with effusion (OME) which is not associated with

Table 6.14 Upper respiratory infections – common etiologic agents and treatment

Classification	Etiology	Treatment
Common cold	Rhinovirus	Symptomatic
	Parainfluenza	
	RSV	
Nasopharyngitis	Adenovirus	Symptomatic
	Enteroviruses (e.g., herpangina)	
	Rhinoviruses	
	Parainfluenza	
	Influenza	
	Respiratory syncytial virus	
Pharyngitis–tonsillitis	Viruses (as with nasopharyngitis)	
	Bacteria	
	Group A streptococci	Penicillin
	Streptococci C and G	Penicillin
	Arcanobacterium hemolyticum	Erythromycin
	Neisseria gonorrhoeae	Penicillin
	Francisella tularensis	Streptomycin
Peritonsillar abscesses	Group A streptococci	Penicillin
	S. aureus	Nafcillin
		Incision and drainage

Table 6.15 Treatment of otitis externa

Acute treatment: otic drops
  Floxacin or ofloxacin 5 drops b.i.d. for 10 days
  Cortisporin (polymyxin B, neomycin, and
    hydrocortisone) or Otobiotic (polymyxin B
    and hydrocortisone) q.i.d. for 10 days
Prophylaxis (swimmer's ear drops) after
  swimming or showering

symptoms, and from chronic suppurative otitis media, which is a persistent inflammatory process with a perforated tympanic membrane and draining exudate for longer than 6 weeks. Identification of AOM is made by direct visualization of the tympanic membrane, using a pneumatic otoscope so that movement of the membrane can be fully evaluated. With AOM, the eardrum may be bulging or retracted, landmarks are distorted and, most importantly, movement is markedly decreased. In difficult to diagnosis cases, particularly in children with scarred tympanic membranes from previous infection, tympanometry and acoustic reflectometry offer simple and accurate means of confirming the presence of fluid. One of these devices should be available to every primary care physician who manages children with otitis media, not only as an aid in the diagnosis of AOM but also to follow children with persistent effusion.

Microbiology

The organisms causing AOM have remained relatively constant during the past two decades (Table 6.16). The aspect of these pathogenic bacteria which has changed dramatically is their susceptibility to previously recommended antimicrobial therapy, particularly increasing resistance to amoxicillin. Beginning a decade ago clinicians were warned that the prevalence of beta-lactamase production by nontypeable *H. influenzae* and *Moraxella catarrhalis* was increasing, and at present 30–40% and 90–100% of these organisms respectively are not susceptible to penicillin by this mechanism. More importantly, *S. pneumoniae* has now developed amoxicillin resistance via an alteration in penicillin

Table 6.16 Etiology of otitis media in infants and children

Pathogen	Mean (%)	Range (%)
S. pneumoniae	39	27–52
H. influenzae (non typeable)	27	16–52
M. catarrhalis	10	2–27
S. pyogenes	3	0–11
None or nonpathogens	20	12–45

binding proteins (PBP) which also renders these organisms non-susceptible to penicillin/ beta lactamase inhibitor combinations such as amoxicillin–clavulanate and ticarcillin– clavulanate.

Selection of first-line therapy for otitis media must be made by the individual physician based on regional susceptibility data of bacterial pathogens and, more importantly, treatment failure rates of previous regimens. Regional differences for these variables make it difficult to offer recommendations that are appropriate for all locations. If a decision is made to change from amoxicillin (or trimethroprim–sulfamethoxazole) as first-line therapy, there are may options (Figure 6.1). Other considerations for selection might include cost and compliance issues. Compliance is enhanced for antibiotics that are better tasting, given once or twice rather than 3 or 4 times a day, and those given for briefer durations. A change to other classes of antibiotics for most outpatient infections also offers the theoretical advantage of reversing the trend to penicillin resistance among these organisms by eliminating the pressure for mutation which always occurs with excessive use of a single agent.

Acute otitis media (AOM)

Spontaneous resolution of signs and symptoms after 48 hours of treatment for AOM in approximately 50% of cases is somewhat organism dependent, lowest for pneumococcus (10%), highest for *Moraxella* (70%) and intermediate for *H. influenzae* (50%). Because there is no way of predicting which children do not require antibiotics, they should be

offered to all cases. Withholding therapy for more than 48 hours, an option to management used by some physicians has been associated with an increase in the incidence of mastoiditis.

Antimicrobial therapy alleviates symptoms within 48 hours in more than 90% of children. Persistence of symptoms at this point is an indication for empiric change to another class of antibiotics. In young children the effusion persists for one month in 40% of patients, two months in 20% and three months in 10%. Therefore additional management is not indicated until after 12 months of follow-up for those with persistent effusion, at which time tympanometry should be obtained. Children with a tympanogram showing a C2, C3, or B pattern should undergo audiometry. If this testing demonstrates a 20dB loss or greater, tympanostomy tubes are indicated. This may be necessary in as many as 2% of all AOM cases, representing 10% of all children less than 3 years of age.

Otitis media with effusion (OME)

A clinical practice guideline for OME was published jointly by the pediatric, family physician, and otolaryngology academies with the review and approval of the Agency for Health Care Policy and Research of the US Department of Health and Human Services. The algorithm in Figure 6.2 is adapted from this document with some modifications.

The option for using antibiotics both initially and after 2 months of persistent effusion was chosen and the addition of steroids at 2 months is included although the practice guideline does not support their use. Regarding the latter decision, although clinical trials have been inconclusive, current practice and the absence of adverse consequences support this modification. The use of antihistamines or decongestants is not recommended at any stage of management because clinical trials have never demonstrated efficacy. Likewise the association between allergy and OME is not clear from available evidence and therefore no recommendation can be made

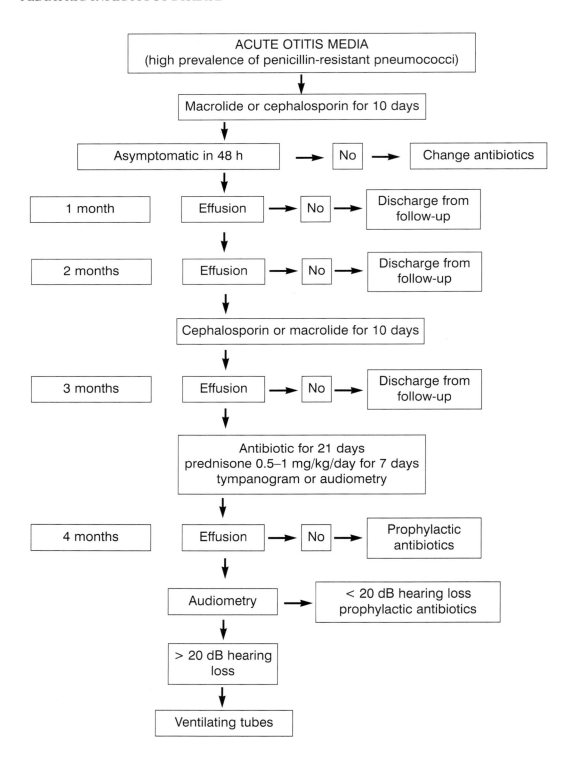

Figure 6.1 Algorithm for management of acute otitis media (AOM) including follow-up of persistent middle ear effusion

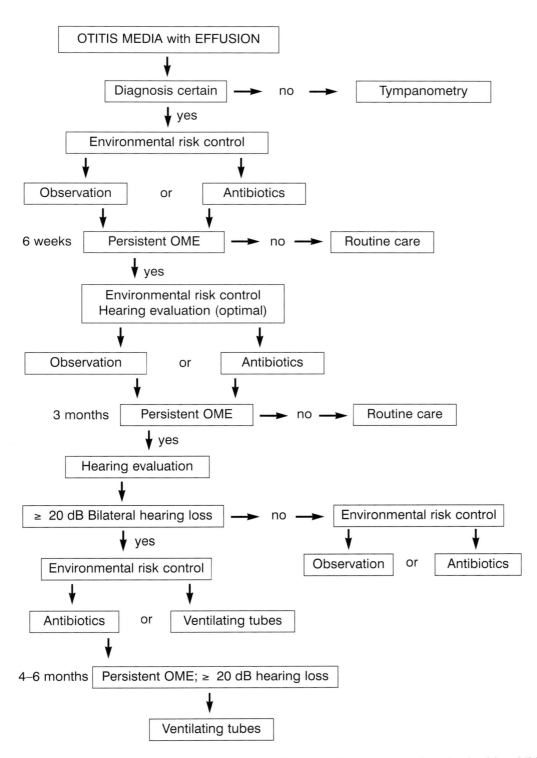

Figure 6.2 Algorithm for managing otitis media with effusion in an otherwise healthy child aged 1 through 3 years

relevant to allergy testing or treatment. The most problematic intervention step pertains to the indications and timing of tympanostomy tube placement. Decisions are guided by the likelihood of persistent effusions resulting in delayed speech and reduction in cognitive development. Age and duration of effusion are both important variables in this assessment. With all data considered, it appears prudent to recommend ventilating tubes in children with effusion of greater than 4–6 months duration who have a hearing loss of ≥ 20dB and for children less than 3 years of age with effusion > 3 months who have recurrent infection while on prophylactic antibiotics.

Chronic suppurative otitis media (CSOM)

Chronic suppurative infection is a sequela of poorly responsive recurrent AOM, particularly when a perforation has occurred. As the perforation heals, squamous epithelium may grow into the organizing abscess material producing a sac-like structure called a cholesteatoma. This frequently disrupts the ossicular chain resulting in a severe conductive hearing loss. It is essential, therefore, to differentiate CSOM without cholesteatoma – which requires aggressive medical management – from CSOM with cholesteatoma which is a surgical disease. Otomicroscopic evaluation by an otolaryngologist of all patients with a perforated drum and otorrhea for more than 6 weeks, particularly with ear pain and hearing loss, is warranted to identify the presence or absence of a cholesteatoma. Risk factors for CSOM, in addition to recurrent AOM are family history of chronic ear disease, crowded family living conditions and large group day care. The incidence has been estimated at one case per 2500 children 0–15 years of age. An algorithm for the management of CSOM is presented in Figure 6.3.

The goal of treatment is a dry ear and healing tympanic membrane. Parenteral therapy may be required in more difficult patients who have failed oral or topical ear drop therapy, selected primarily to eradicate *Pseudomonas aeruginosa*, almost always the causative pathogen, and to a lesser extent to treat *Staphylococcus aureus*. Cultures of exudate will help establish appropriate antimicrobial therapy. Patients require frequent suctioning and debridement of the external auditory canal, usually provided by an ENT consultant.

Parenteral antibiotic therapy in an outpatient setting is preferred, both for cost and convenience, and the option of once daily gentamicin at a dose of 5–7 mg/kg is suggested. With normal renal function, monitoring serum antibiotic concentrations is not necessary. There are no adequate oral agents for CSOM alternatives, but topical quinolones (floxacin and ofloxacin), which represent the only class of antibiotics with adequate antipseudomonal activity, are available for use in children. Many oral antibiotics are available to treat *S. aureus* and most other potential pathogens. Treatment failures following these outpatient options may require combination parenteral antibiotics in an in-patient setting. Tympanomastoid surgery is recommended for the 25% of patients who do not respond to medical management and for any patient who develops a cholesteatoma.

Prevention

Risk factors for recurrent otitis media include many which cannot be controlled, namely male sex, selected racial groups (native Americans, Alaskan and Canadian Inuit, and Africans), winter season, crowded households and age less than 6 months for the first episode of AOM. Other epidemiologic factors can, however, be adjusted for the infant who is felt to be prone to otitis media and might be considered for the routine care of any child. Large group day care attendance for more than 20 hours per week is perhaps the greatest risk factor for frequent infection. Although this cannot be circumvented for many children, alternatives such as care by family members and small group care options could be pursued. Breast feeding is protective and is particularly recommended for the child whose sibling was prone to otitis media. The easiest factor to

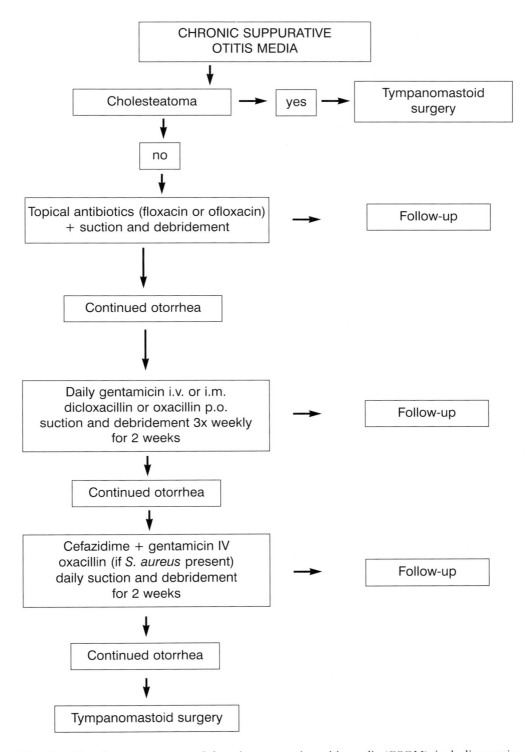

Figure 6.3 Algorithm for management of chronic suppurative otitis media (CSOM), including option of once-daily gentamicin outpatient therapy and indications for tympanomastoid surgery

control is exposure to tobacco smoke, which not only increases the incidence of AOM but is also associated with other respiratory infections in children.

Since the leading pathogen for AOM has always been *Streptococcus pneumoniae*, administration of the 23-valent polysaccharide vaccine was studied shortly after development in the early 1980s for its ability to prevent this disease. Although this vaccine was effective in preventing type-specific infection in children older than 2 years, little benefit was afforded younger recipients. Newer vaccines containing polysaccharide antigens conjugated to protein carriers are immunogenic in infants as young as 2 months, and similar to advances in *Haemophilus influenzae* type b vaccine development, appear to offer significant protection from pneumococcal disease in infants.

Chemoprophylaxis has been shown to reduce the incidence of AOM in children who are otitis media prone. The accepted criterion for this intervention is 3 episodes of acute disease within 6 months or 4 in 12 months. Either amoxicillin or sulfisoxazole may be administered at one-half the usual therapeutic dose divided once or twice a day (amoxicillin 20–30 mg/kg/day and sulfisoxazole 50–75 mg/kg/day). The recommendation for chemoprophylaxis is included in the algorithm for AOM. Studies have suggested benefit with 3 different strategies: chemoprophylaxis during the winter months; chemoprophylaxis for 90 days after the third episode of AOM within 6 months; or antibiotics during the course of each new viral respiratory infection.

Otitis media in neonates

Bacteria causing otitis media in the first 6 weeks of life include Gram-negative coliforms, which are frequently resistant to amoxicillin. A diagnostic tympanocentesis is therefore required to guide therapy. In addition, these patients should be carefully evaluated for evidence of systemic disease, including meningitis (Table 6.17).

PARASITIC INFECTIONS

Most parasitic diseases have virtually disappeared in developed countries as a result of concentrated efforts to improve sanitary conditions. Only pinworm (enterobiasis) and giardiasis are seen with any frequency in pediatric practice, with occasional cases of ascariasis, amebiasis, strongyloidiasis, toxocariasis, hookworm and whipworm (trichuriasis) requiring management. Presenting manifestations are summarized in Table 6.18. This section includes only these more common parasites. Giardiasis and amebiasis are discussed in Chapter 10 because they present with predominantly gastrointestinal symptoms.

The most common parasitic disease, pinworm, should be treated if itching or discomfort interfere with sleep and other activities (Table 6.19). Reinfection is very common but the presence of *Enterobius* is usually of minor clinical consequence. Most important is reassurance of the family that these nematodes are not the result of poor hygiene.

Table 6.17 Etiology of otitis media in neonates

Pathogen	Incidence (%)
Gram-negative enterics	
(*E. coli, Klebsiella, Pseudomonas, Proteus*)	50
H. influenzae	15
S. pneumoniae	15
S. aureus	10
Others	10

Table 6.18 Presenting manifestations of common parasitic infections

Pinworm	Perianal pruritis
Ascariasis	Passage of adult worms
Strongyloidiasis	Marked eosinophilia
	Immunosuppression
	Diarrhea
Toxocariasis	Marked eosinophilia
	Visceral larval migrans
Hookworm	Usually asymptomatic anemia
Whipworm (trichuriasis)	Chronic diarrhea

Table 6.19 Treatment of more common parasitic infections

Ascariasis	Mebendazole 100 mg b.i.d. for 3 days
	Albendazole 400 mg, 1 dose
	Pyrantel pamoate 11 mg/kg (max. 1 g), 1 dose
Hookworm	Mebendazole 100 mg b.i.d. for 3 days
	Albendazole 10 mg/kg (max. 400 mg), 1 dose
	Pyrantel pamoate 11 mg/kg (max. 1 g/day) qd for 3 days
Pinworm	Mebendazole 100 mg, 1 dose (treat all household members)
	Albendazole 400 mg, 1 dose
	Pyrantel pamoate 11 mg/kg, 1 dose (max. 1 g)
Strongyloidiasis	Thiabendazole 50 mg/kg/24 h d.i.v. q.12 h for 2 days
	Invermectin 200 μg/kg qd for 2 days
Toxocariasis	Mebendazole 100–200 mg b.i.d. for 5 days
	Albendazole 400 mg b.i.d. for 3–5 days
	Thiabendazole 50 mg/kg/24 h div. q.12h for 1–4 weeks (depending on symptoms)
Whipworm (trichuriasis)	Mebendazole 100 mg b.i.d. for 3 days
	Albendazole 400 mg, 1 dose

Strongyloides infection in the immuno-compromised patient is associated with a high degree of parasitemia, dissemination, and significant mortality even with early administration of thiabendazole.

Unusual parasitic infections are more likely to be seen in immigrants and individuals who have traveled to areas where such infections are endemic. Presenting symptoms are commonly diarrhea, weight loss, rash, eosinophilia, skin ulcers, or fever. Treatment programs for unusual parasitic infections are summarized in Chapter 20, Table 20.21.

RABIES PROPHYLAXIS

Postexposure rabies management has become much easier now that immunotherapeutic agents of extremely low toxicity have become available (Table 6.20). Rabies immune globulin is prepared from the plasma of human volunteers hyperimmunized with rabies vaccine thereby eliminating serum sickness episodes so common with animal rabies serum, and human diploid cell vaccine is not associated with the encephalitic reactions so characteristic of duck embryo vaccine. The only drawback to this treatment is the high cost.

Table 6.20 Postexposure rabies management

Routine treatment of animal bites (see Table 6.4)
Rabies management
Healthy domestic animal: observe animal for 10 days
Wild rodent (mouse, rat, rabbit, squirrel, etc.): rabies prophylaxis is not indicated
Wild mammal (skunk, raccoon, bat, fox, etc.) or escaped domestic animals (dog or cat):
  HRIG 20 IU/kg total dose
    10 IU/kg infiltrated around wound
    10 IU/kg i.m.
  HDCV
    1 ml i.m. on days 0, 3, 7, 14, and 28
    Follow-up rabies antibody titer on day 42 only for patients who are immunocompromised

SNAKEBITES

Most snakebites are inflicted by nonpoisonous species or result in minimal envenomation where pit vipers (rattlesnakes, water moccasins, and copperheads) are involved. Simple observation for progression of local or systemic symptoms during a 4-hour period following the bite is the only therapy usually required. Emergency procedures are given in Table 6.21. Coral snake bites should always be considered potentially fatal. Large

Table 6.21 Emergency treatment of snakebites

Apply tourniquet loosely, proximal to edema
Splint
Transport to medical facility
For large snakes where transport will take > 1 h
  Clean the bite
  Make 5 mm incision over fang marks
  Apply suction
  DO NOT
    Use tight tourniquet
    Pack on ice

Table 6.22 In-hospital treatment of snakebites

Admit for observation
Laboratory studies
  Complete blood count, urinalysis, electrolytes
  Blood type and crossmatch
  Clotting studies monitored frequently
Antivenin IV for significant envenomation
  Begin within 2 h of bite
  Skin test for hypersensitivity
  Dose is individualized
    Moderate cases – 3–5 vials
    Severe cases – 10–20 vials
  Children – relatively higher doses
  Monitor for allergic reactions
  Serum sickness common at 4–7 days
Fasciotomy if neuromuscular function
  compromised
Tetanus prophylaxis
Severe cases
  Volume expanders, respiratory support, dialysis

rattlesnakes and water moccasins account for the largest number of serious or fatal bites. The greatest number of poisonous bites, however, are inflicted by copperheads, which are small and whose bites almost never result in fatal consequences. A conservative approach is therefore indicated when this species is identified.

Initial assessment of the patient is directed at determining the amount of envenomation and time lapse between the bite and institution of definitive therapy. Antivenin therapy (Table 6.22) should be started within 2 hours of the bite to ensure maximum benefit. Guidelines for amount of antivenin are detailed in the package insert. Surgical consultation should be obtained if the bite is on a distal extremity because a fasciotomy may become necessary to preserve neurovascular function.

Procedures

7

ASPIRATE OF CELLULITIS

Needle aspiration of the leading edge of an area of cellulitis should be obtained for culture, particularly when *Haemophilus influenzae* is a suspected pathogen. The area should be cleansed with an iodine solution and washed with alcohol. A 22- or 23-gauge needle is attached to a syringe containing 0.5 ml of normal saline without bacteriostatic preservative. The needle is advanced 1 cm into superficial subcutaneous tissue, the saline injected and aspirated back into the syringe. The syringe and its contents should be transported to the laboratory for direct plating on appropriate medium. Blood culture bottles should not be used because these do not contain adequate growth nutrients for *H. influenzae* and some other organisms.

BLADDER TAP

The procedure is carried out with the patient lying supine and the lower extremities held in the frog leg position. The suprapubic area is cleansed with iodine and alcohol, and the symphysis pubis is located with the index finger. Using a 20-ml syringe and a 22-gauge, 1/2-inch needle or 2-inch spinal needle in older children, the abdominal wall and bladder is pierced in the midline about 1/2 to 2 cm above the symphysis pubis. The needle is then angled 30 degrees toward the fundus of the bladder. Urine is gently aspirated and the needle withdrawn. No dressing is necessary. As with venipuncture, neither sterile gloves nor local anesthesia is required in carrying out vesicopuncture.

BLADDER WASHOUT

Bladder washout is an excellent procedure for localizing urinary tract infections.

Performed properly, data correlate almost absolutely with those from ureteral catheterization, a much more invasive procedure. Patients must be restrained during bladder washout, nursing personnel should be well trained, and collected urine samples must be carefully labeled as to time and sequence of collection (Tables 7.1 and 7.2).

BLOOD CULTURE

For those infectious processes where bacteremia is associated, blood cultures represent an important source for etiologic diagnosis. These specimens are essential, particularly during the initial workup of sepsis, meningitis,

Table 7.1 Bladder washout methodology

Restrain patient
Catheterize bladder with a Foley catheter
Empty bladder and submit for urinalysis and culture no. 1
Instill 75 ml of 2% neomycin in normal saline plus 2 amps of Elase; clamp catheter for 45 min
Empty bladder; irrigate bladder with 2 l of distilled water in 50 ml aliquots; submit last irrigation for culture no. 2
Collect urine q.10 min × 5 and submit each for culture (nos. 3–7)

Table 7.2 Bladder washout interpretation

Cystitis
  Negative cultures after irrigation
Pyelonephritis
  Progressive increments in colony counts
    1 is positive
    2 is negative
    3–7 (>100 colonies/ml), 10-fold increase from 3–7

endocarditis, pneumonia, cellulitis, osteo-myelitis and septic arthritis. Only one culture is necessary in neonates and young infants because the density of bacteria is higher and the bacteremia more continuous than in older patients. After age 12 months, two cultures should be obtained, and for endocarditis three to six are recommended (Table 7.3).

CENTRAL LINE QUANTITATIVE CULTURES

Often it is difficult to determine whether a catheter is the source of septicemia, particu-larly if there are other potentially infected sites. Although removal of an indwelling catheter is usually simple and provides a definitive diagnosis in catheter-related sepsis, it may be undesirable to remove permanent catheters from patients who have a limited number of sites for infusion or whose parenteral hyper-alimentation central lines are the only source of nutrition. Quantitative blood cultures per-formed with the catheter in place can be compared to quantitative cultures of periph-eral blood, thereby establishing whether the catheter is the source of infection and must therefore be removed (Table 7.4).

LUMBAR PUNCTURE

Cerebrospinal fluid (CSF) should be examined in any child where meningitis is suspected. The only absolute contra-indications to lumbar puncture are increased intracranial pressure or a mass lesion of the central nervous system. In such cases a CT scan should first be obtained. Other relative contraindications are anticoagulation, platelet count of less than 20 000, meningomyelocele, severe scoliosis, suspected abscess in the lumbar area, and instability of the patient. Always perform a fundoscopic examination, obtaining a clear view of the optic disc before performing a lumbar puncture (Table 7.5).

LUNG ASPIRATION

Needle aspiration of the lung is the most useful direct method for establishing the

Table 7.3 Blood culture technique

Wash hands
Clean rubber stopper of culture bottle with alcohol
Clean skin with 2% iodine or Betadine
Wipe skin with alcohol
Perform venipuncture without touching puncture site
Obtain 1–5 ml of blood
Change needles aseptically
Transfer blood to bottles (aerobic and anaerobic)
Volume of sample: a 1:10 to 1:20 dilution (2.5 to 5 ml for 50-ml culture bottle) for routine cul-tures; 1:50 (1 ml) is adequate for Bactec methodology

Table 7.4 Procedure for quantitative blood cultures

Notify laboratory to provide 2 empty sterile petri dishes and 2 melted TSA deeps (in a beaker of hot water)
Flush catheter with 10–20 ml of saline
Aseptically draw 2–6 ml of blood from the catheter and from a peripheral vein
Using a tuberculin syringe, place 0.1 ml of blood from each site in a separate petri dish
Pour TSA over the blood and swirl the dish to evenly suspend the blood
Allow agar to harden and transport to laboratory
Process the remaining blood as for routine blood cultures
Interpretation: quantitative counts from the catheter that are >10-fold those of peripheral blood indicate catheter infection

etiology of pneumonia in children. Because this procedure is associated with a 1 to 5% incidence of pneumothorax, it should not be undertaken unless determining the causative pathogen would alter therapeutic approaches. Such circumstances are most commonly a severely ill or immune compromised host, suspicion of an unusual organism, or failure to respond to initial empiric therapy (Table 7.6).

OSTEOMYELITIS SUBPERIOSTEAL ASPIRATION

Needle aspiration of suspected osteomyelitis should be a routine initial procedure for etiologic diagnosis. This will not alter interpretation of subsequent bone scans and there is no risk of introducing disease into bone if there is an overlying area of cellulitis (Table 7.7).

PERICARDIOCENTESIS

Though pericardiocentesis may be done in almost any setting as an emergency, under ideal conditions it is best done in an intensive care unit or cardiac catheterization laboratory (where fluoroscopic control is possible). Constant ECG monitoring is essential and constant or frequent blood pressure monitoring is also important. The patient is placed in a supine position with the head and chest elevated slightly. The area of the xiphoid is properly prepped and draped. Using sterile technique, the skin and subcutaneous tissue at and just to the left of the xiphoid are infiltrated with a local anesthetic. With a syringe attached, an 18- or 20-gauge needle of 5 to 10 cm length is inserted adjacent to the xiphoid (in the notch between the xiphoid process and the seventh costal cartilage) and advanced slowly toward the middle of the left clavicle. The needle is kept at an angle of 20 degrees off the skin. The needle is passed immediately posterior to the costal cartilage and as it passes through the pericardium a 'pop' may sometimes be felt. An exploring electrode (V lead) may be attached to the metal hub of the needle with a sterile alligator clamp and the ECG so monitored; a 'current of injury' pattern may be noted as the pericardial space is entered and the epicardium encountered. Constant negative pressure is kept on the syringe as the needle is advanced, and pericardial fluid is aspirated as soon as the needle perforates the pericardium. As much fluid as possible should be removed, but in the presence of suppurative pericarditis, the

Table 7.5 Technique for lumbar puncture

Restrain patient in recumbent or upright position (upright preferred for neonates, who may have very low CSF pressure)
Scrub hands, wear surgical gloves and mask
Locate L3-4 interspace at the level of the iliac crest
Clean the back thoroughly with an iodine solution, wash with alcohol or wipe dry
Drape with sterile towels
Insert a 22-gauge spinal needle (B bevel) in the L3-4 interspace, directed toward the umbilicus
Remove the stylet periodically or when the 'pop' of the dura is felt
If blood returns, the procedure may be repeated in the L2-3 interspace

Table 7.6 Needle aspiration of the lung

Determine, by X-ray, the major site of involvement
Clean skin with an iodine solution, wash with alcohol
Use sterile gloves; sterile towels are rarely necessary
Anesthetize skin and soft tissue down to pleura (2% procaine) above a rib
Attach a 22-gauge spinal needle (B bevel) to a 10-ml syringe containing 1 ml of normal saline without bacteriostatic preservative
Time puncture to maximum inspiration; if possible have patient pause in inspiration for 3–4 s
Rapidly advance needle into lung 3 cm, directed toward the hilum, maintaining negative pressure with the syringe; the aspiration should take only 2 s
Transport needle, syringe and their contents to the laboratory for inoculation into enrichment broth or direct plating

Table 7.7 Technique for subperiosteal aspiration

Clean skin with an iodine solution; wash with alcohol
Drape area with sterile towels; use sterile gloves
Anesthetize skin only
Using a syringe containing 0.5 ml of normal saline, aspirate subcutaneous tissue as for cellulitis
Using a second 2.5-ml syringe and 20-gauge needle, advance the needle until the bone is touched and aspirate (saline is not needed)
Transport the needle and syringe to the laboratory for direct plating

purulent material may be difficult to aspirate or may be loculated.

If bloody fluid is obtained, set aside a small sample in a glass tube to observe. Blood that has been in the pericardial space for any significant time will not clot. Blood aspirated from the cardiac chamber will clot normally. Check the hemoglobin content and hematocrit of the fluid aspirated to compare with the patient's peripheral blood values. If the heart has been perforated, remove the needle slowly and observe the patient's vital signs frequently. Perforation of the inferior surface of the right ventricle has rarely resulted in persistent bleeding into the pericardial space.

Some physicians prefer to use a needle-plastic cannula set so that once the pericardial space is entered, the needle can be slipped out of the plastic cannula covering it, and fluid can more easily be aspirated via the cannula. This technique may be safer if a large quantity of fluid is to be removed and considerable time is required to remove it. These plastic cannulas, however, may be stiff enough to perforate the heart of a small child, so great care must still be exercised in manipulating the cannula in the pericardial space.

PERITONEAL TAP

An abdominal paracentesis should be accomplished when primary peritonitis is suspected. Most cases of peritonitis secondary to a perforated viscus require surgery, at which time appropriate cultures can be obtained (Table 7.8).

SUBDURAL TAP

Subdural effusions occurring during or after therapy for bacterial meningitis can be detected clinically by enlarging head circumference, split sutures or fontanels, and lateralizing findings on neurologic examination. Effusions can be evaluated by skull roentgenograms, transillumination of the skull and CT scan. Subdural fluid aspiration,

Table 7.8 Procedure for peritoneal tap

Empty urinary bladder
Sedate patient
Place patient in supine position
Clean skin over rectus muscle with iodine from symphysis pubis to umbilicus
Anesthetize skin, soft issue, and peritoneum just lateral to midline in the lower third between symphysis pubis and umbilicus
Make 5 mm incision in skin
Assure aseptic technique
Using #14F abdominal trocar, insert through incision directed obliquely up and back; continue advancing until release through the peritoneum is felt
Remove stylet and collect fluid for culture, Gram stain, and cell count
Suture incision and apply sterile pressure dressing

when indicated, is easily done on infants with open fontanels. Adequate immobilization of the child is necessary. After shaving the scalp widely around the anterior fontanel, sterile prepping and draping of the scalp, and surgical gloving, an 18- to 20-gauge subdural needle with stylet is introduced into the lateral recess of the anterior fontanel at the coronal suture. Anesthetic agents are generally not required in infants. The subdural needle is introduced 3 to 5 mm through the dura and the stylet removed. Subdural fluid may well from the needle. If no subdural fluid is encountered, suctioning and probing of the subdural space generally is not recommended. Occasionally by rotating or withdrawing the needle and reintroducing it at a slight angle under the convexity of the skull, flow may be established. A thick exudate of purulent empyema or markedly elevated subdural fluid protein may account for lack of flow. Similarly, loculated fluid beyond the reach of the subdural needle may be present. In these cases, a CT scan may be necessary to exclude the possibility of loculated subdural empyema or ventricular enlargement clinically suggesting subdural effusions. If subdural fluid flow is established, 20 to 30 ml of fluid may be removed, and routine studies including cell count, glucose, protein determination, and Gram stain are done. Bilateral subdural taps are indicated in some cases. In general, subdural taps, if done without probing, are innocuous; however, occasionally trauma to the cerebral cortex, bleeding into the subdural space, and prolonged leakage of subdural or subarachnoid fluid following subdural tap may occur. Proper antiseptic preparation precludes infection. Indications for repeated subdural taps are controversial, and these increase the risk of fistula formation and iatrogenic infection. The ready availability of CT scans has decreased the indications for subdural fluid aspirations and permitted a more accurate evaluation of effusion size and localization.

THORACENTESIS

Thoracentesis is performed both for diagnosis and therapeutic purposes. For empyema caused by *H. influenzae*, pneumococcus, or group A streptococci, one or two thoracenteses will often provide adequate drainage, thus avoiding placement of a chest tube. Empyema as a result of *Staphylococcus aureus* almost always necessitates chest tube drainage (Table 7.9).

TYMPANOCENTESIS

This procedure should be considered for any neonate with otitis media where Gram-negative coliform bacteria are commonly recovered, and for older patients who have persistent signs and symptoms of middle ear disease after standard therapy (Table 7.10).

VENTRICULAR TAP

Ventricular taps are generally performed by neurosurgeons; however, the procedure may be useful or mandatory in some emergency situations or in cases where CSF must be obtained without lumbar puncture before beginning antibiotic therapy. Sterile surgical technique is used in all cases. In infants, the

Table 7.9 Procedure for thoracentesis

Place patient in sitting position
Clean skin with iodine solution; wash with alcohol
Anesthetize skin, soft tissue, and pleura in 7th or 8th interspace (level of the tip of the scapula), posterior axillary line
Drape with sterile towels; use surgical gloves
Use 18-gauge needle attached to a 3-way stopcock and syringe; enter pleural cavity above a rib
Remove fluid for culture, Gram stain, and chemistries (see Table 6.13)
Obtain post-thoracentesis chest X-ray
If patient begins coughing, remove needle immediately
If no fluid is obtained, consider repeating under fluoroscopic direction

Table 7.10 Aspiration of middle ear fluid

Remove cerumen
Clean canal with alcohol
Culture external ear canal to monitor contaminants
Restrain patient
Use an 18-gauge, 3 1/2-inch spinal needle bent at a double angle (as a fork) attached to a 2.5-ml syringe
Use an otoscope with an operating head
Advance needle through a speculum that has been sterilized in alcohol
Penetrate the posterior–inferior aspect of the tympanic membrane
Aspirate middle ear exudate and transport to laboratory for culture and Gram stain

ventricular system can be entered by inserting a spinal or ventricular needle through the lateral aspect of the anterior fontanel at the coronal suture, directing the needle toward the midpoint of the orbit on that side. In older children, a burr hole can be drilled in the midpupillary line at the hairline and the needle introduced. Obviously, these facial landmarks vary and experience and a clear mental image of the ventricular system are needed before attempting a ventricular tap. The return of clear or blood-tinged CSF documents correct needle aspiration. Pressure measurements are obtained and sufficient fluid drained both for diagnostic purposes and at times, therapeutic effect. CT and cranial ultrasound are useful in accurately judging the need for and the effects of ventricular tap and should be routinely performed.

VENTRICULOPERITONEAL SHUNT ASPIRATION

Because of the wide variety of shunts currently used in neurosurgery, the surgeon responsible for following the patient's shunt should generally be contacted before aspiration is attempted. Some shunt systems have sites designed for safe aspiration. In other cases, skull radiographs reveal shunt characteristics that help identify the model and specific mechanics. In cases where shunt patency or possible infection is questioned, shunt aspiration is an uncomplicated and safe procedure if sterile technique is used. The goal of the procedure should be not only to obtain CSF, but also to document proximal and distal patency. By elevating the catheter and using a manometer, if necessary, ventricular pressure can be measured. Elevating the catheter and noting drainage of CSF suggests distal patency. Rarely is the quantity of fluid obtained critical. Sufficient fluid should be obtained liberally to carefully and thoroughly perform all cytologic, chemical, and microbiologic cultures and smears (including large amounts of fluid if fungal studies are indicated). Following removal of the needle, CSF may leak and the site should have a sterile dressing and be observed for infection. In general, if the bulb site itself appears infected, no aspiration should be attempted.

Laboratory diagnosis

8

INTRODUCTION

The clinical laboratory is continually striving to meet the needs of both the attending physician and the patient by providing prompt and accurate results. Accomplishing this goal in the most proficient manner necessitates good communication and co-operation between the physician and the laboratory technologist. This chapter attempts to provide the clinician with a simplified review of the available laboratory tests to provide information on which to base clinical decisions. It is the responsibility of the physician to ensure that an appropriate and properly collected specimen is obtained from the patient and promptly delivered to the laboratory. Upon receipt, the submitted specimen will be inspected to determine if it is of sufficient quality and quantity for adequate evaluation.

STAINS

Microscopic examination of unstained and stained smears of specimens from an infected site is the most direct, rapid and least technical of procedures.

Gram stain

Gram-positive and Gram-negative organisms are differentiated on the basis of the cell wall and cell membrane permeability characteristics to organic solvents (Table 8.1). These characteristics are probably due to the glycos-aminopeptide and lipoprotein composition of the bacterial cell wall. Gram-positive organisms, which do not have significant amounts of lipid as an integral part of their cell wall, retain the crystal violet–iodine complex and stain purple, whereas Gram-negative organisms do not retain this complex and stain red from the counterstain.

Acid-fast stain

This stain should be performed if pulmonary tuberculosis or tuberculous meningitis is suspected. It is based on the observation that the staining of mycobacteria with carbol fuchsin resists decolorization with acid alcohol. Other acid-fast organisms such as *Nocardia* sp. may also be detected using this procedure, but must be identified further with special stains and cultures. A technique using auramine and rhodamine fluorescent dyes is easier to read although it is more time consuming compared to the acid-fast stain (Table 8.2).

Methylene blue stain

Methylene blue is a useful stain to establish the morphology of organisms and to differentiate

Table 8.1 Gram stain

Specimen source: Most clinical specimens
Technique
    Air dry smear and fix with methanol (allow to evaporate)
    Flood slide with crystal-violet (60 s)
    Wash, add Gram's iodine (60 s)
    Decolorize with acetone/alcohol (5 s) and wash immediately
    Counterstain with safranin (15 s)
Staining identification
    Gram-positive organisms stain purple
    Gram-negative organisms stain red

cells found in the specimen (neutrophils, lymphocytes, monocytes, red blood cells, and epithelial cells). Intracellular bacteria, such as *Neisseriae*, are often more evident with this stain, as are other bacterial characteristics as demonstrated by the capsules surrounding pneumococci and the metachromatic granules of *Corynebacterium diphtheriae*.

Wright's and Giemsa stains

Both Wright's and Giemsa stains are extremely helpful in demonstrating organisms, inclusion bodies, or cellular differentiation in various specimens (Table 8.3).

WET MOUNTS

Unfixed samples can be examined microscopically as wet mounts for bacterial, fungal, parasitic, and other pathogens (Table 8.4). These commonly used wet mounts are: normal saline, used to detect trichomonads and protozoa; potassium hydroxide (KOH), used primarily for identification of fungal forms; and India ink mounts for identifying encapsulated *Cryptococcus* sp.

SPECIMEN EXAMINATION AND ANALYSIS

Cerebrospinal fluid (CSF)

Collection of CSF is performed under sterile conditions and divided into three 1-ml aliquots for microbiologic cultures, chemistry determinations and cell counts. A fourth sample may be obtained for viral cultures (Table 8.5).

In the bacteriological examination of CSF the Gram-stained smear is an extremely important method for the rapid identification of meningitis. It normally takes approximately 1 to 10×10^4 bacteria per milliliter before detection by a direct smear is possible. Centrifugation of the CSF at 2000 rpm for 10 minutes increases the percentage of positive smears made from the sediment. Caution must be taken to differentiate

Table 8.2 Acid-fast stain

Specimen source
  Sputum
  Cerebrospinal fluid
Technique
  Air dry and fix with methanol (allow to
    evaporate)
  Flood slide with Kinyoun carbol fuchsin (4 min)
  Wash with water and decolorize with acid
    alcohol until faint pink
  Wash, counterstain with methylene blue (30 s)
Identifying organisms
  Acid-fast organisms stain red
    Mycobacterium sp.
    Nocardia sp.
  Nonacid-fast bacteria and cellular elements
    stain blue

Table 8.3 Uses of Wright's and Giemsa stains

Used to stain
  Intracellular organisms in blood (buffy coat)
  Conjunctival scrapings
  Impression smears
  Tissue sections
Used to differentiate
  Multinucleated giant cells in vesicle fluid of
    herpes virus skin or mucosal infections (see
    Tzanck preparation)
  Cell types (polymorphonuclear neutrophils,
    lymphocytes and trachomatis inclusions,
    eosinophils, epithelial cells, monocytes)
Used to detect
  Rickettsiae
  Chlamydiae
  Protozoa (malaria)
  Selected yeast and fungi

artifacts staining similarly to organisms (Table 8.6).

Dark-field examination for spirochetes, if syphilitic or leptospiral meningitis is suspected, is available in most laboratories as well as a variety of rapid immunologic assays that are capable of demonstrating the type-specific polysaccharide capsule antigens of pneumococcus, meningococcus, and *Haemophilus influenzae*.

Table 8.4 Three commonly used wet mounts

Normal saline	Potassium hydroxide	India ink
Specimen source	Specimen source	Specimen source
Cervical secretions	Cervical discharge	Cerebrospinal fluid
Vaginal secretions	Skin scrapings	Urine
Urethral discharge	Sputum	Exudates
Urine sediment	Tissue scrapings	Sputum
Feces		
Technique	Technique	Technique
Mix 1–2 drops of	Mix 1 drop 10% KOH,	Mix 1 drop of
0.9% NaCl and	allow to stand 10–15 min	India ink and
examine microscopically	and examine microscopically	examine microscopically
Identifiable organisms	Identifiable organisms	Identifiable organisms
Trichomonas vaginalis	Fungal forms	Capsule of
Protozoa		*Cryptococcus*
(trophozoites, cysts of		*neoformans* (must
Entamoeba histolytica)		see budding yeast)
Pinworm eggs		

Table 8.5 Processing cerebrospinal fluid (CSF) from meningitis patients

Aliquot	Diagnostic tests	Volume of CSF required
1	Culture for bacteria (and fungi)	1.0–2.0 ml
2	Protein and glucose (compare with simultaneous blood glucose)	1.0 ml
3	Total white blood cell and red blood cell count	1.0 ml
	Sediment for staining	
	Wright's stain cell differential	
	Gram stain (80% positive in meningitis)	
	Acridine orange for rapid detection of bacteria	
	Acid-fast stain	
	India ink (other fungal stains)	
	Antigen detection (Latex agglutination, CoA, etc.)	

CoA, coagglutination A

Table 8.6 Common errors in interpretation of cerebrospinal fluid staining

Gram stain
   Confusing precipitated stain with Gram-positive cocci
   Identifying false capsules because of poor stain
   Misreading of *Haemophilus influenzae* with bipolar staining as overdecolorized pneumococci
India ink preparation
   Cells or artifacts that appear to be *Cryptococcus* sp. causing false-positive results

Urine

The laboratory aid to the diagnosis of a urinary tract infection (UTI) is only as valid as the care given to the collection of a urine specimen for culture and examination. Consequently, the method of collection (see Chapter 12) of urine is important, and it is necessary to know how collection was accomplished in order to interpret results. The volume of urine recommended for a urinalysis is 15 ml or more but as little as 2 ml will suffice for a screen (Table 8.7). Microscopic examination of formed elements must clearly be identified to determine early diagnosis of UTI. This can be done with wet mounts and staining of urine sediment. Practically all uncentrifuged urine with bacterial colony counts of greater than or equal to 10^5/ml will have a positive Gram stain. Several rapid screening methods are available for the identification of bacteriuria. Glucose and nitrite determinations by the dipstick technique to detect bacterial metabolism must be interpreted with caution because dilute urine will result in false-negative results. None of these tests have yet replaced bacterial cultures in the detection of UTIs.

An important aspect of evaluating a patient with suspected UTI is to identify the organism with routine and quantitative cultures (Table 8.8).

Quantitative urine cultures may be obtained by using bacteriologic loops that deliver approximately 0.001 ml of a sample of urine. A sterile loop is dipped into urine from a properly collected specimen and streaked on a blood agar plate. After incubation for 18–24 hours at 37°C the number of colonies of bacteria on the blood agar plate is multiplied by 1000, giving a reasonable approximation of the bacteria per milliliter in the urine specimen. Thus more than 100 colonies on a plate is evidence of significant bacteriuria and a quantitative colony count of 10^5 colonies per milliliter. Urine obtained directly by bladder puncture or catheterization is normally sterile and any growth of urinary pathogens should be considered significant.

Fecal specimens

Fecal specimens should be collected and transported in paper stool cups for evaluation (Table

Table 8.7 Routine screening urinalysis

Test	Volume of urine
Screening for bacteriuria	2–3 drops
Gram stain of uncentrifuged specimen	
Quantitative loop culture	
Specific gravity (performed using a refractometer)	1 drop
Microscopic examination of sediment	1 drop of concentrated sediment from 10 ml urine
Red blood cells, leukocytes, renal epithelial cells, hyaline casts, mucous and excess crystals, microorganisms	
Basic chemical screen (tested with a multiple or single reagent strip)	2 ml
pH ($\geq$ 7.5 in infection)	
Blood	
Protein	
Bilirubin	
Glucose	
Urobilinogen	
Ketone	
Nitrite	

8.9). Care should be taken not to contaminate the stool with urine or water because of the possibility of killing trophozoïtes. The guaiac method represents a suitable test for routine screening of blood in stool specimens (Table 8.10; see also Tables 8.11 and 8.12).

A predominance of polymorphonuclear leukocytes is seen with any inflammatory enterocolitis.

Ova and parasites

When parasitism is highly suspected, a minimum of three specimens should be submitted. The major parasitic species that infect the intestinal tract are protozoa and helminths. The protozoa, which cause amebiasis and giardiasis, have two major forms, trophozoite and cyst. Inspection of the perianal area at night, after the child is asleep, may reveal adult pinworms (thread-like white worms 1/4 to 1/2 inch long) (Table 8.13).

Synovial fluid

Synovial fluid (SF) aspiration may provide information to enable a distinction to be made between joint inflammation due to infectious, immunologic, or traumatic involvement. The specimen should be collected using sterile technique to avoid contamination from exogenous birefringent material; ideally, the patient should fast for 6 to 12 h before taking the specimen to allow equilibrium of glucose between plasma and SF. Infected SF tends to clot spontaneously or within an hour, therefore a specimen to be examined microscopically for cells and bacteria should be placed immediately into a heparinized tube (Tables 8.14 and 8.15).

Pleural, pericardial, and peritoneal fluids

It is important to differentiate these fluids as to whether they are transudates, caused by mechanical factors influencing formation, or exudates that may be caused by infection due to damage of the mesothelial linings (Tables 8.16 and 8.17).

Table 8.8 Bacteriologic cultures for urine

Routine cultures
  Blood agar
  MacConkey agar or EMB for Gram-negative bacilli
  TSA
Special considerations
  Pyuria in the absence of bacterial growth by routine culture might indicate the possible presence of *Mycobacterium tuberculosis*. Sediment from the first morning specimen should be Gram stained and cultured

Table 8.9 Evaluation of fecal specimens

Gross examination
  Consistency, odor, presence of blood, pus, undigested food, mucus, parasites
Microscopic examination
  Fecal leukocytes stained with methylene blue or Wright's stain
  Ova and parasites (wet mounts and Scotch tape preparation)
Routine cultures; fecal specimens are routinely cultured for *Staphylococcus aureus*, *Salmonella*, *Shigella*, *Campylobacter*, and *Yersinia*. It is worth noting that enteropathic *E. coli*, *Vibrio* sp. and viruses require special handling and media
Blood agar
MacConkey or other selective media for Gram-negative enteric bacilli
HE agar, Selenite, SS agar for *Salmonella* and *Shigella*
GN (Gram-negative) broth
CVA plates for *Campylobacter* sp.

Table 8.10 Guaiac method for occult blood

Place about 0.5 g of feces into a test tube
Add 2 ml of water and mix
Add 0.5 ml glacial acetic acid and guaiac solution
Mix 2 ml 3% H_2O_2 with suspension
Observe for 2 min and note maximal blue intensity as 1^+, 2^+, 3^+, or 4^+
Green denotes a negative test

Table 8.11 Staining procedure for fecal leukocytes

Place small fleck of mucus or stool on glass slide
Add 2 drops of Loeffler's methylene blue and mix
Wait 3 min and examine under low-power microscope
Make a rough quantitative count by approximating average number of leukocytes and erythrocytes
Differential is performed under high-power microscopy

Table 8.12 Fecal leukocytes associated with gastrointestinal diseases

Disease	Average predominant leukocyte
Salmonellosis (other than *S. typhi*)	75% polymorphonuclear (PMN) cells, 25% mononuclear cells
Typhoid fever	95% mononuclear cells
Shigellosis	84% PMN cells
E. coli (invasive)	85% PMN cells
Ulcerative colitis (active)	88% PMN cells, 8% eosinophils
Amebic dysentery (active)	Commonly mononuclear cells, unless secondary bacterial infection present
Viral diarrhea, cholera, and healthy controls	

Table 8.13 Simple methods for detecting parasites

Direct wet mounts
  Place fleck of stool on glass slide
  Add 2 drops of 0.9% NaCl for trophozoites and ova or 2 drops of iodine stain for cysts
Scotch tape preparation for pinworm
  Obtain preparation immediately after child awakens
  Cover one end of a tongue depressor with cellophane tape (sticky side out)
  Apply to perianal area with mild pressure
  On a glass slide place one drop of xylol and then transfer tape to slide
  Examine for ova under microscope

CULTURES

It must be emphasized that great care should be taken to ensure proper specimen collection to avoid or minimize unnecessary contamination.

Blood cultures

Whenever there is a reason to suspect clinically significant bacteremia, a blood culture should be ordered. The necessity for strict aseptic technique in the course of obtaining blood for cultures should be stressed. A newer method using the BACTEC 460 system has recently been introduced to the clinical laboratory. The BACTEC 460 is an instrument used to test inoculated BACTEC blood culture vials for the presence of liberated radioactive carbon dioxide ($^{14}CO_2$), a consequence of bacterial growth and metabolism which requires utilization of carbon present as ^{14}C in the medium. Should a high level of $^{14}CO_2$ be present in a vial, it indicates that there are living microorganisms that originated in the initial inoculum. All cultures are read on the BACTEC each day for 7 days. All positive bottles, whether they be aerobic or anaerobic, are subcultured aerobically unless the Gram stain shows a possible anaerobe. The aerobic subculture should include a blood chocolate biplate, and if Gram-negative rods are seen on Gram stain, a MacConkey plate should be set up also. The anaerobic subculture, if done, should include a reducible blood plate and a colistin nalidixic acid-laked kanamycin vancomycin (CNA-LKV) biplate.

Anaerobic cultures

Many anaerobic bacteria of clinical importance are fastidious and oxygen intolerant. Special anaerobic containers must be used in specimen collection and transport, and rapid processing of samples is important in avoiding overgrowth by facultative anaerobes.

Table 8.14 Examination of synovial fluid (SF)

Test	Normal and noninflammatory	Severe inflammatory	Infectious–septic
Color	Clear straw	Yellow to opalescent	Yellow to green
Clarity	Transparent	Opaque*	Opaque
Viscosity	High	Low	Variable
WBC/mm^3	0–5000	500–50 000	500–200 000
Neutrophils	<25%	>50%	≥ 75%
Culture	Negative	Negative	Positive[†]
Mucin clot	Firm	Slightly friable to friable	Friable
Glucose (blood–SF difference in mg/dl)	0–10	0–40	20–100

*Monosodium urate crystals in gout or calcium pyrophosphate dihydrate crystals in pseudogout may be found; [†]positive in about 50% because of low virulence organisms or partially treated disease

Table 8.15 Evaluation of synovial fluid (SF)

Gross examination
 Color, turbidity, viscosity, clotting (observe clot formation after 1 h), organisms, crystals
Cell counts
 Enumerate white blood cells and red blood cells
Stains
 Wright's stain, Gram stain (65% positive in bacterial infected SF), methylene blue, acid-fast stain
Glucose
 SF glucose level is usually <50% of the blood glucose level in septic arthritis. Levels may be normal particularly in gonococcal arthritis
Mucin
 Normal SF forms tight cordlike coagulum clump in 5% acetic acid that is stable for 24 h.
 Fluid from infected joints results in unstable mucin clot
Cultures
 Routine cultures include blood agar, nutrient broth supportive of anaerobes, and chocolate agar or Thayer-Martin for gonococcus. Special consideration for *M. tuberculosis*, fungi, or viral agents
Immunologic tests
 Latex agglutination is helpful in detecting antigens of *H. influenzae* and *S. pneumoniae*, especially during antibiotic treatment

Table 8.16 Evaluation of fluid exudates

Gross appearance (color, clarity, odor)
Total white blood cell and red blood cell counts
Differential (Wright's stain) or cytologic study
Gram stain
Culture (blood agar, medium selective for Gram-negative bacilli, EMB anaerobic and aerobic growth, and chocolate agar for *H. influenzae*)
Chemistry (total protein, LDH, glucose)

Table 8.17 Differentiating transudates and exudates

Pleural fluids (PF)
 90% exudates >3 g/dl total protein
 80% transudates <3 g/dl total protein
 >95% of pleural exudates have at least one of the following characteristics (>95% PF transudates have none of the findings)
  Protein/serum protein ratio >0.5
  Lactic dehydrogenase >600U
  Specific gravity >1.016
  pH <7.2

Peritoneal fluid
 Total protein 2–2.5 g/dl to separate transudates from exudates

Fungal cultures

Scrapings, hairs, or other specimens are planted on Sabouraud agar and incubated for 2 to 4 weeks at room temperature. Positive cultures are examined microscopically by one of the three common wet mounts described in Table 8.4.

Viral cultures

Several innovative methods for the rapid identification of viral infections have been developed because of the renewed interest in useful viral diagnoses. The etiology of a viral syndrome may often be established by viral culture, serologic tests, or both. Table 8.18

shows collection procedures, and Table 8.19 outlines the type of specimen necessary for the isolation of a virus from various clinical syndromes.

Tzanck preparation

The Tzanck preparation is done to distinguish between pustular pyodermas and vesicular lesions due to herpes group viruses, although in many laboratories a fluorescent stain specific for herpes simplex or varicella-zoster has largely replaced this test. Scrapings obtained from the base of a vesicle are air dried onto a glass slide and stained with Wright's stain. Smears demonstrating multi-

Table 8.18   General procedures for viral specimen collection

1. Specimens should be obtained early in the course of illness, when virus shedding is greatest, preferably within 3 days, and generally no later than 7 days after the onset of symptoms
2. The type of specimen and clinical syndrome should be clearly recorded, because different processing steps prior to attempted isolation are necessary for different types of samples, and isolation is only necessary for different types of samples, and only certain viruses are found in some specimen types
3. Samples collected on swabs (conjunctival, pharyngeal, nasopharyngeal, rectal) should be placed quickly in liquid virus transport medium provided by the laboratory
4. Because many viruses are heat labile, samples should be placed in sterile containers, packed in wet, crushed ice, and transported promptly to the virology laboratory. Many specimens can be held at 4°C for up to 24 h (on wet ice or in a refrigerator) without significant decrease in recovery. For prolonged storage, specimens should be frozen at –70°C

Specimen guidelines
1. Nasal secretions: A calcium alginate swab is introduced through the anterior nares into the nasopharynx and plunged into the transport medium after removal from the nares. Nasal washings are collected by instilling 4–5 ml of infusion broth into each nostril while the patient extends the neck slightly and closes the posterior pharynx (by pushing against 'k' sound). The head is tilted forward and a sample collected in a clean container held beneath the nose
2. Pharynx: A swab of the posterior pharynx should be taken by touching the swab to both tonsillar areas and to the posterior pharyngeal wall
3. Blood: Citrated whole blood, 3-5 ml, can be used to isolate viruses from the buffy coat (e.g., HSV, rubella).
4. CSF: Collect 1-3 ml into a sterile container and process immediately. Avoid freezing, particularly for cytomegalovirus
5. Urine: Collect 5–10 ml of a clean catch, midstream urine into a sterile container and process immediately
6. Feces: Place a 2–5 cm sample into a clean specimen container without transport medium. A rectal swab is less satisfactory but can be obtained by inserting a cotton-tipped swab stick 5 cm into the rectum and gently rotating the swab. In contrast to rectal cultures for gonococcus, some fecal material should be obtained when doing viral studies
7. Vesicular fluid: After decontamination of overlying skin, aspirate the lesion with a Pasteur pipette, or a small-gauge needle attached to a tuberculin syringe, or open the vesicle and collect fluids and cellular elements from the base into a swab. If a crust is present, the crust should be lifted off; the fluid beneath the crust can then be swabbed (see Tzanck preparation, below)

Table 8.19   Collections from suspected viral infections

Syndrome	Source of specimen for viral isolation	Most common viral agents
Upper respiratory tract infection	Nasal wash or nasopharynx	Rhinovirus Parainfluenza 1 & 3 Respiratory syncytial virus (RSV) Adenovirus 1, 2, 3, 5, 14, & 21
Lower respiratory tract infection		
Child	Nasal wash	RSV
	Nose or throat swab	Parainfluenza 1, 2 & 3 Influenza A
Adult	Sputum	Influenza A
Pleurodynia	Throat swab Stool	Coxsackie A,B
Central nervous system infection		
Meningitis	Cerebrospinal fluid	Mumps
	Throat swab	Coxsackie A,B
	Stool	ECHO
Encephalitis	Blood	Mumps Herpes simplex 1
Myocarditis and pericarditis	Throat swab Stool	Coxsackie B
Gastroenteritis	Stool	Norwalk, Hawaii agents Reovirus
Urinary tract infection		
Acute hemorrhagic cystitis	Urine	Adenovirus 2, 7 & 11 ECHO 9
Orchitis and epididymitis	Throat swab Stool	Mumps
Parotitis	Throat swab Stool	Mumps
Exanthemata (nonspecific, with fever)	Skin vesicle fluid Throat swab Stool	Coxsackie A9, A16 ECHO 9, 16, 11
Herpangina	Skin vesicle fluid Throat swab Stool	Coxsackie A (1-6, 8, 10, 16 & 22) Coxsackie B
Hand-foot-and-mouth disease	Skin vesicle fluid Throat swab Stool	Coxsackie A
Nonspecific febrile illness	Nose and throat swab Stool Blood	Coxsackie A,B ECHO Influenza A,B

nucleated giant cells with central aggregation of nuclei and/or intracytoplasmic inclusions strongly suggest herpes infection.

Chlamydia culture

Presumptive evidence of *Chlamydia* can be obtained by the examination of stained smears (Giemsa) for the presence of inclusions. Most laboratories today employ a rapid ELISA antigen detection assay or cell culture procedures for the isolation of *Chlamydia*. After inoculation and incubation, the cells are stained with iodine (see Stains in this chapter). Antibodies to *C. trachomatis* are usually measured by complement fixation (CF) (group specific) or microimmunofluorescence (immunotype-specific) methodology (Table 8.20).

ANTIMICROBIAL SENSITIVITY TESTING

Antimicrobial sensitivity testing should be performed only when pathogens have unpredictable susceptibility patterns to the commonly used antibiotics. Sensitivities are not routinely performed on group A streptococci or *Neisseria* sp. because they have relatively predictable susceptibility patterns to antibiotics. The methods available for sensitivity testing include disc diffusion (agar diffusion), agar dilution (plate dilution), and broth dilution (tube or microtiter plate dilution).

Disc diffusion testing

The Kirby-Bauer disc diffusion method is the most commonly used antimicrobial susceptibility test. The technique requires the inoculation of an agar plate with a standard inoculum, addition of disc containing a standardized quantity of antimicrobial agent, incubation for 18 h, and measurement of the zones of inhibition. A three-category system of reporting results of disc diffusion testing is often used: sensitive, intermediate, and resistant.

Dilution susceptibility testing

Dilution susceptibility tests are used to determine the minimum inhibitory concentration (MIC) and minimum bactericidal concentration (MBC) of an antibiotic for an infecting organism. The MIC of the drug is defined as the lowest concentration that prevents visible growth of the test organism under a standardized set of conditions. The MBC of the drug is the lowest concentration that results in complete killing (99.9%) of the test organism. The MIC and MBC are expressed quantitatively in micrograms, international units, or micromoles of antibiotic per milliliter. Dilution susceptibility testing can be done by a broth dilution or agar dilution method.

ß-lactamase test

The development of rapid assays for ß-lactamase permits an assessment of sensitivity to penicillin or ampicillin before standard disc diffusion or broth dilution susceptibility testing results are available. Rapid acidometric, iodometric, and chromogenic cephalosporin methods are currently used to detect ß-lactamase production. Bacteria can be tested after overnight growth in media, and results are usually available within 30 minutes to an hour.

Successful therapy of infections caused by *Haemophilus influenzae*, *Staphylococcus aureus*,

Table 8.20 Specimens and tests used for *Chlamydia* identification

Organism	Specimen	Tests
C. trachomatis	Urethral swabs	Giemsa stain, cell cultures, serology
	Cervical scrapings	ELISA, CIE, IHA (IgM is diagnostic
	Posterior nasopharyngeal	in infants)
	Tracheal secretions	
	Conjunctival scrapings	
C. psittaci	Respiratory secretions	As for C. trachomatis
	Conjunctival scrapings	
	Biopsy of lung (postmortem)	

and *Neisseria gonorrhoeae* may be facilitated by knowing whether the infecting agent is sensitive or resistant to penicillin or ampicillin. Resistance is correlated with the production of the enzyme ß-lactamase.

SEROLOGIC AND IMMUNOLOGIC TESTING

Serologic methods are employed to detect microbial antigen as rapid diagnostic tests or to determine host antibody responses to suspected pathogens. Because of the nature of the immune response patients generally are 10 to 12 days into their clinical illness before most serologic tests are able to measure a response. For conclusive evidence of infection, usually either a conversion from negative to positive or a four-fold rise in titer must be demonstrated. In some cases the titer will decrease. An acute phase serum and a convalescent serum (2 to 4 weeks after the onset of the infection) should be submitted to the laboratory.

Respiratory infections

9

INTRODUCTION

Respiratory tract infections constitute the major complaint for acute care visits to the pediatrician, accounting for an estimated 30 to 40% of all office consultations. The manifestations of the majority of infections are limited to the upper respiratory tract (i.e., ears, nose, throat), but as many as 5% may involve the lower respiratory tract. It should be emphasized that although the symptoms of a respiratory tract infection are fairly well localized, pathologic and physiologic changes may be widespread. Examples include acute exacerbation of asthma, diarrhea, and myalgia associated with viral respiratory disease. More than 90% of upper respiratory infections are viral in origin (excluding otitis media), while approximately half of all cases of pneumonia in children are caused by bacteria and half by viruses. Difficulty documenting etiology of infection in young children unfortunately has required liberal antibiotic use. The age of the patient, localization of the symptoms, and the status of the host's defenses help predict the organism and the need for antimicrobial therapy. In most cases of upper respiratory tract infection, fluids, acetaminophen for fever and bed rest are the only therapies necessary (Table 9.1).

COMMON COLD

The common cold can often be distinguished from the broader category of upper respiratory infections (URIs) by the absence of pharyngitis. Rhinoviruses are by far the most common etiologies, producing primarily nasal symptoms: congestion, mucoid discharge and sneezing. Mild conjunctivitis, throat irritation and low grade fever are occasionally present. For the vast majority of children

with simple rhinovirus infection, no treatment is necessary. Parents should be educated that cold remedies are a waste of money and effort.

PHARYNGITIS

Examination of patients who present with sore throat may reveal tonsillitis, tonsillopharyngitis, or nasopharyngitis. The absence of pharyngeal inflammation or the presence of either rhinorrhea or laryngitis is much more likely to be associated with viral infection. However, no physical findings clearly separate group A beta-hemolytic streptococci (GABHS) from viral, other bacterial, or noninfectious causes.

The primary concern for pharyngitis in children between 3 and 18 years of age is that untreated GABHS may subsequently cause

Table 9.1 Etiology of common upper respiratory tract infections

Common cold	Rhinoviruses
	respiratory syncytial virus (RSV)
	Parainfluenza
	Coronaviruses
Pharyngitis	Viruses
	Adenoviruses
	Enteroviruses
	Epstein–Barr virus
	Group A streptococci
Sinusitis	*Streptococcus pneumoniae*
	Haemophilus influenzae
	Moraxella catarrhalis
Croup	Parainfluenzae
(Laryngitis,	Influenza
laryngotracheitis,	RSV
laryngotracheo-	Adenovirus
bronchitis)	*Bordetella pertussis*

rheumatic fever. To prevent this sequela, adequate antimicrobial therapy should be instituted within 9 days of infection. Rapid antigen detection assays for GABHS are diagnostic if positive since the specificity of such tests is 98–99% (1–2% false positives). However, sensitivity is only 70% (30% false negatives) requiring follow-up cultures for negative tests.

The drug of choice for treatment of group A streptococcus remains penicillin V although many experts recommend a higher dosage than what has been used previously. A minimum of 20 mg/kg/day should be prescribed; larger children would generally receive 500 mg div. b.i.d. for 10 days. Many clinicians prefer amoxicillin because of a more pleasing taste and therefore better compliance. Relapses or failure should be treated with an antibiotic active against beta-lactamase producing organisms, i.e. macrolides, cephalosporins or amoxicillin/ clavulanate. The hypothesis is that colonizing pharyngeal bacteria that produce penicillinase have inactivated penicillin, resulting in treatment failure.

Other bacteria which can occasionally cause pharyngitis and require antimicrobial therapy are the following: gonococcus, *Francisella tularensis*, streptococci groups B, C and G, *Corynebacterium hemolyticum*, and *Treponema pallidum*. No treatment is of any benefit for the usual viral causes of pharyngitis. Throat lozenges, sprays, mouth washes, decongestants and antihistamines should be discouraged.

SINUSITIS

Acute paranasal sinusitis is a more difficult diagnosis to make in children than in adults because the characteristic symptoms are less likely to be present. Furthermore, there is considerable controversy about sensitivity of laboratory methods for documenting this infection. Maxillary or ethmoidal sinusitis usually follows a viral upper respiratory tract infection. Symptoms may include cough, purulent nasal discharge, facial pain and

fever. Diagnosis is most often considered when a URI with purulent nasal discharge lasts longer than 10 days. The diagnosis can be supported by X-ray, but the best radiographic study is a limited CT scan; sinus puncture with culture is the most definitive test, but is infrequently performed owing to its invasive nature. The organisms commonly recovered are considered pathogens when isolated from the sinuses, even though they are part of the normal flora in other parts of the respiratory tract (Table 9-2).

Several antibiotics are effective given orally. The increased resistance to amoxicillin based on beta lactamase production by approximately 50% of *Haemophilus influenzae* and 90–100% of *Moraxella catarrhalis* and an alteration in penicillin binding proteins which occurs in about 50% of *Streptococcus pneumoniae* have questioned the reliability of amoxicillin as first line therapy of sinusitis. If amoxicillin is considered a high dosage (75–90 mg/kg/day) should be prescribed. Alternatives include macrolides, cephalosporins and trimethoprim–sulfamethoxazole.

CROUP (LARYNGOTRACHEOBRONCHITIS)

Laryngotracheobronchitis (LTB) is the most common cause of acute partial upper airway obstruction in children. The terminology describing this disease and that in its differential diagnosis has been confusing.

Table 9.2 Acute sinusitis

Age	Usually > 2 years
Symptoms	Cough, nasal discharge, fever, face pain, prolonged upper respiratory infection
Organisms	*S. pneumoniae* *H. influenzae* *Moraxella catarrhalis*
Complications	Cavernous sinus thrombosis Periorbital cellulitis Meningitis Maxillary osteomyelitis Brain abscess

LTB (or croup) refers to partial airway obstruction due to a viral infection with erythema and edema concentrated mostly in the subglottic area. The organism is usually a parainfluenza virus (in order of frequency types 1, 3, 2), although other organisms can cause croup during periods of increased prevalence (respiratory syncytial virus, influenza, rhinovirus). The peak ages are between 6 months and 2 years. The clinical presentation is that of a child with a few days of upper respiratory tract infection who then develops inspiratory stridor, retractions and a harsh barking cough. The degree of fever depends on the organism and is usually mild with parainfluenza. The severity of the obstruction is variable throughout the day and is often worse at night. The illness gradually resolves spontaneously over several days. No laboratory test is needed for confirmation but neck X-rays show characteristic subglottic narrowing (steeple sign). Therapy at home is symptomatic (i.e., antipyretics for fever) and mist. In-hospital therapy should include steroids, dexamethasone 0.6 mg/kg given as a single dose; management of more severe cases might include mist, oxygen, and racemic epinephrine (1:4 concentration of 2.25%, with increasing concentration to 1:1 as needed) by inhalation. Because of the potential for rebound (i.e. returning to baseline clinical status), the use of racemic epinephrine commits the patient to further observation. It is uncommon for croup to require intubation. Because edema and inflammation are in the narrowest portion of the child's airway, a somewhat narrower endotracheal tube should be selected to decrease the likelihood of postintubation subglottic stenosis (Table 9.3).

Spasmodic croup occurs in the slightly older child and is probably a variant of reactive airway disease rather than an infection, although a viral disease may be a predisposing factor. Characteristically the previously well child awakens suddenly with stridor and coughing, which lasts 45–90 minutes before abating spontaneously. It recurs in an irregular pattern. Steroids,

Table 9.3 Therapy for infectious croup

At home
  Mist-humidity
  Antipyretics
  Observation
In-hospital
  Dexamethasone 0.6 mg/kg i.m., single dose on admission
  Mist-humidity
  Racemic epinephrine
  Oxygen
  Intubation

shown to be helpful in infectious LTB, may also be beneficial in spasmodic croup.

PERTUSSIS

Despite vigorous immunization programs, pertussis continues to be a commonly seen disease in infants and young children. The clinical course is traditionally divided into three phases: coryzal, paroxysmal and recovery. During the coryzal phase the disease is indistinguishable from the common cold. It is during this phase that the organism *Bordetella pertussis* is most likely to be isolated; this is also prior to the time of being suspicious enough to seek it. The subsequent phase is that of paroxysmal coughing, often interspersed with loud inspiratory 'whoops'. Coughing may be triggered by feeding, activity, or crying. Unfortunately, this phase can persist for weeks despite appropriate antibiotic therapy with erythromycin. Cultures are likely to be negative during this phase of the illness when the child is likely to be brought to the physician. Nevertheless, the diagnosis can be made using fluorescent antibody to the organism performed on a posterior nasopharyngeal swab. Diagnosis is strongly suggested by a marked lymphocytosis. Treatment includes erythromycin 50 mg/kg/day divided q.6h for 14 days.

BRONCHITIS

The diagnosis of bronchitis is difficult to make in pediatrics because definition is lacking. If simple inflammation of the trachea and major divisions of the bronchi constituted pathogenesis, bronchitis would be synonymous with the common cold. Chronic or recurrent bronchitis is also difficult to define, but most authors suggest that a productive cough is a prominent feature and that symptoms persist for a period of weeks or recur regularly. As contrasted with adults, bronchitis in children is caused almost exclusively by viral agents (Table 9.4). *Mycoplasma pneumoniae* is the only common pathogen for which antimicrobial therapy is indicated.

BRONCHIOLITIS

Bronchiolitis is a very common lower respiratory tract infection, affecting perhaps as many as 1 to 2% of all infants. The peak age ranges from 2 to 10 months. Respiratory syncytial virus (RSV) is the predominant causative organism, with other viruses being responsible in certain epidemics. The clinical manifestations are preceding coryza, cough, tachypnea and wheezing. The chest X-ray shows hyperinflation, peribronchial thickening and varying amounts of atelectasis. Histologically, there is mononuclear inflammation and sloughing of the bronchiolar epithelium with partial obstruction of the bronchiolar lumen (Table 9.5).

Therapy is primarily supportive with maintenance of adequate oxygenation and appropriate hydration and nutrition. One-third to one-half of children will benefit from albuterol bronchodilator therapy; a therapeutic trial either in the emergency room or shortly after hospitalization should be offered. Treatment should be discontinued if improvement cannot be documented. A small percentage of infants will require mechanical ventilation. Antibiotics are not indicated as this is exclusively a viral illness. Chest physiotherapy may be beneficial to those infants with atelectasis. Steroids have not been beneficial in several large studies. Although bronchiolitis seems to be a self-limited and a generally benign illness, the long-term sequelae may be significant. Up to 50% of the patients have subsequent wheezing or frank asthma. It is yet unclear what role small airway insults early in life have on

Table 9.4 Viruses causing lower respiratory tract infection

Organism	Bronchitis	Bronchiolitis	Pneumonia
Respiratory syncytial virus	+++	++++	++
Influenza virus (A and B)	++	+	++
Parainfluenza virus	++	++	++
Adenovirus	+++	+	+++
Rhinovirus	+	++	++

++++, most frequent; +, occasional

Table 9.5 Bronchiolitis

Age	2–10 months
Organism	RSV predominates, adenovirus, parainfluenza
Symptoms	Wheezing and tachypnea
Therapy	Trial of bronchodilator therapy with aerolized
	β_2 agonists: albuterol 2.15 mg in 3 ml normal saline;
	neonate/infant 0.05–0.15 mg/kg/dose
	children 1.25–2.5 mg/dose q.4–6 h
	Supportive treatment (O_2, etc.)
Sequelae	Recurrent wheezing
	Predilection for chronic obstructive pulmonary disesase

chronic obstructive lung disease in adults. Some children appear to have asymptomatic small airways dysfunction years after the episode of bronchiolitis, suggesting a propensity for progressive dysfunction later in life.

AFEBRILE PNEUMONIA OF INFANCY

Afebrile pneumonia in infants less than 3 months of age is caused by a unique group of pathogens which are acquired during the perinatal period from colonized mothers. Mixed infection is common. The clinical presentation is tachypnea, poor weight gain and inspiratory crackles; wheezing is uncommon. The chest X-ray usually shows interstitial pneumonia hyperaeration, peribronchial thickening, and scattered areas of atelectasis. The diagnosis should be made by culture. *Chlamydia* sp. is suggested by eosinophilia, elevated immunoglobulins, and clinically by the presence of conjunctivitis. Rapid ELISA or fluorescence assays for chlamydia antigen from posterior nasopharyngeal washings or conjunctival exudate can confirm diagnosis. Other agents require culture for identification (Table 9.6).

INFLUENZA

Influenza occurs during well publicized epidemics and is characterized by fever, headache, myalgia, cough and any combination of upper respiratory tract symptoms. Croup or pneumonia are frequently the primary diagnosis. Because disease is spread by direct person to person contact, hospitalized patients require isolation. Etiology is best confirmed by viral culture during the first 3 days of illness. Thereafter the low quantity of virus may result in falsely negative cultures. Rapid antigen detection assays such as immunofluorescence are available but results in the usual office or hospital setting are quite variable.

The antiviral agent of choice for influenza A prophylaxis or treatment is rimantadine or its parent compound, amantadine (Chapter 20, Table 20.18). Influenza vaccine should be mandatory for high-risk children and strongly considered for universal administration, usually given during the month of October (Chapter 3, Tables 3.2 and 3.8).

PNEUMONIA

Although the vast majority of acute pneumonias in children are viral in etiology, standard practice dictates empiric administration of antimicrobial agents for most young pediatric patients. Variables for antibiotic therapy and for hospitalization of infants and children include epidemiologic considerations, clinical symptoms, predisposing host factors, age, and radiographic findings. The virtual elimination of *Haemophilus influenzae* type B as a respiratory pathogen and recent recognition of *Chlamydia pneumoniae* as a common cause of pneumonia in older children have recently changed our selection of initial empiric antimicrobial therapy for lower respiratory tract infections in pediatric patients. New, rapid diagnostic tests are also useful in making clinical decisions and are particularly important for children who are unable to produce sputum for examination and whose small airways limit utilization of bronchoscopy.

In Europe and the USA, pneumonia is diagnosed in approximately 2% of infants

Table 9.6 Afebrile pneumonitis of early infancy: etiology and treatment

Pathogen	Treatment
Chlamydia trachomatis	Erythromycin 50 mg/kg/day div. q.i.d. for 21 days
Cytomegalovirus	Ganciclovir, CMV immunoglobulin
Pneumocystis carinii	TMP/SMX 20:100 mg/kg/day div. b.i.d. for 14 days
Ureaplasma urealyticum	Erythromycin 50 mg/kg/day div. q.i.d. for 14 days

TMP/SMX, trimethoprim/sulfamethoxazole

younger than 1 year and in 4% of children aged 1 to 5 years. The practitioner's primary responsibility is to differentiate upper respiratory tract infections from pneumonia. The practitioner must also decide which patients with lower respiratory tract disease warrant more aggressive management.

Etiology

It is estimated that 90% of pediatric pneumonias are caused by viral agents. Approximately 50% of documented viral lower respiratory infections in children are caused by respiratory syncytial virus (RSV), one-quarter by parainfluenza virus types 3 and 1 and a smaller number of pneumonias result from influenza A and B or adenovirus. Rhinovirus is occasionally implicated. Three of these groups of viral agents (RSV, parainfluenza and influenza) are seen almost exclusively during the winter months. Adenovirus is the more common viral pathogen during the remainder of the year. Such specific seasonal clustering implies a greater likelihood of bacterial causes during the spring, summer, and fall.

Chlamydia pneumoniae is an increasingly recognized pathogen in pediatric community acquired pneumonia (CAP) as well as otitis media. The incidence of this infection varies from 1 to 15%. The symptoms associated with *C. pneumoniae* infection are similar to those seen with *Mycoplasma pneumoniae*; however, sore throat and hoarseness are reported more frequently. Pleural effusions may be seen in as many as 25% of infections. In most studies, the diagnosis has been made by serology but these assays are still not widely available. Bacterial and fungal organisms causing pneumonia are primarily related to the age of the pediatric patient (Table 9.7).

The greatest number of potential pathogens are seen in neonates who require prolonged intensive care, particularly those born prematurely. Group B streptococci (*Streptococcus agalactiae*) and Gram-negative enteric bacilli, particularly *Escherichia coli*, are the most common pathogens causing neonatal pneumonia, often in association with generalized sepsis.

Group B streptococcal respiratory infection usually develops during the first few days of life. Rapidly progressive radiographic findings mimic respiratory distress syndrome. Coliform pneumonia in neonates also occurs during the early neonatal period; it is acquired perinatally from a colonized mother. Pulmonary infection in neonates of 3 to 4 weeks of age is more likely to be nosocomially transmitted during difficult intensive care management. In patients who have been hospitalized for more than 2 weeks, *Staphylococcus epidermidis* is a relatively common cause of sepsis and pneumonia. Infection with *Candida albicans* is a consequence of long-

Table 9.7 Bacterial and fungal causes of pneumonia related to age of the pediatric patient

Age group	Common pathogens
0–48 h	Group B streptococci
1–14 days	*E. coli*, *K. pneumoniae*, other Enterobacteriaceae, *L. monocytogenes*, *S. aureus*, anaerobes, group B streptococci
2 weeks to 2 months (premature neonates)	Enterobacteriaceae, group B streptococci, *S. aureus*, *S. epidermidis*, *C. albicans*, *H. influenzae*, *S. pneumoniae*
2 months to 5 years	*H. influenzae*, *S. pneumoniae*
5–10 years	*S. pneumoniae*
10–21 years	*Mycoplasma pneumoniae*, *Chlamydia pneumoniae* (*TWAR* agent), *S. pneumoniae*

term intravenous catheterization and the administration of broad-spectrum antibiotics. Other data used to determine probable causes include associated clinical signs and symptoms, chest X-ray findings and diagnostic laboratory tests (Table 9.8).

Sputum is rarely produced by children during episodes of pneumonia, so the usual first step in the management of adult pneumonias, Gram's stain examination of sputum, is eliminated.

Clinical appearance

It is not possible to distinguish between viral and bacterial pneumonia on clinical grounds alone. Signs and symptoms together with other assessments, however, allow the practitioner to categorize the correct cause in a majority of cases. Children with bacterial disease have histories suggesting rapid onset, are more likely to appear very sick, and have temperatures above 39°C (102.2°F).

Patients who have viral processes generally have low-grade fever and are usually irritable, although they may not appear toxic. Other important symptoms associated with influenza, parainfluenza and adenovirus infection are headache, photophobia, myalgia and gastrointestinal complaints. In

addition, there is a prodrome of longer than 2 days associated with these 3 viruses, and even more commonly present when rhinovirus is the responsible pathogen.

In older children who are infected with *Mycoplasma pneumoniae*, onset and disease evolution are more suggestive of viral pneumonia because multiple organ systems may be involved. *Mycoplasma* infection may be severe and rapidly progressive in children with sickle cell disease.

Chest roentgenograms

Chest roentgenograms most readily confirm clinical findings that are compatible with pneumonia. In many cases chest X-rays help differentiate viral from bacterial causes. They may even suggest specific pathogens. Viral pneumonias are associated with 4 roentgenographic findings: hyperexpansion, parahilar peribronchial infiltrates, atelectasis, and hilar adenopathy. The latter finding is only commonly associated with adenovirus. Consolidated alveolar or diffuse interstitial infiltrates and large pleural effusions are rarely seen. More severe X-ray changes in young infants suggest respiratory syncytial virus disease. The chest roentgenogram demonstrating infection with *Chlamydia* classically reveals diffuse interstitial infiltrates with hyperaeration, peribronchial thickening and scattered areas of atelectasis. The more extensive diffuse interstitial infiltrates that usually accompany *Chlamydia* infection help distinguish this etiology from viral infections.

Alveolar disease, consolidation, the presence of air bronchograms, and pleural effusions are characteristic of bacterial pneumonia. These roentgenographic findings alone dictate institution of antimicrobial therapy. *Staphylococcus aureus* must be suspected if there is evidence of a consolidated infiltrate accompanied by an effusion or a pneumatocele. This cause is relatively more common in young infants (< 12 months of age) and neonates, and warrants hospitalization and daily roentgenographic monitoring. The primary reason for repeating chest X-rays

Table 9.8 Suggested diagnostic evaluation for pneumonia in children

---

Chest X-rays (posteroanterior and lateral decubitus view if there is consolidation or evidence of effusion)

Blood culture

Complete blood count

Tuberculin skin test

Bedside cold agglutinins (see text)

Afebrile and < 20 weeks of age (in addition to above):

Chlamydia culture, monoclonal fluorescent antibody or ELISA staining of posterior nasopharyngeal swab

Wright–Giemsa stain or rapid antigen assay of conjunctival scraping (for *Chlamydia*) if there is conjunctivitis

---

within 24 to 48 hours is to delineate changes compatible with a staphylococcal cause.

Aspiration pneumonia is often suspected on clinical grounds such as a pre-existing seizure disorder or severe gastroesophageal reflux. Radiographic findings classically include a consolidating infiltrate in the right lower lobe. Young patients who aspirate while recumbent, however, are more likely to develop disease in the upper lobes.

Extensive destruction of lung tissue may result in the formation of multiple small abscess cavities, termed necrotizing pneumonia. This roentgenographic finding should alert the clinician to the presence of less common pathogens, including *Pseudomonas aeruginosa*, *Klebsiella pneumoniae*, *Proteus mirabilis*, other Enterobacteriaceae, and anaerobes. Predominant organisms are often locally unique, and antibiotic sensitivities for such organisms vary considerably from hospital to hospital. Antibiotic regimens generally include a broad spectrum penicillin (for anaerobic coverage) plus an aminoglycoside (for synergistic activity against *Pseudomonas* and other Enterobacteriaceae). Despite early and appropriate antimicrobial therapy, necrotizing pneumonia is often fatal.

Laboratory diagnosis

The 'gold standard' for documenting both bacterial and viral causes of pneumonia is culture. The best source of culture material is a lung aspirate. Published reports have suggested that bacterial pathogens can be isolated in approximately 33% of patients undergoing this procedure. Such studies have been biased, however, because severe cases were more likely to be enrolled. The typical viral pneumonia with a centrally located parahilar peribronchial infiltrate does not safely lend itself to needle aspiration. Bacteremia is only documented in 9% to 10% of all febrile children with pneumonia while more than 50% of community acquired cases are bacterial in origin.

In neonates, pneumonia is frequently associated with generalized sepsis. Organisms recovered are similar to those implicated in other serious infections such as meningitis, septic arthritis, and pyelonephritis. A workup for sepsis, including lumbar puncture, is always indicated in neonates who have febrile pneumonia.

Culture is the only reliable method of identifying influenza viruses. Rapid identification of RSV, however, can be achieved with direct fluorescent staining or ELISA techniques. Likewise, fluorescent staining reagents and ELISA that differentiate other potential viral pathogens, such as parainfluenza virus and adenovirus, are also available. Tracheal aspirates or posterior nasopharyngeal secretions are required as specimens for examination. RSV testing is feasible in community hospitals, but other viral cultures are usually performed in reference laboratories. Unfortunately, because of the time required for isolation and identification of viruses, such tests do not generally provide clinically useful information. *Pneumocystis carinii*, *Ureaplasma urealyticum* and cytomegalovirus must be cultured from tracheal aspirates. *P. carinii* has been successfully recovered in only a few laboratories where investigations of this organism are in progress. Detection of *Pneumocystis* antigen in serum is also performed only in research laboratories. An important rapid diagnostic step for *Mycoplasma* infection is the bedside cold agglutination test. Although it is only 50% sensitive in identifying this cause, a positive result can guide early specific therapy, because specificity is close to absolute. Most critical is that the test be performed correctly. Two to five drops of blood (0.1–0.3 ml) are placed in a 64 mm (small blue top) tube containing sodium citrate anticoagulant. An identical tube with control blood is also obtained. These tubes are refrigerated in an ice bath for 1 min, after which time the tubes are rolled by their ends and blood is observed for agglutination. When the blood is warmed to room temperature, agglutination is no longer apparent. Common mistakes are drawing too much blood, using too large a tube, or using the wrong anticoagulant.

Antimicrobial therapy

Management of children with community acquired pneumonia is presented as an algorithm in Figure 9.1. Early empiric treatment for either bacterial or viral disease is imperative for patients whose condition might take a rapidly progressive course if therapy is delayed. Certainly febrile neonates and infants less than 2 months of age belong in this category. Late institution of antibiotics in these patients is associated with higher rates of mortality and morbidity.

Antibiotics are selected primarily on the basis of age and severity of illness (Table 9.9). Dosages for these agents are listed in Chapter 20. Duration of therapy is 7 to 10 days for uncomplicated pneumonia. Once the causative agent is identified by culture or with one of the rapid antigen detection assays, specific therapy may be readily selected.

Amoxicillin is the drug of choice for outpatient treatment of pneumonia in the 2-month to 5-year age group, even though 25–50% of S. pneumoniae are resistant to penicillins. Half of this is intermediate resistance (MIC 0.06–1.0 µg/ml) so can be managed with the higher dosages of amoxicillin (75–90 mg/kg/day). In areas of the country that report an even higher incidence of highly penicillin resistant (MIC ≥ 2.0 µg/ml) pneumococcus, oral antibiotics active against these organisms may be more appropriate. Such antibiotics include cefprozil, cefpodoxime, azithromycin, clarithromycin, or erythromycin. Selection among these may be made on the basis of relative cost, because all are associated with a very low incidence of significant adverse reactions.

Treatment of pneumonia is usually empiric. If C. pneumoniae is suspected as the responsible pathogen, macrolides should be used as primary therapy. When M. pneumoniae is likely, particularly in the older teenager, newer quinolones or tetracycline-based antibiotics can be considered when macrolides are not tolerated. If a child does not respond to initial antibacterial therapy, the most likely explanation is a viral cause. Other bacterial causes might also be considered, such as S. aureus, multi-resistant pneumococcus, ampicillin-resistant H. influenzae, or anaerobes. If these latter pathogens are probable, hospitalization is warranted. Hospitalization is also based on age, clinical, and roentgenographic factors (Table 9.10).

Antiviral therapy

At the present time there are 2 antiviral chemotherapeutic agents approved for the treatment of pneumonia in children, amantadine and ribavirin. Each offers important therapeutic benefits for specific clinical circumstances. Amantadine is indicated for the prophylaxis and treatment of influenza A virus infection. Unfortunately, central nervous system side-effects occur in 10% to 25% of recipients. These adverse reactions include insomnia, fatigue, difficulty concentrating, nervousness and, to a lesser extent, depression. In published reports 6% to 14% of study patients discontinued therapy because of unacceptable adverse reactions. Rimantadine hydrochloride, an analog of amantadine, is licensed for clinical use in adults. Indications are essentially identical to those for amantadine. Central nervous system adverse reactions associated with amantadine are uncommon with rimantadine; this is in fact the primary reason for its development.

Ribavirin is a broad-spectrum virastatic agent with in vitro and in vivo activity against RSV, influenza A and B, parainfluenza, and adenovirus. It is currently approved by the Food and Drug Administration in its aerosolized form for the therapy of RSV infections in hospitalized children who do not require assisted ventilation. The Committee on Infectious Diseases of the American Academy of Pediatrics has not specifically recommended application of ribavirin for any patient group but suggests that 'some categories should be considered for treatment with ribavirin aerosol'. These essentially include 2 groups: infants at high risk for severe or complicated RSV infection and those in whom prolonged illnesses might worsen an underlying chronic disease.

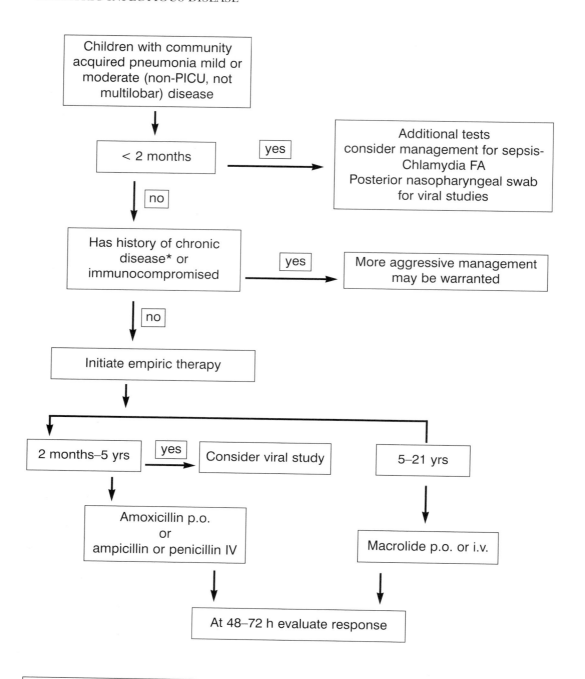

Figure 9.1 Inpatient and outpatient management of children with community acquired pneumonia

Necrotizing pneumonia

Necrotizing bacterial pneumonias are occasionally seen in patients who are debilitated, immunocompromised, or who have undergone prolonged hospitalization. Responsible pathogens are often nosocomial organisms such as *Pseudomonas aeruginosa*, *Klebsiella pneumoniae*, *Proteus mirabilis*, and related species. Penicillins or clindamycin are recommended for these pathogens.

Table 9.9 Empiric antimicrobial therapy for presumed bacterial pneumonia

Age group	Antibiotics
Younger than 2 months	Ampicillin plus Ceftriaxone or cefotaxime (oral erythromycin if *C. trachomatis* is suspected in infants younger than 20 weeks) plus Oxacillin or nafcillin (optional) vancomycin (for multi-resistant pneumococcus) if the illness appears life threatening
2 months–5 years	
Mild	Amoxicillin (oral)
Severe	Ceftriaxone or cefotaxime; add oxacillin or nafcillin if *S. aureus* is suspected, vancomycin (for multi-resistant pneumococcus) if the illness appears life threatening
5–21 years	Macrolide (oral or intravenous depending on severity)

Table 9.10 Children with pneumonia warranting consideration of inpatient management

Toxic appearance
Respiratory distress
Pleural effusion
Age factors
  Less than 2 months
  Less than 3 years with lobar pneumonia
  Less than 5 years with involvement of more than 1 lobe
Those with chronic diseases
  Pulmonary (including asthma)
  Cardiac
  Renal
  Diabetes mellitus
  Anemia (including sickle cell disease)
  Malignancies
Immunocompromised host
Progression during outpatient therapy

Aspiration pneumonia

Pneumonia due to aspiration of gastric contents or oropharyngeal secretions occurs in patients with impaired neurologic function. A depressed level of consciousness, albeit transient, as in seizure disorders, induction of anesthesia, or diabetic coma, or permanent as in mental retardation, is a fairly constant predisposing factor. Chronic aspiration also occurs in patients with an unco-ordinated swallowing mechanism. Careful history and physical examination should uncover the potential for aspiration pneumonitis. The organisms are usually anaerobes, and frequently more than one organism is isolated. The infiltrates on chest X-ray are usually in the dependent lobes; effusions and abscesses are common (Table 9.11).

PLEURAL EMPYEMA

A collection of exudate within the pleural cavity results from the inflammatory response induced by bacterial pneumonia. This empyema progresses through three overlapping stages from initial thin fluid accumulation to organized fibroblast deposition and entrapment of lung (Table 9.12). Decisions to

Table 9.11 Organisms causing aspiration pneumonia

Peptostreptococcus
Peptococcus
Microaerophilic cocci and streptococci
Bacteroides sp.
Fusobacterium sp.
S. aureus
Streptococcus pyogenes
Streptococcus sp.

drain this exudate must be made in a timely manner to prevent pleural thickening and any subsequent need for decortication.

TUBERCULOSIS

Most children are diagnosed because they have a positive tuberculin (IPPD) skin test and are in high risk groups for disease or have an illness compatible with tuberculosis, usually pneumonia. Early morning gastric aspirates may recover *Mycobacterium tuberculosis* for diagnosis and sensitivity testing, but organisms recovered from adult contacts are more commonly used to guide therapy. Short-course chemotherapy has now been shown to be equal to previous regimens of one year or longer (Table 9.13).

Screening for tuberculosis in infants and children

Routine skin testing for tuberculosis in children with no risk factors residing in low-prevalence communities is not indicated. In such settings skin reactions are most likely to be falsely positive. Children at high risk (Table 9.14) should be tested annually using Mantoux tuberculin tests (Table 9.15). All results (positive or negative) should be routinely read by qualified medical personnel. Children with no risk factors but residing in high-prevalence regions, and children whose risk factor history is incomplete or unreliable may be screened periodically for example at 1, 5 and 15 years of age. Such a decision should be made at the local level.

Table 9.12   Empyema in children

Stages of infection
  Exudative: allows needle aspiration
  Fibrinopurulent: may be loculated
  Organizing
Treatment options
  Exudative: repeated needle aspiration (1–5 days)
  Exudative or fibrinopurulent: chest tube drainage
  Organizing: limited thoracotomy after 3–5 days of drainage
  Organized: Decortication
    If > 50% limitation of lung by CT scan
    After 2–4 weeks of medical management
      tachypnea
      asymmetry of chest wall expansion
      fever
      leukocytosis

Table 9.13   Recommended treatment regimens for tuberculosis in infants, children, and adolescents

Tuberculous infection/disease	*Regimen*	*Remarks*
Asymptomatic infection (positive skin test, no disease)		If daily therapy is not possible, twice weekly may be substituted. HIV-infected children should be treated for 12 months
Isoniazid-susceptible	6–9 months of Isoniazid (I) daily	
Isoniazid-resistant	6–9 months of rifampin (R) daily	
Isoniazid–rifampin-resistant	Consult a TB specialist	
Pulmonary	6-months (standard): 2 months of I, R, and pyrazinamide (Z) daily, followed by 4 months of I and R daily	If drug resistance is possible, another drug (ethambutol or streptomycin) is added to the initial therapy until drug susceptibility is determined

Continued

Table 9.13   Continued

Tuberculous infection/disease	Regimen	Remarks
	or	
	2 months of I, R, and Z daily, followed by 4 months of I and R twice a week	Drugs can be given 2 or 3 times per week under direct observation in the initial phase if nonadherence is likely
	9-months alternative regimens (for hilar adenopathy only): 9 months of I and R once a day	Regimens consisting of 6 months of I and R once a day, and 1 month of I and R once a day, followed by 5 months of I and R twice a week, have been successful in areas where drug resistance is rare
	or	
	1 month of I and R daily, followed by 8 months of I and R twice a week	
Extrapulmonary meningitis, disseminated (miliary), bone/joint disease	2 months of I, R and Z and S once a day, followed by 10 months of I and R once a day (12 months total)	Streptomycin (S) is given with initial therapy until drug susceptibility is known
	or	
	2 months of I, R, Z, and S daily, followed by 10 months of I and R twice a week (12 months total)	For patients who may have acquired tuberculosis in geographic locales where resistance to streptomycin is common, capreomycin (15–30 mg/kg/day) or kanamycin (15–30 mg/kg/day) may be used instead of S
Other (e.g. cervical lymphadenopathy)	Same as pulmonary	See pulmonary

Table 9.14   Infants, children and adolescents at high risk for tuberculosis infection: immediate and annual skin testing recommended

Contacts of adults with infectious tuberculosis
Those from or whose parents have emigrated from high-prevalence regions of the world
Abnormalities on chest radiograph
Clinical evidence of tuberculosis
HIV seropositive
Immunosuppressed
Other medical risk factors: Hodgkin's disease, lymphoma, diabetes mellitus, chronic renal
    failure, malnutrition
Children frequently exposed to the following adults:
    HIV infected
    Homeless persons
    Users of intravenous and other street drugs
    Poor and medically indigent city dwellers
    Residents of nursing homes
    Migrant farm workers
Incarcerated adolescents

Table 9.15 Definition of a positive Mantoux skin test (5TU-PPD) in children

---

Reaction size of ≥ 5 mm
    Children in close contact with known or suspected infectious cases of tuberculosis:
        Households with active cases
        Households with previously active cases if:
            treatment cannot be verified as adequate before the exposure
            treatment was initiated after period of child's contact
            reactivation is suspected
    Children suspected to have tuberculous disease:
        Chest roentgenogram consistent with active or previously active tuberculosis
        Clinical evidence of tuberculosis
    Children with underlying conditions which put them at high risk of acquiring severe tuberculosis:
        Immunocompromised conditions
        HIV infection
Reaction size of ≥ 10 mm
    Children at increased risk of dissemination:
        Young age: < 4 years of age
        Other medical risk factors: Hodgkin's diseases, lymphoma, diabetes mellitus, chronic renal failure, malnutrition
    Increased environmental exposure:
        Those from or whose parent have emigrated from high-prevalence regions of the world.
        Children frequently exposed to the following adults:
            HIV infected
            Homeless persons
            Users of intravenous and other street drugs
            Poor and medically indigent city dwellers
            Residents of nursing homes
            Migrant farm workers
Reaction size of ≥ 15 mm
    Children 4 years of age without any risk factors

5TU-PPD, 5 tuberculin units – purified protein derivative

Gastrointestinal infections

10

AMEBIASIS

Amebiasis is primarily an infection of the colon, caused by the protozoan parasite *Entamoeba histolytica*. The organism exists both in trophozoite and cyst forms. Small trophozoites are 10–20 μm in diameter and are not associated with invasiveness. Large forms are usually found in the presence of invasive disease and range from 20 to 60 μm in diameter. The presence of ingested red blood cells in the endoplasm of a large trophozoite is the most reliable morphologic feature in identifying the organism as *E. histolytica*. The cyst form measures 10–20 μm in diameter and contains between 1 and 4 nuclei (as contrasted with *Entamoeba coli* which contains 4–8). Cysts transmit disease and are resistant to drying, cold, and routine chlorination of water.

The pathogenicity of the organism is related to its ability to attach to the colonic mucus layer and disrupt local immune mechanisms. Attachment may be aided by adherence proteins produced by *E. histolytica*. The organism has direct cytotoxic activity toward the intestinal cells as well as toward neutrophils, macrophages and T cells.

Entamoeba histolytica is more common in the United States than had previously been suspected. Its prevalence ranges from 1% in Alaska to 10% in southern states. Worldwide it is more common in tropical and subtropical climates, and affects 10% of the world's population each year. There are approximately 3500 cases reported each year in the United States; it is estimated that an additional 40% of cases go undetected. Transmission is via the fecal–oral route following ingestion of contaminated water, raw fruit, or vegetables. Insects and flies have also been implicated and there is possible sexual transmission. Poor sanitation and crowding account for reported epidemics. More severe infection is seen in pregnant women, younger children, immunosuppressed patients, patients with AIDS and patients on corticosteroid medications. The disease is more common in the third to fifth decade of life but occurrences in all ages, including neonates, have been reported.

Three forms of amebiasis exist (Table 10.1). Asymptomatic carriage of *E. histolytica* is most common and accounts for 90% of infections. Occasional vague symptoms such as abdominal pain, fatigue, headache, or cough are observed but may not be related to the presence of ameba in the bowel. The incubation period is quite variable, 8 to 95 days, and precedes invasion of the bowel mucosa to produce a dysenteric form. Progression of symptoms is usually gradual (over 3 to 4 weeks) and dysentery may not occur until later in the course. Abdominal

Table 10.1 Clinical forms of amebiasis

Asymptomatic carrier
Dysenteric form
  Pain
  Tenesmus
  Diarrhea with blood and mucus
  Fever
  Abdominal distention
Extraintestinal form
  Liver abscess(es)
  Thoracic involvement
  Cerebral abscess
  Cutaneous (perineal)
  Heart and pericardium
  Larynx
  Scapula
  Stomach
  Aorta

117

pain and tenesmus are the most common symptoms. Infants may have a much more rapid and fulminant course with severe watery diarrhea and hematochezia. Blood is present in the stools in over 95% of patients. The leukocyte count is usually elevated with a shift to the left, but eosinophilia is absent.

Endoscopic examination of the colon reveals superficial ulcers surrounded by normal mucosa. A characteristic flask-shaped ulcer is seen in some patients. These ulcerations may then deepen and enlarge with the adjacent mucosa becoming hyperemic and friable. Occasionally, granulation tissue without fibrosis (ameboma) forms. Complications of intestinal disease include necrotizing enterocolitis, toxic megacolon, perforation, abscess formation, stricture and obstruction by amebomas. Amebae spread to the liver via the portal circulation. Although less frequent than in adults, liver abscesses are the most common extraintestinal form of amebiasis in children with invasive disease occurring in 1 to 7% of cases. This process is more fulminating in children. Hepatic involvement is ten times more common in men than women; there is no difference between genders in prepubescent children. Approximately one-half of patients with amebic abscesses have no history of amebic colitis. The right lobe of the liver is more commonly involved than the left lobe and abscesses are usually solitary. Abscess fluid has been typically described as a reddish 'anchovy paste' but can be white or green. Amebae are found in the walls of the abscess but rarely within the fluid. Little inflammatory reaction is evident in the abscess, which explains the normal or minimally elevated level of liver transaminases.

Clinical symptoms of liver abscesses are abdominal pain, fever and tender hepatomegaly. A nonproductive cough, decreased diaphragmatic excursion and pleural effusions may be found but jaundice is unusual. Intestinal disease is found in the majority of children with amebic liver abscesses. Laboratory values of infected patients include a normal or elevated leukocyte count and an invariably elevated sedimentation rate.

Normochromic, normocytic, mild anemia may be present. Other extraintestinal manifestations of amebiasis are thought to occur via spread from the liver. Extension into the thoracic cavity is the most common and occurs in 10% of patients with liver diseases.

Diagnosis of amebiasis is usually made by stool examination (Table 10.2). If a specimen cannot be processed within 1 hour, then it should be put into a preservative (polyvinyl-alcohol or formalin). Identification of *E. histolytica* in stools can be difficult; a survey of public and private parasitology laboratories revealed that 20% were unable to identify trophozoites and 35% could not identify cysts. The cysts of *E. histolytica* resemble those of both *Entamoeba coli* and other non-pathologic forms of *Entamoeba*. Stained material obtained from mucus or scrapings of the base of an ulcer during endoscopic examination may also reveal the organism. Numerous serologic tests are also available. Most public health facilities use indirect hemagglutination (IHA), which is positive in 58% of asymptomatic patients, 61% of those with moderate involvement, and 95% with severe involvement. Almost 100% of patients with extraintestinal amebiasis have positive antibody titers. Serology is less sensitive in newborns and young infants, even in the presence of severe extraintestinal amebiasis. An elevated titer does not differentiate between acute or past infection and titers may remain positive for 6 months to 3 years after the acute infection. A high titer (>1:512) is more suggestive of recent infection. Liver

Table 10.2 Diagnosis of amebiasis

Colonic involvement
Examination of stool or mucus from bowel
Biopsy of colonic ulcer
Serology
Hepatic involvement
Scintigraphy
Computed tomography
Ultrasound
Serology

abscesses may be diagnosed by several methods including liver scans, computed tomography (CT) and ultrasound. Decisions for therapy and its duration are guided by location and severity of disease.

Most liver abscesses do not require needle aspiration. Drainage is indicated for subcapsular hepatic abscesses or abscesses of the left lobe as these can rupture into the pleural cavity or pericardium. If a liver abscess does not respond to medication, closed-needle aspiration under CT or ultrasound guidance may be necessary. If no response is seen, a laparotomy and open drainage should be performed. Other indications for surgery are perforation of the bowel or abscess formation if unresponsive to conservative therapy. Brain abscesses should be treated with early drainage through a burr hole and the abscess residua followed carefully by CT. If a response is not seen, more definitive surgery may be needed. Pericardial abscesses are treated by repeated needle aspirations. Antibiotics are only necessary in patients with secondary infection. Corticosteroids should not be given as this increases the severity of disease (Table 10.3).

CAMPYLOBACTER

Campylobacter gastroenteritis has been identified as one of the leading bacterial infections of the gastrointestinal tract in children. The primary organism causing disease in children was formerly termed *Campylobacter fetus* subspecies jejuni but is currently referred to as *C. jejuni* (Table 10.4).

The incidence of intrafamilial spread of infection occurs at a much lower rate than would be expected. This is probably an indication that the organism is not viable for long periods outside of the body. Several instances of spread from animals to humans have also been recorded and include either direct contact and contamination from the animal or ingestion of contaminated meat that has been inadequately cooked.

Fever, diarrhea, and abdominal pain are the primary symptoms of *Campylobacter* infection;

Table 10.3 Treatment of amebiasis

Asymptomatic	Paromomycin 30 mg/kg/day p.o. div. q.8h for 7–10 days (maximum 1.5 g/day) or iodoquinol 30–40 mg/kg/day p.o. div. q.8h for 20 days (maximum 650 mg q.8h)
Intestinal	Metronidazole 35–50 mg/kg/day p.o. div. q.8h for 10 days (maximum 750 mg t.i.d.) followed by iodoquinol 40 mg/kg/day p.o. div. q.8h for 20 days
Extraintestinal	Same as for intestinal or dehydroemetine 1 mg/kg/day i.m. div. q.12h for 10 days plus Chloroquine 10 mg/kg/day p.o. div. q.24h for 14 days plus Iodoquinol (as above)

Table 10.4 Clinical characteristics of *Campylobacter*

Incubation period	1–10 days (mean 3–5 days)
Peak ages of infection	<1 year old Young adults
Transmission	Contaminated food and water Vertical transmission Person-to-person (family, day care centers) Via animals (chickens, dogs, pigs, cats)
Duration of symptoms	7 days (mean), can be recurrent or chronic

others are headache, hematochezia, malaise, vomiting and toxic appearance. Fever can be quite high and children may appear toxic. Hematochezia has been found in at least half of infected children and typically appears several days after onset of the illness. Abdominal pain may be so severe as to suggest an acute abdomen. Many patients complain of malaise and fatigue (especially in the recurrent form of the illness) and these may be the only symptoms present between bouts of diarrhea. Vomiting is noted in approximately one-third of patients but is usually mild and does not result in dehydration.

There are several presentations of *Campylobacter* gastroenteritis (Table 10.5), the most common being self-limited diarrhea lasting up to 1 week. Recurrent or chronic diarrhea can occur and *Campylobacter* has been implicated as a cause of traveler's diarrhea. *Campylobacter* may cause an exacerbation of symptoms in patients with previously diagnosed inflammatory bowel disease, resembling a relapse of their primary disease. Involvement of the gut can also result in toxic megacolon. Concomitant infection with *Salmonella*, *Shigella*, *Giardia*, and rotavirus has been documented.

The most common extraintestinal manifestation of *Campylobacter* infection is reactive arthritis, which occurs more frequently in men with the HLA-B27 histocompatibility antigen (Table 10.6).

Diagnosis of *Campylobacter* by stool culture is relatively easy to perform with selective medium. Direct examination of the stool is usually positive for red blood cells and leukocytes. Dark-field or phase-contrast microscopic examination reveals the characteristic darting motion of the *C. jejuni* organism. A technique for staining stool smears with fuchsin has been shown to correlate well with stool cultures.

Treatment is not necessary for children with mild disease. Many patients are asymptomatic when the diagnosis by stool culture is made. Treatment beginning later than 4 days after onset of symptoms will not change the natural course of the disease. Studies evaluating treatment instituted prior to 4 days duration of illness have shown conflicting results. However, with treatment, stool cultures become negative within 72 h; without treatment *Campylobacter* can be cultured from stool for up to several weeks. The incidence of intrafamilial spread of *Campylobacter* is low, but antibiotics may be useful in a group setting such as a daycare center. If treatment is initiated, erythromycin, or another macrolide (azithromycin or clarithromycin), is the drug of choice in children, and ciprofloxacin and tetracycline are alternatives for adults. For systemic infection, gentamicin may be added or substituted. Parenteral therapy is probably not needed for asymptomatic bacteremia, except in immunocompromised patients. Table 10.7 provides a summary of treatment for *Campylobacter* infection.

Table 10.5 Gastrointestinal manifestations of *Campylobacter* infection

Recurrent or chronic diarrhea
Traveler's diarrhea
Colitis or enterocolitis
   Ulcerative
   Nodular (Crohn's-like)
   Pseudomembranous
Massive gastrointestinal bleeding
Acute abdomen
   Cholecystitis
   Pancreatitis
   Appendicitis
   Mesenteric lymphadenitis
Exacerbation of inflammatory bowel disease
Toxic megacolon

Table 10.6 Extraintestinal manifestations of *Campylobacter* infection

Reiter's syndrome
Guillain–Barré syndrome
Septic arthritis
Bacteremia
Glomerulonephritis
Reactive arthritis
Meningitis
Urinary tract infection
Hemolytic uremic syndrome
Carditis

Table 10.7 Treatment of *Campylobacter* infection*

Enteritis
   Erythromycin, azithromycin, or clarithromycin p.o.
Systemic
   Intravenous erythromycin, azithromycin, clarithromycin or gentamicin
Alternatives
   Tetracycline
   Doxycycline or clindamycin
   Ciprofloxacin

*For dosage see Tables 20.11 to 20.16

DIARRHEA AND DEHYDRATION

One of the most common diseases encountered in pediatrics is gastroenteritis, most episodes being mild and self-limited. Young infants are particularly vulnerable to dehydration as a consequence of diarrhea, and this may require hospitalization for rehydration and correction of acid–base or electrolyte disturbances. Acute infectious diarrheal illnesses may be caused by bacteria, viruses, or protozoa. Some of the more common causes of acute infectious diarrhea may be differentiated on clinical grounds (Table 10.8).

Treatment of diarrhea is predominantly supportive with correction of fluid and electrolyte abnormalities. Antibiotic therapy is recommended in some forms of bacterial or protozoan diarrhea (see individual sections). Treatment of dehydration requires recognition of the type of dehydration present, as well as its severity.

ESCHERICHIA COLI

Escherichia coli is the most common coliform bacteria found in the bowel. Several strains are capable of producing enteric disease, and are classified according to their virulence, resulting symptoms and epidemiology. Virulence factors are found in plasmids, and each classification group has a characteristic mechanism by which it interacts with the intestinal mucosa. Antigens expressed by these bacteria are called O, H and K antigens. O and H antigens are used to classify bacteria in the O:H system of which there are 171 O and 56 H currently identified serotypes.

Enterotoxigenic *E. coli* (ETEC) binds to mucosa in the small bowel and produces an enterotoxin which results in secretory diarrhea. It is a frequent cause of traveler's diarrhea and infant diarrhea in developing nations, but is rare in the United States. ETEC is acquired by ingestion of contaminated food or water, and causes nausea, watery diarrhea, abdominal pain, and mild fever. Traveler's diarrhea usually lasts for 4–5 days. Treatment with trimethoprim/sulfamethoxazole or ciprofloxacin for 5 days is usually adequate, but the disease is often mild and self-limited.

Enteropathogenic *E. coli* (EPEC) attaches to the intestinal mucosa and destroys its microvilli, yet it is not invasive and does not produce a toxin. EPEC causes watery diarrhea (chronic and acute), nausea, abdominal pain, vomiting, fever, malaise and polymorphonuclear leukocytes in the stool. It is more severe in infants and has been implicated in outbreaks of diarrhea in nurseries. Treatment with trimethoprim/sulfamethoxazole may be helpful.

Enterohemorrhagic *E. coli* (EHEC) also attaches to the intestinal mucosa, but then produces cytotoxins. These result in the destruction of microvilli in a manner

Table 10.8 Comparison of clinical findings in acute infectious diarrhea

Finding	Shigella	Salmonella	Campylobacter	Rotavirus
Vomiting	Rare	Common	Uncommon	Common
Fever	Present	Variable	Present	Variable
Stool				
Volume	Small	Moderate	Moderate	Large
Consistency	Viscous	Slimy	Watery	Watery
Odor	Odorless	Foul	Foul	Odorless
Blood	Very common	Variable	Common	Uncommon
Mucus	Very common	Moderate	Variable	Absent
White blood cells	Very common	Very common	Present	Uncommon
Bronchitis	Common	Absent	Uncommon	Uncommon

distinctive from EPEC. The most common serotype found is O157:H7, which has been associated with several outbreaks in the United States (through contaminated beef which was improperly cooked). Cattle are the normal reservoir for this organism. Initial symptoms of EHEC are diarrhea, progressing to bloody diarrhea, abdominal pain, fever (low grade), and nausea. Severe cases result in hemorrhagic colitis and serotype O157:H7 is associated with hemolytic uremic syndrome (HUS), thrombotic thrombocytopenic purpura, and intussusception. Children less than 5 years of age are more commonly affected and more likely to develop HUS than older patients. The use of antimotility drugs also predisposes patients to developing HUS. A limited number of prospective studies have been performed on the treatment of EHEC but there are no current antibiotic recommendations. Initial reports of HUS being more commonly seen in patients taking antibiotics have been refuted. A vaccine to prevent *E. coli* O157:H7 is in the early stages of development.

Enteroinvasive *E. coli* (EIEC) causes a dysenteric profile similar to that of *Shigella*. Colonic mucosal cells are invaded by EIEC, with proliferation of the bacteria and resulting cell death. Clinical findings are diarrhea with blood and mucus, abdominal pain, fever (often high) and a toxic appearance. A stool smear may reveal sheets of polymorphonuclear leukocytes and blood. Treatment recommendations are the same as for *Shigella* (see individual section).

Escherichia coli are grouped as enteroadherent (EAEC) according to their ability to adhere to HEp-2 cells in tissue culture. EAEC do not produce toxins nor invade the mucosa; their exact method of pathogenicity is not defined. They have been identified as a cause of chronic diarrhea in children, especially in developing nations. Treatment with neomycin (100 mg/kg per day for 5 days) may be useful.

The diagnosis of enteric *E. coli* infections can be difficult. Clinical information, such as recent travel to an underdeveloped nation or a dysenteric profile with a negative culture for *Shigella*, is useful. Other more easily identifiable enteropathogens should be looked for, and a stool smear for white blood cells performed. EPEC and EHEC do not ferment sorbitol, and this observation is used to help identify these organisms. A sorbitol screen and definitive latex agglutination test for serotype OH:157 are readily available. EIEC does not ferment lactose, a finding that can aid its diagnosis. DNA probes are available for several types of *E. coli*. Serotyping is used primarily for epidemiologic studies (Table 10.9).

FOOD POISONING

Bacterial food poisoning may be caused by a variety of organisms, the most common being *Salmonella* and *Staphylococcus aureus* (Table 10.10). At least 300 outbreaks of food-borne disease are reported each year in the US, with this likely to be only 1–10% of the true figure. The majority of patients experience self-limited disease. Disease may be caused by ingestion of preformed toxin, elaboration of toxin into the gastrointestinal tract, or direct invasion of mucosa by organisms. Ingestion of preformed toxin is associated with a shorter incubation period. Most patients with food poisoning only require supportive therapy (Table 10.11), the major exception being botulism, which represents a medical emergency (see Chapter 1).

GIARDIASIS

Giardia lamblia is second only to *Enterobius vermicularis* (pinworm) as the most common parasite found in the United States, but

Table 10.9 Classification of diarrheagenic *Escherichia coli*

Enterotoxigenic *Escherichia coli* (ETEC)
Enteropathogenic *Escherichia coli* (EPEC)
Enterohemorrhagic *Escherichia coli* (EHEC)
Enteroinvasive *Escherichia coli* (EIEC)
Enteroadherent *Escherichia coli* (EAEC)

Table 10.10 Epidemiologic aspects of food poisoning

Organism	Pathogenesis	Source	Prevention
Salmonella	Infection	Meats, poultry, eggs, dairy products	Proper cooking and food handling, pasteurization
Staphylococcus	Preformed enterotoxin	Meats, poultry, potato salad, cream-filled pastry, cheese, sausage	Careful food handling, rapid refrigeration
Clostridium perfringens	Enterotoxin	Meats, poultry	Avoid delay in serving foods, avoid cooling and rewarming foods
Clostridium botulinum	Preformed neurotoxin	Home-canned foods, uncooked foods	Proper refrigeration
Vibrio parahaemolyticus	Infection enterotoxin	Sea fish, seawater, shellfish	Proper refrigeration
Bacillus cereus			
Vomiting type	Preformed toxin	Cooked or fried rice, vegetables, meats, cereal, puddings	Proper refrigeration of cooked rice and other foods
Diarrheal type	Sporulation enterotoxin	Many prepared foods	Proper refrigeration

Table 10.11 Clinical aspects of food poisoning

Organism	Incubation	Symptoms	Duration	Treatment
Salmonella	8–72 h average 12–18 h	Diarrhea (blood), abdominal pain, fever, chills, nausea, vomiting	3–5 days	None unless severe
Staphylococcus	1–6 h	Severe vomiting, abdominal pain, diarrhea	6–8 h	None
Clostridium perfringens	8–24 h	Watery diarrhea, crampy abdominal pain, nausea, vomiting rare	≤ 24 h	None
Clostridium botulinum	12–36 h	Nausea, vomiting, diarrhea, dysphagia, dysarthria, muscle weakness, respiratory paralysis	Death within several days unless treated	Supportive
Vibrio parahaemolyticus	4–48 h	Severe watery diarrhea, abdominal cramps, nausea, vomiting, fever, chills, can produce dysentery	2 h to 10 days	None
Bacillus cereus				
Vomiting type	1–6 h	Vomiting, abdominal pain	8–24 h	None
Diarrheal type	6–12 h	Diarrhea, abdominal pain, vomiting	20–36 h	None

owing to the benign nature of pinworm infestation, *Giardia* is regarded as the most significant parasitic pathogen. Giardiasis is especially prevalent in day-care centers, institutional care facilities, areas with overcrowding and in the tropics. Children are more often affected than adults, with person-to-person transmission being most common. Infants and toddlers may be an important reservoir for infection as up to 50% are asymptomatic. Transmission may also occur through contaminated water and food. Prevalence rates in children attending day-care centers range from 17 to 90% with an average of 20 to 30%. Clinical symptoms vary with age and include diarrhea (which may be episodic), weight loss/failure to thrive, anorexia, vomiting, abdominal cramps, belching and malodorous stools; on occasion no symptoms are seen, but young children are more likely to be symptomatic.

Diagnosis of giardiasis is most readily achieved by antigen detection in stool using commercially available enzyme immunoassay (EIA) techniques. These assays have a sensitivity of 92% and specificity of 98% for a single stool sample and have largely replaced microscopic identification. Direct examination of three stool samples by a laboratory with expertise in parasitology will establish the diagnosis in 85% of cases. Medications (such as antacids) or concurrent diagnostic testing (such as upper gastrointestinal radiographs with barium) may obscure these organisms. Detection of trophozoites requires examination of fresh stools (within 1 h) or stools preserved in polyvinyl alcohol (PVA). Cysts are quite hardy and will survive at room temperature. However, as infection with more than one parasite is frequently encountered, fixatives to preserve both trophozoites and cysts allow for detection of other parasites. These tests also have the convenience of home collection of samples as the bottles containing fixatives can be mailed to the laboratory (Table 10.12).

Two medications are primarily used for treatment of *Giardia* infection, furazolidone and metronidazole (Table 10.13). The major

Table 10.12   Diagnosis of giardiasis

Antigen in stool – enzyme immunoassay (EIA)
Stool examination (fresh or with fixatives)
Duodenal fluid examination
  Entero-test capsule*
  Intubation of small bowel
Biopsy of duodenum or jejunum
Serology – antibodies to *Giardia*

*Health Development Corporation, Palo Alto, CA

Table 10.13   Treatment of giardiasis

Drug	Dosage
Furazolidone	6–8 mg/kg per day p.o. div. q.6h for 7–10 days (maximum 400 mg/day)
Metronidazole	15 mg/kg per day p.o. div. q.8h for 5 days (maximum 750 mg/day)
Albendazole	7–10 mg/kg/day div. q.d. for 5 days
Quinacrine	6 mg/kg per day p.o. div. q.8h for 7 days (maximum 300 mg/day)
Tinidazole	50 mg/kg p.o. single dose (maximum 2 g) not available in US
Ornidazole	40 mg/kg p.o. single dose (maximum 1.5 g) not available in US

advantage of furazolidone is that it is in liquid form. Other agents have also been shown to be effective in older children and adults but data are limited for younger patients. Many of these medications produce an antabuse-like effect, so those containing alcohol should not be given concomitantly. Quinacrine and metronidazole must be compounded into solution, and have a bitter taste. Persistent symptoms after therapy may indicate small bowel bacterial overgrowth or incomplete eradication of the pathogen, requiring a second course of medication.

HELICOBACTER

Gastric infection with *Helicobacter pylori* has been associated with gastritis, duodenal ulcer disease and gastric ulcers. The organism is a multiflagellate, unipolar, spiral bacterium. It can assume a dormant coccoid form in unfavorable environments, making it more resistant to eradication. *Helicobacter pylori* is more often found in developing countries. However, some areas of the United States have similar prevalence rates. In the United States, prevalence in healthy adults is 20–45% and 4–31% in children. Many factors influence these rates including age, race, ethnicity and occupation (Table 10.14).

Transmission is thought to be via the fecal–oral route (person-to-person and possibly by contaminated food or water). Humans are the only natural host and there is no known animal reservoir. Gastric and duodenal inflammation results from infection by the organism, but the exact mechanism is undetermined. *Helicobacter pylori* produces several enzymes which may allow penetration into the gastric mucosa. It also produces urease which converts urea (present in the gastric epithelium) to ammonia and bicarbonate. This raises the pH around the organism and allows back diffusion of H$^+$ ions into the mucosa resulting in epithelial damage. *Helicobacter pylori* is found almost exclusively in gastric mucosa, including areas of gastric metaplasia in the duodenum or esophagus.

The extent to which *H. pylori* causes disease (Table 10.15) is still under investigation. Colonization does not uniformly result in development of peptic disease; however, infected adults and children have a much higher incidence of duodenal ulcers and gastritis. It also appears that colonization may more frequently result in upper gastrointestinal pathology in children than in adults.

Approximately 90–100% of adults with duodenal ulcers and 60–90% with gastric ulcers are found to have *H. pylori*. Children with peptic disease are less likely than adults to have *H. pylori* isolated. In reported studies about 50% of children with gastritis and 60% with duodenitis were found to be colonized by *H. pylori*. Symptoms of peptic disease associated with *H. pylori* do not differ from that without the organism.

Table 10.14 Epidemiologic factors associated with *Helicobacter pylori*

Increasing age
Lower family income
Family member in home with *Helicobacter pylori*
Patients in institutions for the mentally retarded
Contaminated water supplies
Meat handlers
Doctors and nurses involved in endoscopy
Black races
Hispanic ethnic groups

Table 10.15 Clinical disease associated with *Helicobacter* infection

Gastritis and gastric erosions (primarily of antrum and fundus)
Atrophic gastritis
Antral nodularity in children
Nonulcerative dyspepsia
Duodenal ulcers and duodenitis
Gastric cancer

Diagnosis can be made by several methods, including serologic testing (Table 10.16). In an untreated patient, high titers of antibody to *H. pylori* are likely to represent current infection. Titers usually decline after treatment but may be slow to fall and difficult to interpret. A positive ^{14}C urea breath test is present only with infection; however, these tests are not readily available and the ^{14}C test causes low radiation exposure. Other methods are invasive and require endoscopy. However, many patients with gastrointestinal symptoms and suspected infection will undergo endoscopy during evaluation of their symptoms. Histologic stains of the gastric mucosa, usually the antrum, or biopsy culture are sensitive and specific. The rapid ^{14}C urea breath test is less expensive and has excellent ability to detect the organism.

Treatment protocols are still a matter of discussion and research. Most often, patients are treated with a combination of bismuth and two antibiotics in addition to an H_2 antagonist (Table 10.17). Omeprazole plus amoxicillin and clarithromycin for 10–14 days is the preferred regimen in adults. Many new treatment protocols are under investigation.

HEPATITIS

The clinical presentation of jaundice, following a prodrome of anorexia, nausea, vomiting and right upper quadrant pain, suggests a diagnosis of acute hepatitis and dictates a serologic evaluation for etiology (Table 10.18). Hepatitis is often asymptomatic in children, particularly hepatitis C in all ages and hepatitis A in infants under 18 months of age.

Hepatitis A virus (HAV) is the most common cause of hepatitis in children in the United States. Transmission through the fecal–oral route often occurs in day-care centers, schools, institutional settings and among household members. The incubation period is 30 days and the virus is excreted for one week before clinical symptoms occur. Patients often remain anicteric but other symptoms last approximately two weeks. The presence of anti-HAV IgM confirms the diagnosis. Treatment is supportive, although acute fulminant hepatitis can occur. Patients with hepatitis A may be contagious for as long as 1 week after the onset of jaundice. Chronic liver disease does not occur. A hepatitis A vaccine is now available and in some states is required routinely (Chapter 3).

Hepatitis B virus (HBV) infection is less common in the United States, but endemic in many parts of the world, particularly Southeast Asia. About 300 000 new cases of hepatitis B occur each year in the United States. Transmission occurs by percutaneous exposure to contaminated blood, through sexual transmission, and vertically from mother to child. The incubation period is 60–180 days. Serologic testing detects various parts of the virus which include:

Table 10.16   Diagnosis of *Helicobacter* infection

Serology by ELISA (IgG and IgA)
^{13}C or ^{14}C urea breath tests
Histology of gastric biopsy with Giemsa stain or
   Warthin-Starry silver stain
Culture of gastric biopsy
Rapid urease test

Table 10.17   Treatment of *Helicobacter* infection

H_2 antagonist for 6–8 weeks
plus
Amoxicillin 40 mg/kg per day p.o. div. q.8h (maximum 1.5 g/day) or tetracycline 40 mg/kg per day p.o. div. q.6h for 3 weeks (maximum 2g/day)
plus
Metrondiazole 20 mg/kg per day p.o. div. q.8h for 3 weeks (maximum 1.5 g/day)
plus
Bismuth subsalicylate 2 tablets p.o. q.6h for 3 weeks (1 tablet or liquid for smaller children)

Table 10.18   Differential etiology of hepatitis

Hepatitis, A, B, C, D, E
Epstein–Barr virus
Cytomegalovirus
Leptospirosis
Noninfectious
   Drug induced (INH, erythromycin)
   Obstructive jaundice

HBsAg (surface antigen, the outer shell, indicates infectivity), HBcAg (inner core antigen), HBeAg (a nonstructural core antigen which indicates replication), and DNA polymerase (a DNA repair enzyme that indicates replication). Antibodies to HBc and HBs are found at a later stage of infection, and the patient has eliminated the virus when antibodies to Hbs appear. Infection with HBV can also be confirmed by polymerase chain reaction (PCR) detection of hepatitis B DNA. Individuals with hepatitis B are infective while they are seropositive for HBsAg or have antibodies to HBc but lack antibody to HBs. Chronic hepatitis B occurs in <5% of adult infections, but is found in 50% of children with infection acquired during the first year of life, and in 80–90% of perinatal infections. Chronic liver disease consists of chronic antigenemia, chronic persistent hepatitis, chronic active hepatitis, cirrhosis and hepatocellular carcinoma. Interferon alfa-2b may be used to treat chronic active hepatitis. Recommendations for HBV immunization in high-risk groups and for childhood immunization are reviewed in Chapter 3.

Hepatitis C virus (HCV) infection is becoming an increasing concern in the United States and is responsible for the majority of cases of post-transfusion hepatitis. Whether sexual or perinatal transmission occurs is still under investigation, although many clinicians feel that both methods of transmission occur. The incubation period is 6 to 12 weeks. A pattern of fluctuating liver transaminases is common. Diagnosis can be difficult, as ELISA only confirms the presence of antibody to the virus, not the stage of disease as with HBV infection. An ELISA is usually performed first, with confirmation by recombinant immunoblot assay (RIBA) or PCR as there are many false-positives. Knowledge of the clinical course of HCV is growing slowly, but it appears that chronic infection is very common and progression to cirrhosis or hepatocellular carcinoma may be high. Treatment with a combination of interferon alfa-2b and oral ribavirin is available for chronic active hepatitis but results are variable. Because this therapy is largely investigational in children, patients should be managed by experienced pediatric gastroenterologists.

Hepatitis D virus (delta, HDV) is a defective virus that only coinfects with HBV. It is endemic in the Middle east and Mediterranean areas and seen epidemically in other parts of the world. HDV infection is more commonly associated with fulminant or chronic hepatitis B. Serologic markers include anti-HDV IgM and IgG, HDAg, and HDV RNA.

Hepatitis E virus (HEV) is transmitted by the fecal–oral route via contaminated water or food. It is more common in North Africa, Asia, India and Russia. The incubation period is approximately 6 weeks and clinical symptoms are usually mild. More severe forms of acute hepatitis particularly in pregnant women can occur. Detection is by identification of HEAg.

The serologic markers available to detect many forms of hepatitis are given in Table 10.19. Etiologic diagnosis is made by serologic evaluation and should be accomplished rapidly so that decisions for prophylactic administration of hepatitis A or B vaccine or hyperimmune human immunoglobulin (for HBV) to family members can be made (see Chapter 3). If a delay in laboratory testing is anticipated, family members should receive hepatitis A vaccine because this is inexpensive and must be given early to protect against HAV.

Therapy for patients with acute hepatitis is supportive and can be managed at home. Indications for hospital admission include intractable vomiting, an elevated prothrombin time and altered neurologic status. While contagious, patients should be advised as to stool and/or blood precautions and sexual transmission of disease.

PSEUDOMEMBRANOUS COLITIS (PMC)

Pseudomembranous colitis (PMC) is an inflammatory condition of the colon associated with

Table 10.19 Serologic diagnosis of acute hepatitis

Hepatitis A virus	Anti-HAV IgM
Hepatitis B virus	HBsAg, anti-HBcIgM
Hepatitis C virus	Anti-HCV (ELISA)
Epstein–Barr virus	Heterophil test; anti-VCA*, anti-EA† anti-EBNA‡ for younger children
Cytomegalovirus (CMV)	Anti-CMV IgM

*VCA, viral capsis antigen; †EA, early antigen; ‡EBNA, Epstein–Barr nuclear antigen

antibiotic use. The etiology has been determined to be *Clostridium difficile* toxin.

Virtually all antibiotics have been associated with PMC. In children, more cases have been reported following administration of ampicillin or amoxicillin, but this probably reflects the widespread use of these antibiotics and their broad-spectrum coverage. The route (parenteral, enteral and topical antibiotic use), dose and length of treatment for the antibiotic are not related to the development of PMC. The diarrhea associated with PMC is usually of rapid onset and patients may experience 10–20 stools per day, although children tend to have less severe diarrhea. At least half of patients have blood and/or fecal leukocytes in the stool. Abdominal pain and tenderness can occur and may mimic an acute abdomen. Fever, anorexia, nausea and vomiting are also part of the symptom complex (Table 10.20).

The onset of disease is usually within 4 to 10 days of initiation of antibiotics. Onset has occurred within 4 h of starting an antibiotic, and as late as 10 weeks after stopping the antibiotic. At least one-third of these patients have onset of disease after the antibiotic has been stopped. The exact incidence of PMC is unknown, but it appears to be less common in children than in adults.

Diagnosis is usually established by testing the stool for the presence of *C. difficile* toxin or by endoscopic examination of the colon. The distribution of PMC is predominately in the descending and sigmoid colon and rectum, and is easily viewed by colonoscopy or flexible sigmoidoscopy. Pseudomembranous colitis has a characteristic profile of raised, well-circumscribed lesions. Toxin is present in 97–100% of patients with endoscopic evidence for PMC. *Clostridium difficile* produces two toxins: toxin A, an enterotoxin that causes colitis and toxin B, which is less enterotoxic. Newer ELISA techniques detect both toxin A and B, but their sensitivity is relatively low. Demonstration of *C. difficile* toxin in the stool is important in confirming a diagnosis, but does not allow detection of all cases of PMC. Stool cultures are of little

diagnostic use because asymptomatic colonization with this organism is common, particularly in neonates and infants.

General supportive care with fluids is an important aspect of treatment (Table 10.21). Antiperistaltic medications should not be used as they may prolong colonization with *C. difficile*. If the patient is hospitalized, simple isolation or enteric precautions should be observed. If possible, the offending antibiotic should be discontinued and in one-third to one-half of cases this is the only intervention necessary. Metronidazole and vancomycin

Table 10.20 Clinical and laboratory findings in pseudomembranous colitis

Symptoms
  Watery stools
  Hematochezia
  Fever
  Tenesmus
  Nausea and vomiting
  Anorexia
  Abdominal pain and tenderness
  Dehydration
  Toxic megacolon
  Perforation of the bowel
Laboratory findings
  Guaiac-positive stools
  Fecal leukocytes
  Elevated white blood cells with elevation of
    polymorphonuclear leukocytes

Table 10.21 Treatment of pseudomembranous colitis

Fluids, supportive care
Avoidance of antiperistaltic medications
Discontinue offending antibiotic
Simple isolation
Metronidazole 15–25 mg/kg/day (maximum 2 g) p.o. div. q.6h for 7–14 days
Vancomycin 50 mg/kg/day (maximum 2 g) p.o. div. q.8h for 7–14 days should only be considered for patients who have not improved with metronidazole
or
Lactobacillus
Cholestyramine

are effective in the elimination of *C. difficile* for patients who do not respond to simple discontinuation of the offending antibiotic. However, drugs used in the therapy of PMC are efficacious even when used concurrently with the offending antibiotic. Drugs may be given intravenously in the presence of an ileus or in patients who are critically ill. Oral vancomycin is minimally absorbed and very effective for treatment of PMC but is expensive, and induces antibiotic resistance, particularly among enterococci. For mild to moderate forms of PMC metronidazole is usually adequate. Cholestyramine has also been used to bind the toxin in mild cases of the disease.

The relapse rate is 12 to 20% and usually begins 4 to 20 days after the initial treatment. Clinically, the patients experience the same signs and symptoms as during their initial bout of PMC. *Clostridium difficile* and its toxin can again be isolated, even though during the period between initial treatment and relapse they may not have been detectable. Patients who have diverticulitis or who are granulocytopenic are more likely to relapse. The ability of the organism to undergo sporulation is probably the most important factor in relapse as the spore form is less sensitive to antibiotics and therefore may not be eradicated with treatment. Reinfection from the environment is also a possibility as *C. difficile* can readily be cultured in the room of patients hospitalized for PMC. It can also be found in their home environment and on the hands of hospital personnel. *Clostridium difficile* inoculated into a carpet can be recovered for up to 5 months and is resistant to many routine methods of cleaning.

Treatment for relapse involves a second course of antibiotics at the original dosage but continued for a longer duration, generally 2 to 3 weeks. Use of foods or preparations containing *Lactobacillus* can help suppress the growth of *C. difficile*. Also, vancomycin can be used at one-half of the original dose, or on an alternate day schedule. This allows regrowth of normal bowel flora while suppressing the growth of *C. difficile*, which is extremely sensitive to vancomycin. In Europe, *Saccharomyces boulardii*, a nonpathogenic yeast which may be taken in capsule form, has been used to help prevent the growth of *C. difficile*.

ROTAVIRUS

Rotavirus is most common in infants, accounting for up to one-half of all cases of viral gastroenteritis. Rotavirus strains are divided into 7 antigentic groups A-G, with group A being responsible for the majority of human infections. There are also subgroups and serotypes within this grouping system. Rotavirus is an RNA virus with two outer layers which contain antigens detectable by immunologic techniques. These glycoprotein antigens allow classification of the rotavirus into subgroup types. Polyacrylamide gel electrophoresis patterns can also separate rotavirus strains and are used in epidemiological studies. Rotavirus is spread by the fecal–oral route. Children can have asymptomatic shedding of the virus which enhances its spread. A respiratory route of infection has also been postulated.

Rotavirus may be a clinically significant infection in young infants, while older children are less severely affected. As infants are more likely to have both vomiting and diarrhea, dehydration is common. Patients may also become intolerant of their formula secondary to disaccharidase deficiency or protein intolerance. Up to 13% of hospitalized patients with rotavirus infection have another infectious agent identified (e.g. *Salmonella* or *Shigella*). Tables 10.22 and 10.23 show clinical aspects of rotavirus infection.

Table 10.22 Clinical aspects of rotavirus gastro-enteritis

Incubation	48–72 h
Seasonality	Winter
Peak age of illness	6–24 months
Transmission	fecal–oral, possibly respiratory
Duration of illness	5–8 days
Diagnostic tests	ELISA, latex agglutination

Diagnosis of a rotavirus infection is usually made by detection of the virus (antigen) in the stool. Several commercial kits, using ELISA or latex agglutination methodologies, are available and are the most clinically applicable. Other techniques include electron microscopy, immunoelectron microscopy, and antibody titers performed by several methods. Treatment is symptomatic and usually based upon correction or maintenance of body fluid balance. A live, oral, tetravalent vaccine is now available and is recommended for routine administration to infants (Chapter 3).

SALMONELLOSIS

Salmonella sp. are pathogens which commonly cause bacterial gastroenteritis in children. Although there are over 2000 serotypes, 10 of these account for approximately two-thirds of total isolates. Clinically, *Salmonella* sp. are divided into those strains that cause enteric fever, such as *S. typhi*, *S. paratyphi A*, *S. paratyphi B*, and *S. cholerae-suis*, and those more commonly associated with other forms of disease, such as gastroenteritis, bacteremia (possibly occult), localized infection and the possibility of a person being a chronic carrier. Gastroenteritis is the most common form and accounts for most *Salmonella* infections in the United States. In other countries, enteric fever (typhoid) is more common as *S. typhi* is the predominant species. Bacteremia tends to occur in the young and the old, with approximately 40% of cases arising in children under 5 years of age. Neonates account for the highest proportion of this group, despite breast feeding providing protection against salmonellosis. Localized infections (Table 10.24) are frequently due to *S. cholerae-suis*.

A chronic carrier state can also be established. This predominantly occurs following enteric fever in adults with gallbladder disease. One study demonstrated that a chronic carrier state (defined as excretion for over 1 year) was seen in 2.6% of patients who were infected with nontyphi *Salmonella*. Most chronic carriers were under 5 years of age.

Table 10.23 Clinical signs and symptoms of rotavirus infection

Signs and symptoms
Vomiting
Diarrhea
Fever
Dehydration (usually isotonic)
Pharyngeal redness
Rhinitis
Otitis media
Irritability
Complications
Intussusception (also associated with vaccine)
Necrotizing enterocolitis (also assocaited with vaccine)
Sudden infant death syndrome

Table 10.24 Focal infections of salmonellosis

Meningitis	Abdominal abscess
Brain abscess and empyema	Cholecystitis
	Salpingitis
Prosthetic valve endocarditis	Urinary tract infection
Endocarditis	Arthritis
Pericarditis	Osteomyelitis
Mycotic aneurysm	Reiter's syndrome
Myocardial abscess	Pharyngeal abscess
Septic thrombophlebitis	Pneumonia and empyema
Necrotizing enterocolitis	
Appendicitis	Endophthalmitis

Salmonella may be introduced into food by a food handler or processor. It is resistant to mild refrigeration, thus undercooked food is a potential source of contamination and transmission of the disease.

Symptoms can begin quite abruptly (Tables 10.25 and 10.26). The distal small bowel and colon are the predominant sites of involvement. Salmonellae invade the lamina propria, induce an inflammatory reaction and release of prostaglandins; this stimulates cyclic AMP, which in itself causes secretory diarrhea. An endotoxin of *Salmonella* can be isolated but may not be associated with the pathogenesis of the disease. The damage to cells is not as extensive as with *Shigella*, thus the resulting colitis and enteritis are not as destructive. The organism is limited to the superficial layers of the gut mucosa; therefore, normal mechanisms of elimination allow clearance of *Salmonella* in a rapid manner.

Salmonella gastroenteritis is, in general, a self-limited disease. However, there are several conditions that may influence its ability to cause sepsis or other complications (Table 10.27).

Neonates and infants under 3 months of age are more prone to sepsis and meningitis than other age groups. Patients with sickle cell anemia have a higher incidence of osteomyelitis due to *Salmonella*. The ability of *Salmonella* to cause extraintestinal and focal infections is partly dependent upon the state of the host, the species of *Salmonella* involved, and the inoculum dose. Studies of febrile children in emergency departments have documented *Salmonella* in as many as 10% of blood cultures. Although gastroenteritis and localized infections are by far the most common forms of salmonellosis, enteric fever still occurs in the United States (Table 10.28). The term 'typhoid fever' has been mostly abandoned since organisms other than *S. typhi* can cause identical symptoms.

Salmonella typhi is very unusual in that there is no natural host in nature other than humans. The main route of transmission is via food or water contaminated by human fecal material. There are some instances of possible transmission by insect vectors; however, this has not been firmly established.

There are four phases of salmonellosis. The first is a flu-like illness, during which the patient may also have symptoms of gastroenteritis. The second phase reflects multisystem invasion by the organism. Patients show encephalopathic changes, bronchitis and evidence of reticuloendothelial system involvement with hepatosplenomegaly and lymphadenopathy. Relative bradycardia usually occurs during this period, which begins approximately 2 to 3 weeks after ingestion of the organism. High fever may be seen and without treatment can persist for 2

Table 10.25 Characteristics of salmonella gastroenteritis

Incubation	8–72 h
Seasonality	Warm weather
Transmission	Via food, animals, marijuana, fomites, flies insects, person-to-person
Sites of involvement	Distal small bowel, colon
Duration of symptoms	2–7 days

Table 10.26 Symptoms and laboratory findings in *Salmonella* gastroenteritis

Symptoms
  Diarrhea
  Fever > 38.9°C (102°F)
  Abdominal pain
  Abdominal distension
  Vomiting
  Constitutional symptoms
  Tenesmus
  Hematochezia
Laboratory findings
  Elevated white blood cell count
  Guaiac-positive stools
  Polymorphonuclear leukocytes in stool smears (85%)
  Positive stool culture

Table 10.27 Factors associated with severe salmonellosis

Age below 12 months
Decreased gastric acidity
Stress (cold, malnutrition)
Antibiotics
Depressed immune function
Hemolysis

to 3 weeks. Owing to gastrointestinal involvement, perforation or hemorrhage is a risk. If the disease does not abate a third phase is entered, during which metastatic phenomena such as myocarditis occur. The fourth phase is the carrier state, which occurs in approximately 3% of patients. The presence of gallbladder disease markedly enhances the chances of becoming a chronic carrier. Chronic carriage is more common in adult women, but this may be related to the fact that gallbladder disease is more common in this group.

Diagnosis of enteric fever is made on clinical grounds, serologic measurement (salmonella O and H antibodies) and cultures. During the initial phases of enteric fever, stool cultures may be positive; however, there is an increasing yield from the stool culture between 3 and 4 weeks of disease. Initially, blood cultures are positive in 80–90% of patients. Other sites that can be cultured are bone marrow and rose spot biopsies. Antibody titers for febrile agglutinins become positive after the first week of illness.

Salmonella gastroenteritis is not usually treated as antibiotics are ineffective in improving the course and may prolong excretion of the organism. However, there are specific instances when treatment is indicated (Table 10.29). These include patients who are highly prone to invasive disease or already have established severe disease.

Ampicillin, amoxicillin, chloramphenicol and trimethoprim/sulfamethoxazole are all effective for susceptible organisms (Table 10.30). Amoxicillin or trimethoprim/sulfamethoxazole are the drugs of choice but selection is dependent upon local sensitivities. Third generation cephalosporins and ciprofloxacin, for patients over 18 years of age, are also effective against most strains of *Salmonella*. Patients with AIDS or altered immunity are best treated with ampicillin or a third generation cephalosporin. Eradication of the chronic carrier state is often unsuccessful even after 4–6 weeks of therapy. Detection of *Salmonella* in stool cultures following therapy does not necessitate a second course of treatment unless the patient remains symptomatic. The local public health department should be notified of all cases of *Salmonella* infection.

Table 10.28 Enteric fever in salmonellosis

Organism	*Salmonella typhi* and paratyphoid strains
Transmission	Via human reservoirs, contaminated food or water, insect vectors
Seasonality	All
Incubation	3–56 days (mean 10 days)
Symptoms	Fever, headache, chills, diarrhea, vomiting, abdominal pain, cough
Signs	Rose spots, hepatosplenomegaly, neurologic signs, relative bradycardia

Table 10.29 Indications for treatment of *Salmonella* gastroenteritis

Infants under 3 months of age
Toxic or severe disease
Bacteremia
Immunodeficiency (acquired, primary, or secondary)
Malignancy
Patients on immunosuppressive medications

SHIGELLOSIS

Shigella is a nonmotile Gram-negative rod. It has 32 serotypes divided into four groups: group A, *Shigella dysenteriae*; group B, *S. flexneri*; group C, *S. boydii*; and group D, *S. sonnei*. In the United States and many developed nations *S. sonnei* is responsible for the majority of gastrointestinal infections. Virulence is related to genetically determined properties that allow the organism to invade gastrointestinal cells, multiply within a cell, escape from host defenses and spread from cell to cell. Plasmids code for proteins on the organism's outer membrane, permitting these activities by the bacteria.

Toxins also contribute to pathogenicity. The toxin of *S. dysenteriae* (the most intensely studied) is an exotoxin and produces transudation of fluid in ileal loops of experimental animals. It is also a cytotoxin, inducing cell death by suppression of cell protein synthesis. Damage to intestinal villus cells inhibits

Table 10.30 Treatment of salmonellosis

Gastroenteritis (if indicated)	Ampicillin 100 mg/kg per day p.o. or i.v. div. q.i.d. (maximum 6 g) for 5–7 days
	Amoxicillin 40 mg/kg per day p.o. div. t.i.d. for 5–7 days
	Trimethoprim/sulfamethoxazole 10 mg/kg per day TMP/50 mg/kg per day SMX p.o. div. b.i.d. (maximum 320 mg TMP/1600 mg SMX) for 5–7 days
Enteric fever or bacteremia	Ceftriaxone 50–75 mg/kg per day (maximum 2 g) for 14 days
	Trimethoprim/sulfamethoxazole 20 mg/kg per day TMP/100 mg/kg per day SMX p.o. or i.v. div. b.i.d. (maximum 320 TMP/1600 mg SMX) for 14 days
	Chloramphenicol 80–100 mg/kg per day p.o. or i.v. div. q.i.d. (maximum 4 g) for 14 days
	Cefotaxime 200 mg/kg per day i.v. div. b.i.d. (maximum 12 g) for 14 days
Localized or focal infection	As directed by infectious process and location

sodium and water absorption and leads to accumulation of fluid in the intestinal lumen.

Transmission of *Shigella* occurs via the fecal–oral route. Humans are the major reservoir for these bacteria and, unlike other enteric pathogens, only a very small number of organisms (200) are needed to produce disease. Contaminated food and water are the primary sources associated with epidemics of shigellosis; however, houseflies may also transmit disease. *Shigella* can be cultured from toilet seats for up to 17 days post-inoculation. There may also be asymptomatic carriers that contribute to the spread of the disease.

The incubation period of *Shigella* is 1 to 3 days and the duration of illness, if uncomplicated, is 3 to 7 days. There is an increased incidence during winter months in the United States, but in other countries more cases are reported during hot, dry weather. The majority of patients are under 10 years of age with a peak incidence at 2 years (Table 10.31).

In children, the diarrhea is watery and voluminous with blood usually noted 24–48 h after initial symptoms (Table 10.32). Stool volume may then decrease with a frequent stooling pattern. Respiratory symptoms and fever are prominent features. Endoscopic examination of the colon reveals intense inflammation with crypt abscesses most prominent in the rectum and decreasing

Table 10.31 *Shigella* gastroenteritis

Criterion	Characteristic
Incubation	1–3 days
Seasonality	Varies depending upon worldwide location
Age of illness	Before 10 years of age (peak at 2 years)
Transmission	Person-to-person, food, water, housefly
Site of involvement	Colon (primarily distal segment)
Duration of illness	3–7 days

Table 10.32 Clinical signs and symptoms of *Shigella* infection

Symptoms
  Watery stools (10–25 times per day)
  Blood and mucus in stools
  Abdominal cramps and tenesmus
  Fever
  Malaise
  Anorexia
Laboratory findings
  White blood cells in stool smear
  Guaiac-positive stools
  Leukocytosis with increased absolute band count
  Positive stool culture
  Protein loss in stools

proximally. In severe dysentery, a pseudo-membrane can be seen.

There are several culture media able to support the growth of *Shigella*; stool specimens should be plated as soon as possible to achieve optimum results. The stool smear typically shows a large number of white blood cells, with predominant polymorphonuclear leukocytes and bands. Leukocytosis is also seen with the band count greater than the neutrophil count in 32–85% of patients. A high absolute band count may also be seen with *Campylobacter* and *Salmonella* infection.

There are many complications of shigellosis (Table 10.33); however, the majority of complications are associated with *S. dysenteriae*. Dehydration can be seen with shigellosis due to any of the *Shigella* species. Protein loss in stools can contribute to the development of clinically significant malnutrition in the child with a marginal premorbid nutritional state. Hemolytic uremic syndrome with progression to renal failure can develop, usually after 1 week of clinical disease, when the patient may have shown improvement.

The incidence of bacteremia is quite low but clinical sepsis with shigellosis ranges from 0.6 to 7%. The majority of children affected are under 5 years of age and there is 35–50% mortality with bacteremia. Children with bacteremia more frequently present with dehydration, and are afebrile and malnourished. Blood cultures are most often positive during the first two days of disease. Another complication is seizures, which are associated with all species of *Shigella*. Seizure incidence varies from 10 to 45% in children up to 7 years of age. The mechanism for the seizure is most probably fever-related, and not due to a neurotoxin as previously thought.

There is at present a high incidence of ampicillin resistance among isolates of *Shigella*. Drug selection, therefore, depends on local sensitivities to ampicillin and trimethoprim/sulfamethoxazole (Table 10.34); however, some isolates have become resistant to both of these medications. Nalidixic acid is often used in developing nations, and third generation cephalosporins are frequently effective

Table 10.33 Complications of shigellosis

Dehydration	Hemolytic uremic syndrome
Hyponatremia	Urinary tract infection
Bacteremia-sepsis	Pneumonia
Toxic megacolon	Eye involvement
Intestinal perforation	Seizures
Rectal prolapse	Reiter's syndrome

for treatment of multiply-resistant strains. Additionally, quinolones are excellent options for adults, but their potential toxicity to epiphysial cartilage in children must be considered.

Fever should defervesce within 12–20 h with therapy and improvement of diarrhea should be seen in 1 to 3 days. *Shigella* is eliminated within the first two days of therapy but, if therapy is not instituted, it can be cultured from stools for up to 1 month. This finding may influence the decision to treat children with mild enteritis. Anti-diarrheal drugs should be discouraged as they prolong fever, diarrhea and excretion of the organism. Mortality in uncomplicated gastroenteritis is less than 1% and chronic carriage of *Shigella* in stools is very unusual unless the patient was initially malnourished.

VIRAL GASTROENTERITIS

Viral gastroenteritis is one of the most common illnesses in childhood, with numerous etiologic agents identified in sporadic and epidemic cases (Table 10.35). Rotavirus (see individual section) and enteric adenovirus are most identified as the cause of infection.

Enteric adenovirus gastroenteritis usually occurs in children under 2 years of age and at any time of the year. The incubation period is up to 7 days and transmission is through the fecal–oral route. Respiratory symptoms and vomiting are common, and diarrhea can last up to 2 weeks. Viral detection kits using techniques similar to rotavirus detection are available. Treatment is symptomatic and supportive. Norwalk viruses usually affect school-age children and adults throughout the year. Incubation is 18–48 h and symptoms usually last only 1–2 days. Vomiting is the most common symptom in children, often with concomitant diarrhea, nausea and abdominal pain. Treatment is supportive.

YERSINIA

Yersinia enterocolitica is a small Gram-negative facultative anaerobic coccobacillus responsible for large numbers of gastroenteritis cases in Europe and Canada, but less commonly in the United States. There are numerous serotypes with types 0:3 and 0:9 being most common in human infections in Europe. Serotype 0:3 is most common in Canada and 0:8 in the United States, although many cases of serotype 0:3 have now been reported in the United States. The pathogenicity of this organism is genetically determined by the presence of plasmid-encoded proteins on its outer membrane. These proteins permit resistance of *Yersinia* to several host defense

mechanisms including opsonization and neutrophil phagocytosis. Iron is a growth requirement for several bacteria and it appears to play an important role in the development of infections with *Yersinia*. Treatment of experimental animals with iron, or deferoxamine (which allows iron to be more readily utilized by the bacteria), significantly increases the virulence of *Y. enterocolitica*.

The mode of transmission in sporadic cases is unclear. In epidemic cases, person-to-person transmission (within families or hospital personnel) and food-borne transmission have been identified (Table 10.36).

Clinically, there are several forms of the disease which include enterocolitis, pseudo-appendicitis, autoimmune-like disease, sepsis and metastatic disease. Younger children have a milder form of disease with diarrhea being the predominant symptom (Table 10.37); however, several cases of sepsis and metastatic disease have been reported in infants.

Table 10.34   Treatment of shigellosis

Strain	Treatment
Susceptible strains	Trimethoprim/sulfamethoxazole 10 mg/kg per day TMP/50 mg/kg per day SMX p.o. or i.v. div. b.i.d. (maximum 320 mg TMP/1600 mg SMX)
	Ampicillin (not amoxicillin) 80–100 mg/kg per day p.o. or i.v. div. q.i.d. (maximum 2 g)
Resistant strains	Ceftriaxone 50–75 mg/kg/day div. q.i.d.
	Nalidixic acid 55 mg/kg per day p.o. div. q.i.d.
	Ciprofloxacin 1 g (total daily dose) p.o. div. b.i.d. (for patients >17 years of age)
	Norfloxacin 800 mg/kg per day (total daily dose) p.o. div. b.i.d. (for patients >17 years of age)

Table 10.35   Viral etiology of gastroenteritis

Rotavirus
Enteric adenovirus
Norwalk virus
Coronavirus
Astrovirus
Calicivirus

Table 10.36   Characteristics of *Yersinia* infection

Incubation	1–11 days
Seasonality	Cool weather
Peak age of illness	Any
Transmission	Food, milk, oysters, raw chitterlings, water, wild and domestic animals, person-to-person, blood transfusion
Duration of illness	5–14 days (longer for systemic disease)

A profile of pseudoappendicitis is usually seen in older children and young adults and is due to acute mesenteric adenitis. Older adolescents and young adults may also have symptoms of an acute enteritis resembling Crohn's disease with localization of disease to the terminal ileum. Several groups of patients are at higher risk of developing systemic infection with *Y. enterocolitica* (Table 10.38). A group somewhat uniquely affected by this organism are patients with iron overload, such as in thalassemia or hemochromatosis.

Yersinia is readily isolated from uncontaminated sources such as joint fluid or blood. It is difficult to isolate on routine stool cultures because it appears as a very small colony which is easily overgrown. Selective media have been developed to facilitate identification of the organism. Serologic techniques for diagnosis are available, including radioimmunoassay and ELISA, but have their limitations.

Acute gastroenteritis is usually a self-limited disease that does not require therapy except in immunosuppressed patients. Patients with chronic gastrointestinal symptoms have responded to antibiotics, but controlled studies have not been performed. Metastatic infections, such as osteomyelitis or hepatic abscesses, should be treated with antibiotics and the duration of treatment dictated by the site of involvement. Antibiotic therapy has not been proven beneficial in mesenteric adenitis; however, septicemia is an absolute indication for therapy.

Yersinia is generally sensitive to trimethoprim/sulfamethoxazole and tetracycline, and most strains are resistant to the penicillin group and first generation cephalosporins owing to the production of β-lactamase by *Yersinia*. Other useful drugs include amino-

Table 10.37 Clinical signs and symptoms of *Yersinia* infection

Diarrhea
Blood in stools
Vomiting
Abdominal pain
Fever
Signs and symptoms of appendicitis
Increased absolute band count on complete blood count (infants under 6 months of age)
Guaiac-positive stools
White blood cells on stool smear

Table 10.38 Risk factors for development of systemic disease in *Yersinia* infection

Infants under 3 months of age
Disease associated with iron overload
Hemoglobinopathies
Hemosiderosis
Hemochromatosis
Accidental iron overdose
Immunodeficiency
Malignancy

glycosides, chloramphenicol, quinolones and third generation cephalosporins. Focal or gastrointestinal infections in susceptible hosts may be treated with a single drug, such as trimethoprim/sulfamethoxazole or tetracycline. Septicemia is generally treated with aminoglycosides, doxycycline, chloramphenicol, or trimethoprim/sulfamethoxazole. Combination therapy, such as doxycycline plus an aminoglycoside, may be needed. The necessary duration of therapy in septicemia has not been established; several weeks of therapy may be needed (see Chapter 20 for dosages of antibiotics).

Bone and joint infections

11

INTRODUCTION

Infectious agents are introduced into bone by: (1) hematogenous infection from bacteremia, (2) local spread from contiguous foci such as cellulitis or infected varicella lesions, and (3) direct inoculation following trauma, invasive procedures, or surgery. The incidence of osteomyelitis is greater in males (2.5 times more often than females) and approximately 40% of cases occur in patients under 20 years of age.

HEMATOGENOUS OSTEOMYELITIS

The pathogenesis of hematogenous osteomyelitis begins in the metaphysis of tubular long bones adjacent to the epiphyseal growth plate. Thrombosis of the low velocity sinusoidal vessels due to trauma or embolization is considered the focus for bacterial seeding in this process. This avascular environment allows invading organisms to proliferate while avoiding the influx of phagocytes, the presence of serum antibody and complement, the interaction with tissue macrophages, and other host defense mechanisms. The proliferation of organisms, release of organism enzymes and by-products, and the fixed volume environment contribute to progressive bone necrosis. The signs, symptoms and pathologic progression vary by age (Table 11.1).

Tubular long bones are primarily involved, especially of the lower extremities; the common sites of bone involvement in children demonstrate this predilection (Table 11.2).

The bacterial etiology of hematogenous osteomyelitis demonstrates an age-specific pattern (Table 11.3). Other epidemiologic factors, predisposing chronic diseases and exposure history may suggest unusual pathogens (Table 11.4).

The differential diagnosis of hematogenous osteomyelitis includes: septicemia, cellulitis, toxic synovitis, septic arthritis, thrombophlebitis, or, in a sickle cell disease patient, a bone infarction. The diagnosis of osteomyelitis is confirmed with isolation of organisms from bone, subperiosteal exudate, or contiguous joint fluid. Needle aspiration through normal skin over involved bone at a subperiosteal site or at the metaphyseal area combined with a potentially involved joint aspiration should be performed by an orthopedic surgeon. Aspirates of involved focal areas yield positive cultures in 80 to 85% of cases that have not been pretreated with antibiotics. However, because early institution of antimicrobial therapy is so common, only 50% of suspected cases are culture positive. Blood cultures have been reported to be positive in as many as 50% of cases so should be obtained routinely before initiation of antimicrobial therapy.

Diagnosis

A technetium bone scan remains the procedure of choice for establishing a diagnosis of osteomyelitis and localizing disease. However, routine plain X-rays are initially obtained since they are readily available and may identify other etiologies of bone pain. The diagnosis of osteomyelitis on routine roentgenographs can be subtle to obvious (Table 11.5) depending on the duration of disease and are adequate for differentiating patients with trauma, including physical abuse. X-rays are also fairly sensitive for identifying leukemic infiltrates, which represent one important cause of bone pain.

Diagnosis of bone infection is enhanced with the use of technetium scanning, which can be completed in 1–2 hours. This study

Table 11.1 Hematogenous osteomyelitis: signs and symptoms

Sign	Newborn	Older infant and young child (2 wk–4 yr)	Older child and adolescent (4–16 yr)
Systemic symptoms*	Clinical sepsis, irritable, especially to touch; pseudo-paralysis	Pain, limp, refusal to use affected limb	Focal symptoms, less restriction of movement; local pain; mild limp; fever, malaise
Signs	Red, swollen, discolored local site; massive swelling	Marked focality; point tenderness; well localized pain	Focal signs; point tenderness very localized
Pathology	Thin cortex; dissects into surrounding tissue	Cortex thicker; periosteum dense	Metaphyseal cortex thick; periosteum fibrous and dense
Progression	Nidus (purulent) rapidly progresses†; subperiosteal purulence spreads; secondary septic arthritis	Subperiosteal abscess and edema; metaphyseal involvement	Cortical rupture (rare)
Roentgenograph	Useful early periosteal and bony changes	Later findings confirmatory; early changes – deep soft tissue swelling	Bony changes apparent only after 7–10 days of of involvement

*May be subclinical; constitutional symptoms (fever, malaise, anorexia, irritability) are no different among the different age groups; also no correlation with severity of constitutional symptoms and ultimate severity of subsequent osteomyelitis; †Residual effects may be anticipated in up to 25% of newborns

Table 11.2 Site of bone involvement

Site	Frequency (%)
Femur	36
Tibia	33
Humerus	10
Fibula	7
Radius	3
Calcaneus	3
Ilium	2

should be obtained for any patient who has obvious evidence of focal bone pathology, fever of undetermined etiology with bone tenderness on physical examination and an elevated C reactive protein or sedimentation rate, or suggestive findings on routine radiographs. The bone scan can also aid in directing aspirate procedures for diagnosis and culture.

In situations where osteomyelitis is suspected on physical examination but the technetium bone scan is equivocal or non-diagnostic, secondary radionuclide imaging or magnetic resonance imaging (MRI) may be performed. In selected cases, including pelvic, vertebral or small bone (hands/feet) osteomyelitis, the use of MRI or computerized tomography (CT) can be useful in establishing a diagnosis or directing surgical intervention. A technetium or indium labeled white blood cell (WBC) scan, using tagged autolgous leukocytes, requires 24 h of imaging for completion and has only limited usefulness. Gallium scanning requires 24 to 48 h, may be difficult to read (midline scans) owing to uptake in the bowel, and has been replaced by MRI, CT and WBC scans.

Table 11.3 Bacterial etiology in hematogenous osteomyelitis

Neonates		Infants and children	
Organisms			
Staphylococcus aureus	40%	S. aureus	80%
Group B streptococci	30%	Group A streptococci	7%
Coliforms	10%	Salmonella sp.	6%
Others	20%	Others	7%
Neisseria gonorrhoeae		Coliforms	
Pseudomonas aeruginosa		Streptococcus pneumoniae	
Candida sp.		Candida sp.	
		Anaerobes	

Table 11.4 Specific etiologies of osteomyelitis

Clinical circumstances	Probable etiology
Human bite	Anaerobes
Dog or cat bite	Pasteurella multocida
Puncture wound of foot	Pseudomonas aeruginosa
Sickle cell disease	Salmonella sp.
Rheumatoid arthritis	Staphylococcus aureus (from joint)
	P. multocida
Diabetes mellitus	Fungi
Newborns	Group B streptococci
	Escherichia coli
	Salmonella sp.
Uncommon etiologies	
Facial and cervical area; in the jaw; sinus drainage; lytic bone changes with 'egg shell' areas of new bone	Actinomyces sp.
Age 3 months to 6 years (uncommon compared to staphylococci)	Haemophilus influenzae*
Vertebral body or long bone abscesses; systemic signs and symptoms	Brucella Salmonella
Regional distribution; systemic findings; vertebral body, skull, long bone involvement	Coccidioides
Skin lesion; pulmonary involvement; skull and vertebral bodies most common, but long bone involvement is reported	Blastomyces
Very distinct, slowly progressive bony lesions can occur	Cryptococcus
Exposure to cats, FUO, liver granulomas, chronic adenitis	Bartonella henselae (cat scratch disease)

*Reduced incidence with use of conjugate vaccine

Table 11.5 Roentgenographic diagnosis of hematogenous osteomyelitis

Day	Changes
0–3	Local, deep soft tissue swelling; near metaphyseal region or with localized findings
3–7	Deep soft tissue swelling; obscured translucent fat lines (spread of edema fluid)
10–21	Variable, bone-specific; bone destruction, periosteal new bone formation

NONHEMATOGENOUS OSTEOMYELITIS

Bone involvement arises through spread from a contiguous focus of infection or direct inoculation. The following are the more common types of nonhematogenous osteomyelitis.

Pseudomonas osteochondritis

The predilection of *Pseudomonas* to involve cartilaginous tissue and the relative amount of cartilage in children's tarsal–metatarsal region are the reasons for this infection being classified as an 'osteochondritis'. The classic history is a nail puncture through a tennis shoe. This entity is seen as early as 2 days postinjury but frequently requires up to 21 days to manifest clinically. The proper initial management of this trauma is vigorous irrigation and cleansing of the puncture wound in conjunction with tetanus prophylaxis. Upon diagnosis of *Pseudomonas* osteochondritis from wound, drainage culture or surgical curettage culture, intravenous antibiotics should be initiated and guided by antibiotic sensitivity testing. The crucial factor in successful therapy is complete evacuation of all necrotic infected bone and cartilage. If this is accomplished, only 7 to 10 days of parenteral antibiotics are necessary (depending on soft tissue healing and appearance) for completion of therapy. *Pseudomonas* osteochondritis of the vertebrae or pelvis should lead one to suspect intravenous drug abuse as an etiology.

Patellar osteochondritis

Patellar osteochondritis is seen in children 5 to 15 years of age when the patella has significant vascular integrity. Direct inoculation via a puncture would yield symptoms within 1 week to 10 days. Constitutional symptoms are uncommon. *Staphylococcus aureus* is the most common etiology. Roentgenographs may take 2 to 3 weeks to show bone sclerosis or destruction.

Contiguous osteochondritis

Infection is uncommon in children compared to adults. It is associated with nosocomial-infected burns or penetrating wounds. The clinical course characteristically includes two to four weeks of local pain, skin erosion, ulceration, or sinus drainage. Multiple organisms are common and draining sinus cultures correlate well with bone aspirate or biopsy cultures. *S. aureus*, streptococci, anaerobes and nosocomial Gram-negative enterics are the etiologic organisms; peripheral leukocyte count or erythrocyte sedimentation rates are usually normal. It is important to be aware of predisposing conditions (Table 11.6).

PELVIC OSTEOMYELITIS

The frequency of bone involvement (highest to lowest) is: ilium, ischium, pubis, and sacroiliac areas. The tendency for multifocal involvement is high in the pelvis compared to other sites. The symptoms may be poorly localized with vague onset; hip and buttock pain with a limp are frequently the only findings. Tenderness to palpation in the buttocks, the sciatic notch, or positive sacroiliac joint findings suggest this diagnosis. The differential diagnosis includes mesenteric lymphadenitis, urinary tract infection and acute appendicitis. Patients with inflammatory bowel disease have an increased risk for the development of pelvic osteomyelitis.

Table 11.6   Predisposing conditions for contiguous osteochondritis

Closed fractures
   Osteomyelitis one to several weeks postfracture; after postfracture pain subsides, the pain recurs with progression; local erythema, warmth, and fluctuation; fever common; osteomyelitis applies to this circumstance
Open fractures
   Thorough debridement and wound cleansing paramount; lower infection rates have been reported in patients receiving prophylactic first generation cephalosporin for open fractures; the consequence of infection can be significant; staphylococci, streptococci, anaerobes and *Clostridia* sp. or Gram-negative enterics depending on the environment related to the trauma should be considered; tetanus prophylaxis vital (see Chapter 3)
Hemodialysis
   Increased risk owing to multiple procedures with intravascular cannulae; ribs, thoracic spine and bones adjacent to indwelling catheters; *Staphylococcus aureus* and *S. epidermidis* commonly found

VERTEBRAL OSTEOMYELITIS

The vertebral venous system is valveless with a low velocity bidirectional flow, probably the predisposing factors for vertebral body osteomyelitis. It is common for two adjacent vertebrae to be involved while sparing the intervertebral disc. Spread to the internal venous system (epidural abscess) or the external venous system (paraspinous abscess) are complications of this infection. The symptoms of vertebral osteomyelitis include constant back pain (usually dull), low-grade fever and pain on exertion; the signs may include paraspinous muscle spasm, tenderness to palpation or percussion of the spinal dorsal processes and limitation of motion. The symptoms can frequently be present for 3 to 4 months without overt toxicity or signs of sepsis. Roentgenographs show rarefaction in one vertebral edge as early as several days and progress to marked destruction, usually anteriorly, followed by changes in the adjacent vertebrae and new bone formation.

Staphylococci are the infecting organisms in 80 to 90% of cases with Gram-negative enterics (associated with urinary tract infections), *Pseudomonas* sp. (i.v. drug abusers), and a small percentage of miscellaneous organisms (see Table 11.3). Parenteral antibiotic therapy for presumed staphylococcal involvement should be initiated with consideration for a needle aspirate or bone biopsy for culture and sensitivity testing.

Antibiotic therapy should be continued for a minimum of 6 weeks but no data are available for the optimal duration; the clinical course should be considered for decisions of therapy beyond this limit. Treatment should also include surgical drainage (especially if cord compression is present) and immobilization (bed rest versus casting).

DISCITIS

Noninfectious disc necrosis versus bacteremic seeding of the disc space during the loss of blood supply are difficult to separate clinically. Intervertebral disc infection demonstrates some important characteristics: male sex predominance, peak incidence under 5 years of age, occurrence nearly always in the lumbar area (L4–L5 then L3–L4 most common), peripheral leukocytosis in only one-third of patients and consistently elevated erythrocyte sedimentation rate (ESR). The symptoms include backache, progressive limp, irritability and refusal to sit (nonambulatory infants), hip pain and low-grade fever. These can be present 1 to 18 months (median 10 to 12 weeks) before diagnosis. Signs include back stiffness, tenderness to spine palpation, and limitation of movement. *S. aureus* is the most frequent causative organism; needle aspirate and bone biopsy have been reported as culture positive in up to 50% of cases. Less common isolates include pneumococcus and

Gram-negative organisms. Roentgenographs (lateral view of lumbar spine) may show disc space narrowing by 2 to 4 weeks after onset of symptoms. This is followed by destruction of adjacent vertebral edges; vertebral body compression is rare.

The benfit of antimicrobial therapy remains controversial. Oral antibiotics may be given following a short course (3–5 days) of parenteral therapy, depending on the organism and the clinical situation. Prolonged periods (4 to 6 months) of oral antibiotics may be prudent for patients with extensive disc damage. The prognosis varies but, in general, young children reconstitute and heal the disc space whereas older children are more likely to have spontaneous spinal fusion.

TREATMENT OF OSTEOMYELITIS

The treatment of hematogenous osteomyelitis should be guided initially by Gram stain and subsequently by susceptibilities of organisms recovered from bone or joint aspirates. Empiric therapy on an age- and disease-related basis administered parenterally should be initiated once a diagnosis is confirmed and cultures have been obtained (Table 11.7).

Parenteral antibiotics in acute bacterial hematogenous osteomyelitis are indicated initially because: physiologic and constitutional changes are not ideal for oral antibiotic absorption; there is a propensity for dissemination and abscess formation (especially for *S. aureus*); and compliance must be assured during early treatment. Although the route of administration of antibiotics remains controversial, oral absorption is adequate for the continuation of therapy (Table 11.8). Parenteral therapy should be continued until a clinical response is documented, usually 3 to 5 days. The duration of antibiotic therapy (parenteral and oral) should generally be 3 weeks and may have to be extended longer depending on the sites of infection and clinical response. The use of home intravenous antibiotics for selected cases can substitute for part of the initial therapy or for the entire course if oral continuation therapy is felt to be suboptimal for age, site or severity (*Pseudomonas* osteochondritis following

Table 11.7   Simplified management of osteomyelitis

Phase	Management
Initial: Day 0–3 inpatient	Obtain complete blood count (CBC) and C reactive protein (CRP) Begin i.v. antibiotics (e.g. cefazolin) Repeat CBC and CRP when afebrile and clinical response observed CBC and CRP returning to normal (CRP < 20 mg/l): proceed to next phase
Continued therapy: Days 4–21 outpatient	p.o. antibiotics (e.g. cephalexin) at 2–3 times the usual dose
Completion: Day 21 (ESR < 30 mm/h)	Obtain erythrocyte sedimentation rate (ESR); if < 30 mm/h stop antibiotics
Delayed response: Days 21–42 (ESR > 30 mm/h)	ESR > 30 mm/h Obtain MRI. Surgical debridement if bone inflammation and destruction identified Continue p.o. antibiotics Repeat ESR at 42 days < 30 mm/h: stop antibiotics > 30 mm/h: repeat MRI consider continued surgical and/or medical management for 6 weeks

Table 11.8 Antimicrobial therapy for osteomyelitis and septic arthritis

Infection	Antimicrobial agents		
Osteomyelitis and septic arthritis			
Empiric therapy			
Neonate (0–28 days)	Oxacillin	plus	cefotaxime or ceftriaxone
Infant (1–12 months)	Oxacillin, nafcillin or cefazolin	plus	ceftriaxone or cefotaxime
Children (> 1 yr)	Cefazolin, clindamycin, oxacillin or nafcillin		
Puncture wound to foot	Gentamicin*, tobramycin or amikacin or	plus	ceftazidime
	ticarcillin	plus	cefazolin**, clindamycin or nafcillin
Specific therapy†			
Staphylococcus aureus	Cefazolin, clindamycin, oxacillin, nafcillin, vancomycin (methicillin resistant)		
Group B streptococci	Penicillin		
Group A streptococci	Penicillin		
Haemophilus influenzae	Ampicillin (sensitive) or cefotaxime, ceftriaxone, chloramphenicol, (ampicillin resistant)		

Streptococcus pneumoniae	Penicillin
	    Penicillin resistant – ceftriaxone, cefotaxime
	    Penicillin/cephalosporin resistant – vancomycin		

Enterobacteriaceae	Aminoglycoside; if resistant, azlocillin, aztreonam, mezlocillin, piperacillin or third generation cephalosporins, depending on sensitivities		
Neisseria gonorrhoeae	Penicillin or ampicillin; if penicillin resistant, cephalosporin (third generation) or spectinomycin		
Pseudomonas aeruginosa	Aminoglycoside plus ticarcillin;		
Salmonella sp.	Chloramphenicol; third generation cephalosporins		
Candida albicans	Amphotericin B with or without 5-flucytosine		
Anaerobes	Penicillin, clindamycin, or metronidazole		
Continuation oral therapy††			
S. aureus	Cephalexin, cefadroxil, dicloxacillin, oxacillin, nafcillin, or clindamycin		
Streptococci (group A)	Penicillin or amoxicillin		
S. pneumoniae	Penicillin or amoxicillin; third generation cephalosporins		
Enterobacteriaceae	Ampicillin or trimethoprim/ sulfamethoxazole		

Continued over

Table 11.8 Continued

Infection	Antimicrobial agents
Neisseria gonorrhoeae	Cefixime
Pseudomonas aeruginosa	Ciprofloxacin or other quinolones; not approved for children < 18 yr unless there are no safer alternatives
	Carbenicillin
Salmonella sp.	Amoxicillin, chloramphenicol, or third generation cephalosporins
Candida albicans	Fluconazole
Anaerobes	Penicillin, metronidazole or clindamycin
Culture negative	Coverage for Staphylococcus aureus (see above)

*Aminoglycoside choice guided by Pseudomonas sensitivities in your hospital; **Concomitant wound infection, Gram stain positive; †Inpatient or home intravenous therapy; ††Oral continuation (modified by sensitivity testing)

puncture wound of the foot and surgical debridement is an exception). Surgical drainage or debridement of subperiosteal abscesses or soft tissue abscesses should be considered. Immobilization of an affected extremity is necessary for pain relief and to enhance healing.

Duration of treatment

Most cases of hematogenous osteomyeltis are culture negative after 21 days of therapy (Table 11.7). Exceptions are vertebral osteomyeltitis, which should be treated for 6 weeks, and puncture wound osteochondritis caused by Pseudomonas which only requires 7–10 days of antimicrobial therapy following adequate surgical debridement.

SEPTIC ARTHRITIS

With the production of joint fluid by the synovial membrane, the kinetics of capillary diffusion of fluid into the joint space and the effective blood flow of the joint space, the relatively high frequency of joint infections is not surprising. Bacteria can enter the joint space by direct inoculation (kneeling on a needle, trauma), contiguous extension (osteomyelitis), or via a hematogenous route. In children the lower extremities account for over 80% of cases (Table 11.9).

Table 11.9 Joint involvement in septic arthritis

Joint*	Involvement (%)
Knee	38
Hip	32
Ankle	11
Elbow	8
Shoulder	5
Wrist	4
Small joints	2

*2–5% of cases have multiple joint involvement

The diagnosis of septic arthritis is made earlier than in osteomyelitis owing to the onset of constitutional symptoms within the first few days of the infection. Patients almost always have fever, focal findings in the joint (swelling, tenderness, heat, limitation of motion), and placement of the joint in a neutral, nonstressed position. In infants the hip may have an absence of focal findings with the exception of positioning. Infants are observed with the involved leg abducted, slightly flexed and externally rotated. Resistance to movement or pain should be evaluated for a possible septic hip. There is often an associated dislocation in this setting. An obvious portal of entry in septic arthritis is uncommon.

The diagnosis of suspect joint infection by roentgenograms depends on finding evidence of capsular swelling. In the case of hip involvement, roentgenograms can be valuable; placement of the child in the frog-leg position for an anteroposterior radiograph shows displacement of fat lines. Obliteration or lateral displacement of the gluteal fat lines or a raised position for Shenton's line with widening of the arc are consistent with hip joint effusion under pressure. The presence of a significant joint effusion by hip ultrasound is adequate to dictate a joint aspiration. Radionuclide imaging or MRI (see osteomyelitis in this chapter) may be a useful adjunct in a complex or uncharacteristic case for early diagnosis. The use of hip ultrasound followed by a technetium bone scan (or CT/MRI) in selected cases is a reasonable progression of tests based on usefulness, cost and radiation exposure.

The confirmatory procedure for diagnosis is a joint aspiration with Gram stain, culture, and cytology–chemistry evaluation. Joint aspiration of knees (the most common joint involved) should be a procedure for all primary care physicians; aspiration of hips or shoulders should be limited to an experienced orthopedist (under fluoroscopic control for hip aspirations). Joint fluid should be processed for Gram stain and aerobic and anaerobic cultures. The fluid should be analyzed for glucose concentration (compared to a concomitant blood glucose), leukocyte count and differential, ability to spontaneously clot and mucin clot test (Table 11.10). Joint fluid

should be obtained in a heparinized syringe to assure leukocyte analysis. To perform the mucin clot test, glacial acetic acid is added to the joint fluid while stirring; normal fluid reacts with a white precipitate (rope) that clings to the stirring rod, with a clear supernatant.

Etiologic diagnosis of septic arthritis can be aided by blood cultures; some series have reported up to 20 to 30% of sterile joint fluids with concomitant positive blood cultures. Additional laboratory studies include a hemogram to screen for anemia (hemoglobinopathy), ESR (usually elevated in septic arthritis), serum or urine for bacterial antigen detection (only in partially treated cases with suspect group B streptococci, *Haemophilus influenzae*, pneumococcus, or meningococcus), and accessory cultures: wound, infected skin lesions (secondarily infected varicella lesions over the involved joint), cellulitis, or urethral–cervical–rectal cultures in sexually active adolescents (gonorrhea). Cerebrospinal fluid analysis should be included when meningitis is clinically suspected, and in newborns.

The differential diagnosis of septic arthritis includes joint fluid inflammation due to a variety of etiologies (Table 11.11).

The causative bacteria in most cases of septic arthritis are Gram-positive aerobic organisms particularly since the introduction of *H. influenzae* vaccine. *S. aureus* remains the most frequent single pathogen. The causative organisms differ for neonates, infants, and older children (Table 11.12).

Table 11.10 Joint fluid analysis

	Septic arthritis	Juvenile rheumatoid arthritis	Reactive arthritis
Spontaneous clotting	Large clot	Large clot	Small clot
Mucin clotting	Curdled milk	Small friable masses	Tight rope; clear supernatant
Glucose concentration (% of blood glucose)	30	75	75–90
Leukocytes, total	≥ 70 000	15 000	15 000–30 000
Leukocytes, % PMNs	90	60	50

Table 11.11 Differential diagnosis of septic arthritis

Infectious	Viral, mycobacterial, fungal or mycoplasma, bacterial endocarditis, deep cellulitis, Lyme disease, congenital syphilis
Hypersensitivity	Serum sickness (drug, postinfectious), anaphylactoid purpura
Oncologic	Leukemia, neuroblastoma, pigmented villonodular synovitis, primary bone tumor
Metabolic	Gout, hyperparathyroidism
Immunologic	Agammaglobulinemia, Behçet's syndrome, hepatitis
Neurogenic	Diabetes mellitus, peripheral nerve or spinal cord injury, leprosy
Bleeding	Trauma (to include physical abuse), skeletal trauma due to birth, hemophilia
Orthopedic	Toxic synovitis, aseptic necrosis, osteochondritis, bursitis
Miscellaneous	Kawasaki's syndrome, collagen vascular disease, polyarthritis nodosa, sarcoidosis, inflammatory bowel disease, familial Mediterranean fever, Tietze's syndrome, reactive arthritis

Table 11.12 Etiology of septic arthritis

	Newborns and infants		Older children
	Community acquired	Nosocomial	Combined series
Staphylococcus aureus	25%	62%	77%
Staphylococcus epidermidis		4%	
Group B streptococci	50%	4%	
Group A streptococci	3%	1%	7%
Pneumococcus	5%	1%	6%
Enterobacteriaceae	5%	9%	7% (predominantly immuno-compromised patients)
Candida sp.		17%	
Neisseria gonorrhoeae	10%		
Miscellaneous	2%	2%	3%

TREATMENT OF SEPTIC ARTHRITIS

The empiric choice of antimicrobial therapy in septic arthritis should be guided by the age of the patient, site of involvement, underlying disease and the Gram stain of joint fluid but should consider: *S. aureus* in all cases; declining incidence of *H. influenzae* in fully immunized children; group B streptococci, and to a lesser extent Gram-negative organisms and *Candida* sp. in neonates, and *Neisseria gonorrhoeae* in newborns and sexually active adolescents (Table 11.8). The other etiologies and age-related incidence include *Mycoplasma* (> 10 years), *Ureaplasma* (> 5 years), Lyme arthritis (Borrelia-type organism; > 6 months), hepatitis B (> 1 year), rubella (> 10 years), mumps (< 12 years), varicella (< 5 years), herpes simplex virus, cytomegalovirus, and parvovirus (all ages).

Antibiotic therapy should be directed in cases with negative Gram stains and negative bacterial antigen assays for the most likely organisms for age (see Table 11.8). Nearly all antibiotics that have been studied penetrate readily into joint fluid, averaging 30 to 40% of peak serum concentration. The penicillins, cephalosporins (first, second and third generation), macrolides, aminoglycosides and chloramphenicol attain effective concentrations in joint fluid. Intra-articular antibiotics add no benefit. Larger joints may require

146

open drainage. The duration of antibiotic therapy should be 3 weeks minimum with the first 3 to 5 days administered parenterally followed by oral continuation therapy as long as the following criteria are met: no gastrointestinal disorder due to underlying disease that would diminish oral absorption, clinical response to parenteral antibiotics and surgical management has been established; the organism is sensitive to a class of antibiotic in oral form and compliance can be guaranteed. Some experts administer a trial dosage of oral antibiotics during inpatient management.

To evaluate the effectiveness of antibiotic therapy in more difficult cases, serial joint aspirations can be performed. Although cultures may be positive for up to 5 to 7 days in nonsurgically drained joint fluid, a decrease in leukocyte density should be seen by 1 to 2 weeks of therapy. In studies using serial joint aspirations, by days 1 through 10 of antibiotic therapy those patients who subsequently recover had less than 5000 cells/mm^3 compared to those with recrudescent infection who had more than 60 000 cells/mm^3. The best predictor of outcome and complications is the duration of signs and symptoms prior to diagnosis and effective therapy.

Septic arthritis in neonates and infants and most cases of hip or shoulder involvement should be drained as soon as the diagnosis is established. Any joint should be considered for open drainage when loculation, high fibrin content, or tissue debris prevents adequate drainage by needle aspiration.

Table 11.13 shows special considerations that should be taken into account when evaluating arthritis.

Table 11.13   Special considerations in evaluating arthritis

Neonatal septic arthritis	Subtle presentation
	Unusual organisms
	Use of umbilical catheters
	Difficulty in evaluating hips, shoulders
	Potential catastrophic outcome
Adolescents, monoarticular	Sexual contact history due to arthritis increases possibility of gonococcal etiology
	Disseminated gonorrhea (perihepatitis, endocarditis, meningitis, sepsis)
Reactive arthritis	Predisposition in HLA-B27 positive individuals
	Occurs following *Shigella* sp., *Salmonella* sp., *Yersinia*, and *Campylobacter* enteric infections
	May mimic rheumatic fever, collagen vascular disease, or serum sickness
Reiter's syndrome	Urethritis, conjunctivitis, with or without rash and arthritis (ankles, knees) associated with *Chlamydia* infection
Lyme disease	Clinical suggestion that early diagnosis and treatment with penicillin or amoxicillin may prevent arthritis
Kawasaki's syndrome	Arthritis, most common noncardiac complication
	Occurs in 20–30% of cases
	Large joints most common
	Multiple joints
	Responds to salicylates

Urinary tract infections 12

INTRODUCTION

Over the previous decade considerable progress has been made in the management of urinary tract infections (UTIs), resulting from a better understanding of host factors and bacterial virulence. Additionally, radiographic imaging of the urinary tract has advanced, simplifying evaluation of the child with documented infection. Covert (asymptomatic) bacteriuria, discussed later in this chapter, should be distinguished from symptomatic UTI, which is of major clinical significance. On screening, bacteriuria has been identified in 1–1.5% of neonates, with a high male predominance. This male preponderance of UTI, during infancy, is potentially related to poor retractability of the foreskin and a higher incidence of urinary tract anomalies. In school-age children, both covert bacteriuria and symptomatic UTI are more commonly encountered, with an aggregate risk of 3.0–7.8% for girls and 1.1–1.7% for boys. The shorter urethra and greater potential for perineal colonization accounts for this higher incidence in girls. The predominant mechanism of UTI for both sexes is ascent of bowel organisms but, during the neonatal period, hematogenous seeding of the kidney from bacteremia may also play a role.

Pyelonephritis may lead to irreversible renal scarring. Successful diagnosis involves a high index of suspicion and awareness of optimal techniques to diagnose UTI. It is possible to prevent renal damage with prompt diagnosis and treatment. The American Academy of Pediatrics, Subcommittee on Urinary Tract Infection, has published guidelines for the diagnosis, treatment and evaluation of the initial UTI in febrile infants and children aged 2 months to 2 years. The 11 recommendations contained in this document are summarized in Table 12.1 and represent an appropriate starting point for discussing management of urinary tract infections in children.

CRITERIA FOR DIAGNOSIS

Clinical criteria

Cystitis classically presents with urgency, frequency, dysuria, secondary enuresis, and foul-smelling urine. Spiking fever, flank or abdominal pain, and irritability suggest pyelonephritis. The clinical manifestations of chronic pyelonephritis are most commonly recurrent abdominal pain, unexplained febrile episodes and failure to thrive.

A higher index of suspicion is necessary to diagnose UTI in the infant in whom fever, sepsis, lethargy, and jaundice may be initial symptoms. It is important to recognize that many children with urethral or perineal irritation may present with voiding symptoms (Table 12.2) in the absence of UTI.

Laboratory testing

A positive dipstick or microscopic urinalysis result is suggestive of UTI (Table 12.3), but confirmation must be obtained by culture with a quantitative colony count. Identification of the organism is essential, especially with recurrent UTI. Pyuria is poorly correlated with UTI. Approximately 40% of children with UTI have a white blood cell count < 10/high-power field in centrifuged sediment. Conversely, children with pyuria frequently do not have bacteriuria (Table 12.4).

Specimen collection greatly influences the accuracy of UTI diagnosis. When a specimen is carefully collected by clean-catch midstream technique, catheterization, or suprapubic

Table 12.1 American Academy of Pediatrics, Subcommittee on Urinary Tract Infections (UTI): recommendations on the diagnosis, treatment and evaluation of the initial UTI in febrile infants and young children*, 1999

1. The presence of UTI should be considered in children with unexplained fever.
2. In children with unexplained fever, the degree of toxicity, dehydration, and ability to retain oral intake must be carefully assessed.
3. If a child with unexplained fever warrants immediate antimicrobial therapy, a urine specimen should be obtained by suprapubic aspiration (SPA) or catheterization; the diagnosis of UTI cannot be established by a culture of a bagged urine.
4. If a child with unexplained fever does not require immediate antimicrobial therapy, there are 2 options:
   i: Obtain and culture a urine specimen collected by SPA or catheterization.
   ii: Obtain a urine specimen by the most convenient means and perform a urinalysis. If the urinalysis is positive, culture a urine specimen collected by SPA or catheterization; if urinalysis is negative, it is reasonable to follow closely, recognizing that a negative urinalysis does not rule out a UTI.
5. Diagnosis of UTI requires a urine culture.
6. If the child with suspected UTI is assessed as toxic, dehydrated, or unable to retain oral intake, initial antimicrobial therapy should be administered i.v. and hospitalization should be considered.
7. In the child who may not appear ill but who has a culture confirming a UTI, antimicrobial therapy should be initiated, i.v. or p.o.
8. Children with UTI who have not defervesced within 2 days of antimicrobial therapy should be re-evaluated and recultured.
9. Children, including those whose initial treatment was administered i.v., should complete a 7 to 14 day course of p.o. antibiotics.
10. After a 7 to 14 day course of antibiotics and sterilization of the urine, children should receive antibiotics until imaging studies are completed.
11. Children with UTI who do not defervesce within 2 days of antimicrobial therapy should undergo ultrasonography and cystography promptly. Children who have the expected response to antimicrobials should have a sonogram and cystography performed at the earliest convenient time.

*Refers to infants and children 2 months to 2 years of age

Table 12.2 Causes of urinary tract symptoms in the absence of bacteriuria

Urethritis
Meatal irritation
Vulvovaginitis
Balanitis
Topical irritants
  Bubble bath or soap
  Laundry detergents
  Lotions
  Dyes/scents in clothing or toilet tissue
Medications
Vaginal foreign body
Pinworms
Emotional stress
Trauma (including masturbation and sexual abuse)
Daytime frequency syndrome
Candida
Trichomonas

aspiration, substantial bacteriuria on urinalysis usually correlates with a high colony count of a single organism (Table 12.5). Multiple organisms or a low colony count suggest a contaminated specimen rather than a true UTI.

Urine specimens collected by bag technique carry a high risk (50%) of contamination, especially in female infants and uncircumcised males with nonretractable foreskins. A positive urinalysis on such a specimen must be confirmed by catheterization or suprapubic aspiration, but a negative specimen collected by bag technique is helpful in excluding UTI. Girls should be instructed to carefully cleanse the perineum and to straddle the toilet facing backwards in order to abduct the labia and reduce voiding of urine into the vagina. A midstream specimen can then be obtained. In uncircumcised boys,

Table 12.3   Screening tests for urinary tract infections

Routine urinalysis
    White blood cell count ≥ 10/high-power field
        Urine (10 ml) centrifuged for 5 min at 3000 rpm and viewed at 45 x magnification
    Leukocyte esterase
        Correlates with pyuria
        Positive predictive value of 50%
Nitrite
    Bacteria slowly reduce nitrate to nitrite
    Overnight or concentrated urine optimal
    Negative result with high fluid intake or frequency
    Negative result with *Pseudomonas* UTI
Bacteria
    Presence in unspun urine correlates with 10^5 bacteria/ml
White blood cell casts
    Indicative of pyelonephritis
Serum C-reactive protein
    Elevated with pyelonephritis

Table 12.4   Causes of pyuria without bacteriuria

Febrile systemic illness
Concentrated urine (dehydration)
Irritation from catheter or instrument
Inflammation of neighboring structures (e.g. acute appendicitis)
Calculi
Acute glomerulonephritis
Interstitial nephritis
Nonbacterial infection (e.g. *Candida, Mycobacterium tuberculosis, Ureaplasma*)
Previous reconstructive surgery using an intestinal patch

Table 12.5   Criteria for culture diagnosis of urinary tract infections (single organism)

Specimen collection	Intermediate result (colonies/ml urine)	Positive result (colonies/ml urine)
Suprapubic aspiration	Any growth	> 100
Catheterized urine	10 000–50 000	> 50 000
Clean-voided (male)	≥ 10 000 (foreskin retracted or absent, glans penis cleansed)	> 100 000
Clean-voided (female)	> 50 000	> 100 000
Bagged urine	> 100 000	Indeterminate

the foreskin should be retracted sufficiently to allow cleansing of the meatal region. Urine culture should be plated within 30 min, or refrigerated if the culture will be delayed. Storage of urine at room temperature promotes bacterial multiplication, resulting in higher colony counts. On a temporary basis, urine specimens may be stored in a refrigerator or in a basin of ice water to reduce bacterial multiplication.

RISK FACTORS FOR URINARY TRACT INFECTION

Failure of host defenses resulting in UTI may arise from defects at the cellular, organ, or functional level. Increased bacterial adherence to the urothelium of children with recurrent UTI has been attributed to a mucin layer deficiency. The nonsecretor phenotype for blood group antigens is an additional, hereditary risk factor. Nonsecretor status is associated with reduced excretion of water-soluble glycoproteins and alteration of the terminal oligosaccharide configuration on the exterior of epithelial cells. This deficiency facilitates bacterial adherence and results in an increased incidence of recurrent UTI. Other host defenses such as urinary inhibitory glycoproteins have been identified.

Organ-specific risk factors include poor vulvar hygiene in females or the presence of a foreskin in males (Table 12.6), both of which predispose to bacterial colonization of the perimeatal region and subsequently the urethra. Numerous studies have documented the increased risk (5–20-fold) of UTI in the uncircumcised male. In one study, 95% of male infants with UTI were uncircumcised, and the majority of these were under 3 months of age. Multiple studies have confirmed the beneficial aspects of circumcision in reducing the risk of UTI in early infancy.

Table 12.6 Factors predisposing to urinary tract infection

Urothelial deficiency
  Increased bacterial adherence owing to
    nonsecretor phenotype
Organ-specific deficiencies
  Anomalies with hydronephrosis or obstruction
  Nephrolithiasis
  Vesicoureteral reflux
  Indwelling catheter or foreign body
  Nonretractable foreskin
  Fecal incontinence
  Poor perineal hygiene
Functional factors
  Bladder dysfunction with detrusor hypertonicity
  Constipation

Of all the structural abnormalities, vesicoureteral reflux is the most frequent and significant predisposing abnormality for recurrent UTI and renal scarring.

Obstruction of the ureter may occur at the upper end (ureteropelvic junction) or the lower end (ureterovesical junction). Significant dilatation of the upper urinary tract will result in stasis which predisposes to infection. Duplication of ureters is commonly associated with reflux into the ureter which drains the lower segment of the kidney. Obstruction of the ureter draining the upper kidney segment (ectopic ureter/ureterocele) also occurs. With an ectopic ureter, which drains outside the bladder, the abnormal renal segment may become infected. In such cases, urine collected directly from the bladder by catheterization or suprapubic aspiration may show reduced colony counts, delaying the diagnosis of UTI. In males, obstruction is most commonly caused by posterior urethral valves which highly predispose these children to UTI; the initial indication of this anatomic anomaly is most commonly infection.

Functional factors which protect against UTI include regular, complete bladder emptying and low-pressure bladder filling. Bacterial multiplication may be increased by voluntary postponement of voiding owing to children's normal lack of interest in routine bodily functions. When bladder capacity is increased, or the child interrupts urination, bladder emptying may be incomplete and residual urine predisposes to UTI. Two main categories of lower urinary tract dysfunction may result in UTI with or without incontinence: bladder instability with increased intravesical pressure and incomplete sphincter relaxation during voiding. Neurogenic bladder due to spinal cord injury, spina bifida, or cerebral palsy can result in either or both of these types of lower urinary tract dysfunction.

After toilet training, the pattern of an 'unstable bladder' may persist owing to a maturational delay and may be associated with involuntary bladder contractions. Other children demonstrate inappropriate voiding habits with voluntary contraction of the sphincter during micturition and higher residual urine. Both of these functional abnormalities occur in association with vesicoureteral reflux. Unless these dynamic problems are identified and treated, UTI is likely to recur. Severe constipation or fecal retention with soiling are associated with bladder dysfunction. Improvement in bowel habits is necessary to prevent recurrence of UTI.

LOCALIZATION OF URINARY TRACT INFECTION

The location of UTI may influence the type of therapy required (intravenous versus oral) but does not alter the need for radiologic investigation. Although current methods of localization for pyelonephritis versus cystitis are imprecise, differentiation is rarely essential. Based on clinical features, the diagnosis of cystitis and pyelonephritis can often be accomplished. Symptoms of renal infection (fever, flank pain) with leukocytosis and white blood cell casts in the urine suggest pyelonephritis. Bladder washout testing is not feasible on a routine basis in children with UTI. Ureteral catheterization or percutaneous aspiration of the renal pelvis is rarely necessary except when an organism cannot be identified or when infection in a specific renal moiety may influence subsequent management; for example the need for surgery with a congenital anomaly. If documentation of renal infection is required in a patient with a fever of unknown origin, radionuclide scans, using dimercaptosuccinic acid (DMSA) or gallium, may be useful.

BACTERIAL ETIOLOGY

Escherichia coli is the primary uropathogen, both in neonates and in older children. Other organisms of the Enterobacteriaceae group, such as *Proteus, Klebsiella, Enterobacter, Pseudomonas, Acinetobacter* and *Serratia*, also cause infection (Table 12.7). These less common organisms may be seen in cases of recent antibiotic exposure. Enterococcus is seen in

Table 12.7 Etiology of urinary tract infection

Organism	Incidence (%)
Escherichia coli	80
Klebsiella sp.	10
Proteus	3
Pseudomonas	1
Enterococcus	1
Staphylococcus aureus	1

5–15% of UTI in adults and sexually active adolescent females but is rare in young children.

A positive urine specimen will have a high colony count of a single bacterium. Specimens showing intermediate growth may be confirmed by repeat culture of a sample obtained by catheterization or suprapubic aspiration before starting antibiotic therapy. Falsely low colony counts in the presence of true UTI are encountered with high fluid intake (dilute urine), severe urinary frequency, concomitant intake of antibiotics or sequestered UTI (e.g. obstructed, infected segment or abscess).

TREATMENT

The goals of treatment of UTI are to provide relief of symptoms as well as to prevent future episodes and renal damage. Untreated, symptomatic patients with a history of fever for 3 days or longer are at risk of developing renal scarring. More intensive therapy with parenteral antibiotics should be considered in cases of vomiting with inability to retain oral medications, suspected sepsis, dehydration, poor parental compliance with oral treatment, or a urologic anomaly with poor response to oral therapy. Gram stain of urine assists in the selection of an antibiotic having a predominant Gram-negative or Gram-positive spectrum. In children with compromised renal function, nephrotoxic antibiotics should be used with caution and serum creatinine and peak and trough concentrations of antibiotics monitored.

In the outpatient setting, UTI is usually treated with amoxicillin, sulfonamide antibiotics, or a cephalosporin (Table 12.8).

Table 12.8 Oral antibiotics for the treatment of lower urinary tract infection

Antibiotic	Dosage
Amoxicillin	20–40 mg/kg per day div. q.8h
Trimethoprim/sulfamethoxazole	6–12 mg TMP/30–60 mg SMX/kg per day div. q.12h
Sulfisoxazole	120–150 mg/kg per day div. q.6h
Cephalosporins	
Cefixime (Suprax)	8 mg/kg per day div. q.12h
Cefpodoxime (Vantin)	10 mg/kg per day div. q.12h
Cefprozil (Cefzil)	30 mg/kg per day div. q.12h
Cephalexin (Biocef, Keflex, Keftab, generic)	50–100 mg/kg per day div. q.6h
Loracarbef (Lorabid)	15–30 mg/kg per day div. q.12h

Emerging resistance of *E. coli* to ampicillin may render this drug less effective. In infants under 2 months of age, sulfonamide antibiotics or nitrofurantoin should be avoided as they have the potential to displace bilirubin from albumin. Antibiotics that are excreted in high concentrations in urine but do not achieve therapeutic concentrations in the bloodstream, such as nalidixic acid or nitrofurantoin, are less effective in acute pyelonephritis. Antibiotic sensitivity is most commonly determined by the disk method, using the usual serum antibiotic concentrations. Antibiotics are excreted in urine in extremely high concentrations, thus an intermediately sensitive organism may be fully eradicated. Antibiotic susceptibility testing is required to confirm the appropriateness of an empiric regimen.

With initiation of appropriate antibiotic therapy, a clinical response is usually seen within 24 to 48 h. The optimal duration of treatment in uncomplicated cystitis is controversial. Parents should be cautioned that single-dose or short-course antibiotic therapy may be associated with a higher risk of recurrence, thus a course of 7 days, in uncomplicated UTI, is appropriate. With pyelonephritis, effective treatment should be instituted as soon as possible. With a delay in treatment of more than 3 days, the risk of renal scarring is increased. For acute pyelonephritis, therapy should be continued for 7 to 14 days (Table 12.9).

Any toxic appearing child or infant with suspected pyelonephritis should be hospital-

Table 12.9 Parenteral antibiotics for the treatment of pyelonephritis

Antibiotic	Dosage*
Ceftriaxone	75 mg/kg per day div. q.24h
Cefotaxime	150 mg/kg per day div. q.6h
Ceftazidime	150 mg/kg per day div. q.6h
Cefazolin	50 mg/kg per day div. q.8h
Gentamicin	7.5 mg/kg per day div. q.8h
Tobramycin	5 mg/kg per day div. q.8h
Ticarcillin	300 mg/kg per day div. q.6h
Ampicillin[†]	100 mg/kg per day div. q.6h

*See Chapter 20 for dosages in neonates;
[†]Ampicillin should be added to cephalosporin or aminoglycoside for coverage of enterococci in adolescent females

ized for intravenous antibiotic treatment. Oral antibiotics may be substituted for intravenous therapy when the patient has been afebrile for 24–48 h.

ASYMPTOMATIC BACTERIURIA

Management of patients with asymptomatic bacteriuria remains controversial since routine antimicrobial therapy has not been shown to alter the rate of recurrence, the incidence of symptomatic episodes, nor the long-term outcome. The following groups are theoretically at higher risk for long-term sequelae and warrant consideration for antibiotic therapy once the pathogen and its sensitivities have been defined: children under 5 years of age; patients with polycystic kidney disease, medullary sponge kidneys, partial obstruction or presence of calculi, vesico-ureteral reflux; immunosuppressed patients; and patients who are to undergo genitourinary instrumentation or surgery.

Children identified as having asymptomatic bacteriuria or 'screening UTI' often have a history of previous UTI, enuresis, or voiding symptoms. On further investigation a significant percentage are found to have vesicoureteral reflux and renal scarring; therefore, asymptomatic bacteriuria should be evaluated radiographically similar to any child with a symptomatic UTI. Asymptomatic bacteriuria is common in children who have lower urinary tract dysfunction necessitating intermittent catheterization. In this population, a urine culture is only obtained and positives treated once symptoms develop.

RECURRENT URINARY TRACT INFECTION

Recurrence is observed in 30–50% of children with UTI, with approximately 90% of recurrences occurring within 3 months of the initial episode. Eighty per cent of recurrences are new infections by different fecal–colonic bacterial species that have become resistant to recently administered antibiotics. The recurrence rate is not altered by extending the duration of initial treatment. A daily prophylactic dose is recommended until imaging studies are obtained.

The anatomic status of the upper urinary tract or the presence or absence of vesicoureteral reflux can have an important bearing on the long-term treatment chosen in recurrent UTI (Table 12.10).

Children having more than two UTI episodes in a 12-month period and who have normal X-rays may need chronic prophylactic antibiotic therapy for 3–6 months to allow repair of intrinsic bladder defense mechanisms. Girls with frequent UTI tend to have asymptomatic recurrences. Resistance to antibiotics commonly develops owing to R_1 factors in fecal–colonic bacteria in patients on long-term suppressive therapy. Children with recurrent UTI and anatomic defects or reflux may need prophylactic antibiotics as long as the defect exists (Table 12.11).

During antimicrobial prophylaxis for recurrent UTI, girls, and less commonly boys, may experience breakthrough infections. There is a high incidence of voiding dysfunction or constipation in these children. The number of breakthrough infections can be reduced by placing these children on a regimen of frequent, timed voiding and double antimicrobial prophylaxis consisting of nitrofurantoin 2 mg/kg each morning and trimethoprim/sulfamethoxazole 2/10 mg/kg

Table 12.10 Long-term management of recurrent urinary tract infection

Clinical findings/management	Prophylaxis
With vesicoureteral reflux	
Surgical correction	Prophylaxis until resolution of reflux
No surgical correction	Prophylaxis until 10 years of age, and risk of renal scarring is reduced, or until reflux resolves
Without vesicoureteral reflux	
Investigate other genitourinary abnormalities: obstructive uropathy, neurogenic bladder, bladder dysfunction, ureter duplication, calculi	
Investigation findings positive	Prophylaxis for at least 1 year or until surgical correction
Investigation findings negative (with three or more episodes of urinary tract infection over past 12 months)	Prophylaxis for 6 months and assess any dysfunction of the lower urinary tract

at bedtime. Other methods for reducing reinfection of the lower urinary tract in girls include: intense therapy of any constipation, avoiding bubble bath and detergents in bath water, wiping perineal area from front to back after voiding or defecation, ingesting 1–2 liters of water per day, emptying the bladder every 3–4 h during the day, and wearing cotton rather than nylon underwear.

PERSISTENT URINARY TRACT INFECTION

Failure to eradicate an organism from the urine suggests an anatomic or physiologic defect (Table 12.12). Such patients require continuous antibiotics until the underlying abnormality resolves or is corrected surgically.

INDICATIONS FOR RADIOGRAPHIC EVALUATION

Guidelines for radiographic evaluation of the upper and lower urinary tract following UTI differ among authoritative sources; however a reasonable approach is to evaluate the urinary tract after the first culture-proven infection in all boys and younger girls (Table 12.13). The only exception is for cystitis in older females, especially if sexually active. Renal scarring and damage are most common before 5 years of age in children with recurrent infection associated with anatomic or functional abnormalities. In girls with vesicoureteral reflux, the incidence of renal

scarring is increased 3–4-fold if a second urinary tract infection has occurred prior to recognition and management of reflux.

Cystography, either radiographic or radionuclide, is the only way to detect reflux with certainty. A standard contrast voiding cystourethrogram (VCUG) is preferred for the initial study, especially in males because it best defines the anatomy of the bladder and urethra and detects posterior urethral valves. Renal ultrasound will demonstrate hydronephrosis of one pole or the entire collecting system and will show ureteral dilatation with a high degree of accuracy. If both of these tests are negative, a structural defect is unlikely.

If the child has symptoms of incontinence with or without constipation, a fluorourodynamic study (FUDS) may be done in place of the VCUG. FUDS will elucidate any detrusor or sphincter dysfunction as well as demonstrate reflux and urethral anatomy (Figure 12.1).

Appropriate timing of radiographic studies is variable. A child hospitalized with pyelonephritis should undergo renal ultrasound as early as possible, since results might influence management. A voiding cystogram can be obtained at any convenient time during treatment. Antimicrobial therapy should be continued in therapeutic or prophylactic doses as the radiographic assessment is being performed and evaluated. Any degree of vesicoureteral reflux is sufficient to warrant treatment and long-term observation (Table 12.10). Obtaining the cystogram in closer proximity to the episode of UTI may reveal marginal vesicoureteral reflux, since some

Table 12.11 Antibiotic prophylaxis for recurrent urinary tract infections

Antibiotic	Dosage
Trimethoprim/sulfamethoxazole	2 mg TMP/10 mg SMX/kg per day as a single bedtime dose or 5 mg TMP/25 mg SMX twice per week
Nitrofurantoin	1–2 mg/kg per day div. q.24h
Sulfisoxazole	10–20 mg/kg per day div. q.12h
Nalidixic acid	30 mg/kg per day div. q.12h
Methenamine mandelate	75 mg/kg per day div. q.12h
Amoxicillin	10 mg/kg per day
Cephalexin	15 mg/kg per day

Table 12.12 Factors causing persistent urinary tract infections

Anatomic defects (obstruction or vesicoureteral reflux)
Foreign bodies (catheters, stones)
Dysfunction of the lower urinary tract
Constipation

Table 12.13 Recommendations for radiographic evaluation

Upper urinary tract
  Renal ultrasound
Lower urinary tract
  Radiographic contrast voiding
    cystourethrogram in males
  Contrast voiding cystourethrogram or
    radionuclide cystogram in females
Special studies
  Intravenous pyelography (IVP)
    Anatomical detail
  Dimercaptosuccinic acid (DMSA) scan
    Early diagnosis of pyelonephritis
    Vesicoureteral reflux
    Scar detection
    Assessment of renal function
  Computerized tomography
    Suspected abscesses
  Fluorourodynamic study (FUDS)
    Assess associated lower urinary tract
      dysfunction

children only demonstrate reflux while infected. Renal scintigraphy to confirm pyelonephritis by demonstration of a photopenic area is not necessary unless it would alter the management of the patient.

VESICOURETERAL REFLUX

The path of the ureter through the bladder wall and submucosa follows an oblique course. This configuration creates a flap-valve mechanism which normally prevents the reascent of urine into the upper urinary tract. When the ureterovesical junction is deformed owing to a congenital defect or high bladder pressure, a bladder contraction will cause urine to ascend into the ureter and pelvis. Vesicoureteral reflux therefore allows bacteria access to the kidney. The different configurations of the renal papillae include both simple and compound types. Compound papillae have more circular openings to the collecting ducts, which allow easier access of bacteria into the renal parenchyma.

Vesicoureteral reflux is graded according to the degree of filling of the ureter, renal pelvis and calyces and the presence of dilatation – a scale of I to V has become standard (Figure 12.2). The majority of children will show low-grade reflux (I or II) and 85% of these cases resolve spontaneously over a period of several years. Those children with higher grade reflux show lower rates of resolution. All children with vesicoureteral reflux should initially be maintained on prophylactic antibiotic therapy until the reflux resolves, in order to reduce the risk of renal scarring. In older children who have not demonstrated break-through urinary tract infection, a period of observation without antibiotics may be considered, provided that compliance is optimal. Cystograms with X-ray contrast material or radionuclide agents should be obtained every 1–2 years to monitor the resolution of reflux. Renal growth, as well as any degree of renal scarring, should be assessed on an annual basis with renal ultrasound or radionuclide scanning. Children with recurrent UTI, poor renal growth, progressive renal scarring, or persistent high-grade reflux (IV–V) are candidates for ureteral reimplantation. The inheritance of vesicoureteral reflux has not been defined, but it is a familial disorder. One third of asymptomatic siblings will also have this disorder and should be evaluated for vesicoureteral reflux.

LOWER URINARY TRACT DYSFUNCTION

Bladder dysfunction, as already outlined, may be due to maturational factors, or neurogenic

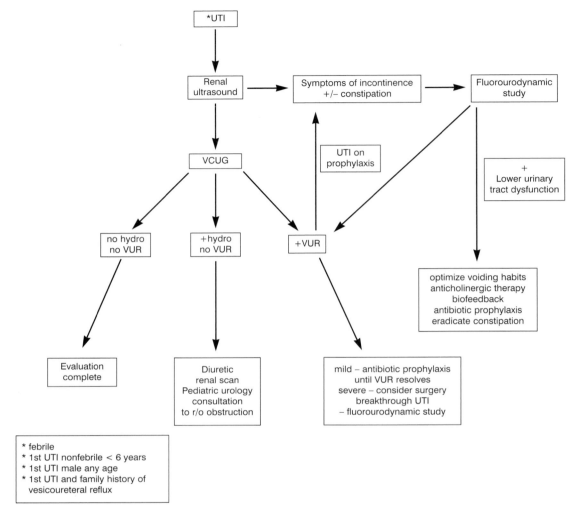

Figure 12.1 Algorithm for the evaluation of initial febrile urinary tract infection (UTI); VCUG, voiding cystourethrogram; VUR, vesicoureteral reflux

disorders, or the dysfunctional elimination syndrome. Children with recurrent UTI should be questioned carefully about voiding habits, daytime incontinence, posturing to defer voiding, or constipation. Unstable bladder contractions should be suspected in children with symptoms of detrusor instability, urgency incontinence, squatting or posturing to defer voiding. Anticholinergic therapy (oxybutinin, propantheline, or imipramine) may be required for long-term control of UTI in addition to prophylactic

antibiotic therapy. Causes of fecal soiling or constipation should also be addressed.

Dysfunctional elimination syndrome is a relatively new term established to describe the interplay between functional constipation and bladder dysfunction, and should be considered in children with recurrent UTI. Any child being evaluated for recurrent UTI should be questioned specifically about bowel habits. No standard definition of constipation exists, but symptoms indicative of constipation include a greater than 72 h interval between

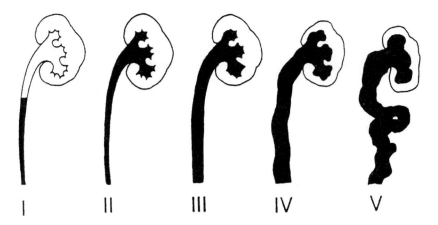

Figure 12.2   The grading of vesicoureteral reflux as defined by the international study classification; blacked-out areas show extent of reflux

bowel movements, encopresis, small hard stools, fecal retention as determined by rectal exam after defecation or the appearance of stool throughout the colon on X-ray. Constipation has been implicated as a major cause of failure of medical treatment of UTI. In addition, constipation has been found to cause uninhibited bladder contractions that result in incontinence or enuresis.

Constipation should be aggressively treated with dietary fiber supplementation. The amount of fiber needed daily can be calculated by the simple formula of grams of fiber needed daily = age + 5, which is approximately 0.5 grams per kg per day. Laxatives, enemas, and reconditioning of normal bowel habits by timed toilet sitting are also used to treat constipation. Progressively, as constipation resolves, medications may be titrated down and eventually discontinued. Physicians should be aware that anticholinergic therapy, which may be used for bladder instability, can predispose to constipation. Several studies have found that successful treatment of constipation can cure recurrent UTI in patients without anatomic abnormalities.

Clean intermittent catheterization

In children with neurogenic bladder dysfunction requiring clean intermittent catheteri-

zation, asymptomatic bacteriuria may persist. In such cases repeated treatment of positive urine cultures in the absence of symptoms may result in selection of progressively more resistant organisms. Treatment should thus be reserved for symptoms of UTI, such as new onset of wetting between catheterizations, fever, or abdominal pain.

URINARY TRACT OBSTRUCTION

Hydronephrosis may be detected on initial ultrasonography following a UTI. If VCUG fails to demonstrate vesicoureteral reflux, a diuretic renal scan should be obtained to assess the degree of obstruction at the ureteropelvic junction (UPJ) or ureterovesical junction (UVJ). When hydronephrosis is detected prenatally, asymptomatic infants with certain categories of milder urinary tract obstruction and good renal function may be observed for spontaneous improvement. Close urologic surveillance with frequent imaging studies of the upper urinary tract and prophylactic antibiotics is recommended. Accurate documentation of any episodes of UTI is essential to determine whether corrective surgery may be required. In patients with severe urinary tract obstruction, sufficient antibiotic concentrations may not be achieved in the urine owing to poor renal function. In such cases, failure to respond to antibiotics suggests the need for retrograde or percutaneous drainage of the infected system.

CANDIDURIA

Immunosuppression, prematurity, debilitation, prolonged antibiotic therapy and catheterization are risk factors for candiduria. Infection may present with tissue invasion or obstruction of the urinary tract secondary to fungus balls. Urine culture containing 10 000 colonies/ml of *Candida* defines significant infection, and visualization of hyphae on urinalysis suggests tissue invasion. Investigation of candiduria consists of ultrasound of the kidneys and bladder to detect any fungus balls. *Candida* spreads to the kidneys hematogenously as well as by ascending infection from the bladder. Asymptomatic candiduria occurs as a consequence of isolated colonization of the urinary tract. Any predisposing factors should be removed and the urine should be alkalinized to a pH of 7.5 because *Candida* grows best in acidic urine.

If candiduria is confined to the bladder, both oral fluconazole and irrigation with amphotericin B (100–300 ml solution, 5–15 mg/100 ml D_5W) have been shown to sterilize the bladder. Removal of an indwelling catheter is required to eradicate *Candida* and intermittent catheterization is an option in patients needing continued bladder drainage. Bladder irrigation should not be performed in the presence of vesicoureteral reflux with high bladder pressures, as systemic absorption of amphotericin B may result. Systemic therapy for *Candida* may be required if multiple sites of infection are documented (Table 12.14). In cases of systemic candidiasis, the renal parenchyma is involved in 88% of cases.

Table 12.14 Treatment of candiduria

Removal or change of catheter
Fluconazole 3–6 mg/kg/day p.o. for 2–5 days
Bladder irrigation with amphotericin B, 5–15 mg/100 ml D_5W
Intravenous antifungal agents
Fluconazole 12 mg/kg/day d.i.v. q.12 h
Amphotericin B 0.3 mg/kg/day i.v. div. q.d. for 2–5 days

PERINEPHRIC AND RENAL ABSCESSES

A renal abscess may be caused by ascending infection of mainly Gram-negative organisms or hematogenous seeding by Gram-positive infections during episodes of bacteremia. Patients present with spiking temperatures, flank pain, abdominal distention, or other abdominal symptoms. Renal abscess is often a difficult diagnosis to make, but it should be considered in cases of prolonged fever refractory to antimicrobial therapy. Computed tomography is the diagnostic test of choice in cases of renal abscess because it delineates the extent of the abscess. Confirmation of a renal abscess warrants continued intravenous antibiotic therapy until full resolution of the abscess is documented by repeat radiographic studies. If there is no concomitant infection in the renal collecting system and the pathogen has not been determined, percutaneous aspiration of the abscess may be performed to obtain a specimen for culture. Failure to respond to continued intravenous antibiotics dictates the need for drainage of the abscess. A cortical abscess may rupture into the perinephric space, and remain confined within the fascia surrounding the kidney. The evaluation and treatment of a perinephric abscess is similar to that of a renal abscess. Multiloculated perinephric abscesses usually require surgical drainage.

Skin and soft tissue infections

13

INTRODUCTION

Skin and soft tissue infections occurring in the normal child are usually easily managed with debridement and good personal hygiene. When therapy is considered necessary, local care (topical) and/or systemic antibiotics are the treatments most commonly used. Persistent or severe infections should alert the physician to the possibility of other underlying conditions.

ACNE

The pathogenesis of adolescent acne involves a combination of sebaceous follicle obstruction, increased sebum production and overgrowth of the common skin bacterium, *Propionibacterium acnes*. Therapy is directed at skin cleansing, drying, removal of comedones, and reduction in bacterial colonization (Table 13.1).

ADENOPATHY

Lymph node enlargement in children may reflect either a localized or a generalized systemic process (Table 13.2). Adenitis (Chapter 6) should be differentiated from adenopathy since etiologies and management vary considerably. Multiple bacteria have been recognized as etiologic agents of adenitis and therapy should be aimed at these organisms (see Tables 6.2 and 6.3). Diagnosis may require needle aspiration or biopsy. When adenopathy is persistent, there are other important diagnostic considerations, both infectious and noninfectious. Most important is ruling out diagnoses where early intervention is of major clinical benefit (Table 13.3).

In persistent adenopathy the primary concern centers around the possibility that an oncogenic process may be the etiology. If the

Table 13.1 Treatment of acne

Initial:
    Topical benzoyl peroxide 2.5% q.d. (morning) or b.i.d.

plus

    Topical antibiotic b.i.d. (morning and afternoon)
        Clindamycin
        Erythromycin
        Tetracycline or
        Meclocycline

After response seen:
    Add tretinoin q.d. (at night before bed)
        0.025% cream or 0.01% gel
    Stop topical antibiotics
    Begin p.o. antibiotics

Inflammatory acne:
    Prednisone 40 mg q.d. for 10 days (or improvement) then 30 mg q.d. for 7 days; decrease 5 mg/wk until 20 mg then 30 mg q.d. decreasing 5 mg q.4 days until off.
    Doxycycline 100 mg q.d. or b.i.d.
    or
    Erythromycin 250–500 mg q.d. or b.i.d.

patient is younger than 8 years of age, leukemia is the most likely malignancy and this can be screened with a simple complete blood count (CBC). If the child is older than 8 years, lymphoma is a possibility and can only be ruled out with a fine needle or excisional biopsy. Before this procedure, other aspects of the differential diagnosis may be evaluated during a 30-day observation period as outlined in Table 13.3.

BLEPHARITIS

Recurrent inflammation of the eyelid margins frequently occurs in persons with poor personal hygiene or hypersensitivity. Complaints include redness, irritation and burning.

Table 13.2 Causes of persistent generalized adenopathy

Infectious
  Tuberculosis (scrofula)
  Infectious mononucleosis
  Cat scratch disease
  Cytomegalovirus
  Toxoplasmosis
  Other viruses
  Tularemia
  Kawasaki disease
  Syphilis
  Hepatitis
  Brucellosis
Noninfectious
  Leukemia
  Lymphoma
  Neuroblastoma
  Other malignancies
  Sarcoidosis

Table 13.3 Approach to persistent adenopathy

Initial evaluation
  History (pertinent exposure)
  Physical examination (measure lymph nodes; if fluctuant see Table 6.3)
  Complete blood count (CBC)
  Bartonella henselae serology (if exposure to kittens)
  Mono spot test (if CBC supportive)
  TB skin test
  Throat culture
  Chest X-ray
  Serum to hold (acute serum)
Initial management (if above laboratory results are negative)
  Penicillin or other p.o. antibiotic for 14 days
  Remeasure node in 14 days
14 days
  Node smaller: no further evaluation
  Node unchanged, larger or additional nodes:
    Serum (convalescent, paired with acute) for EBV, CMV and toxoplasma
30 days (all tests negative)
  Fine needle biopsy
  If not definitive, excisional biopsy

Diagnosis may require culture and scrapings from the inflamed eyelid margins. Gram stains demonstrate polymorphonuclear leukocytes and bacteria (Table 13.4).

Treatment consists of daily debridement with warm, moist compresses and generalized improved personal hygiene. Topical antibiotic ophthalmic drops (sulfacetamide, bacitracin, chloramphenicol, or gentamicin) may be used three to four times per day. Local corticosteroids are employed for allergic blepharitis. Systemic antibiotics are only necessary in resistant cases. For *Pediculus* sp. infestation, remove the parasites and ova with forceps and apply 3% ammoniated mercury ointment or 1% physostigmine ointment four times per day for 7 days. Another alternative is petrolatum, two or three times daily for 7 to 8 days. Other areas of infestation must also be treated.

Table 13.4 Etiologic agents of blepharitis

Staphylococcus aureus
Moraxella lacunata
Pediculus pubis
Pediculus capitis
Demodex folliculorum

ses, bacterial colonization and subsequently deeper invasion occur. Bacterial etiology can be determined by standard culture techniques, but occasionally biopsy is required to obtain meaningful culture material. Causative agents are *Staphylococcus aureus*, *S. epidermidis*, Gram-negative enteric bacteria, *Pseudomonas* and anaerobic organisms; treatment follows Table 13.5.

DECUBITUS ULCERS

Decubitus ulcers occur when soft tissues have suffered prolonged pressure, friction, and shearing force. Pressure over body sites first results in erythema most commonly at the sacrum, heel, ischium or lateral malleolus. Once skin and soft tissue breakdown progres-

EXANTHEMATOUS DISEASES

The exanthematous diseases may be difficult to diagnose. Features to consider include: immunization history, exposure, prodromal period, nature and distribution of rash,

Table 13.5 Treatment of decubitus ulcers

Relieve pressure, friction and shearing force
Remove devitalized tissue, whirlpool for large
    or deep areas
Keep surrounding areas of skin clean and dry
Topical and systemic antibiotics should be
    selected on the basis of culture and sensitivity
    patterns, and used only for more severe cases
Ciprofloxacin plus clindamycin when multiple
    pathogens recovered

Table 13.6 Classification of rashes

Maculopapular lesions
    Miliaria
    Measles
    Rubella
    Scarlet fever
    Enteroviral infection
    Infectious mononucleosis
    Erythema infectiosum
    Exanthem subitum
    Toxoplasmosis
    Kawasaki disease
    Scalded-skin (staphylococcus)
    Meningococcemia
    Rocky Mountain spotted fever and other tick
        fevers
    Typhus
    Toxic erythemas
    Drug eruption
    Sunburn
Papulovesicular lesions
    Varicella-zoster virus infection
    Coxsackie virus infections
    Rickettsialpox
    Disseminated herpes simplex
    Impetigo
    Insect bites
    Gianotti-Crosti syndrome (Hepatitis B in 25%
        of cases)
Petechial lesions
    Rocky Mountain spotted fever
    Meningococcemia
    Ehrlichiosis
    Infectious mononucleosis
    Haemophilus influenzae sepsis
Papular urticaria lesions
    Drug eruptions
    Molluscum contagiosum

diagnostic and pathognomonic signs and laboratory confirmation (Table 13.6).

HORDEOLUM AND CHALAZION

A hordeolum is an infection of the glands of Zeis. Most frequently it results from a staphylococcal infection of the ciliary follicle and associated sebaceous glands. A chalazion is a granulomatous process caused by retention of Meibomian gland secretions. Although it usually resolves spontaneously, excision is occasionally required (Table 13.7).

IMPETIGO

Impetigo is a superficial infection of the skin caused primarily by *Staphylococcus aureus*. Group A streptococcus is also recovered in 20–30% of cases. The localized skin infection may follow minor trauma. Disease first appears as discrete papulovesicular lesions surrounded by erythema which become purulent and form an amber-colored crust. These lesions are only mildly contagious but care must be taken to prevent spread to other individuals (Table 13.8).

Table 13.7 Treatment of hordeolum and chalazion

Hordeolum	Warm compresses
	Topical antistaphylococcal ointment
	Resistant cases may require incision and drainage and systemic antibiotics
Chalazion	Similar to hordeolum but may require excision

Table 13.8 Treatment of impetigo

Careful cleansing with soap and water
Erythromycin 35–50 mg/kg/day div. q.6h
    (maximum 1 g/day) for 10 days
or
Mupirocin ointment q.i.d. for 10 days

LACERATIONS AND PUNCTURE WOUNDS

Trauma to the skin and soft tissues, particularly lacerations or puncture wounds, have the potential of developing secondary bacterial infection. Often the most probable bacterial etiology depends on the nature of the wound and location (i.e. *Staphylococcus* and *Streptococcus* with lacerations and *Pseudomonas* with puncture wounds to the feet). Initial antibiotic therapy depends on assessment as to the most likely organisms, while definitive therapy is guided by culture results. Treatment consists of careful cleansing and removal of foreign material, along with suturing as indicated for cosmetic repair and to prevent fluid collection; antibiotics should only be used if infection occurs, but tetanus prophylaxis should be initiated as indicated.

LUDWIG'S ANGINA

Ludwig's angina is an extensive, rapidly progressing cellulitis of the floor of the mouth and neck. Although rarely seen today, it can be a serious infection leading to sepsis and/or airway obstruction. Culture from needle aspiration is recommended (Table 13.9).

Treatment involves controlling the infection and maintaining an airway. Intravenous antibiotics (penicillinase-resistant penicillin or clindamycin and a third generation cephalosporin) can be used and surgical drainage is indicated if fluctuation is present.

MOLLUSCUM CONTAGIOSUM

Molluscum contagiosum is a disease of the skin caused by a pox virus. It appears that the virus is spread by direct contact, and sexual abuse is one consideration in the infected child. Diagnosis is established by biopsy, stained smears of the expressed molluscum body, or viral cultures. Often no treatment is necessary, as mild cases usually resolve without medical intervention. In more severe cases, extraction or curettage, liquid nitrogen freezing and topical application of cantharidin collodion are appropriate treatments.

MYOSITIS

Myositis is inflammation of a large muscle, which may be preceded by local trauma. Muscle pain is usually the initial symptom, followed by local swelling. Diagnosis may be made by needle aspiration, blood cultures, or muscle biopsy (Table 13.10). The treatment of myositis is determined by the etiologic agent, and is usually systemic penicillinase-resistant penicillin, though nafcillin (or oxacillin) and cephalosporin are alternatives. Incision and drainage may be necessary, with concomitant analgesics as needed.

SCABIES

Sarcoptes scabiei, the itch mite, causes a pruritic rash classically involving the sides and webs of the fingers, flexor surface of the

Table 13.9 Etiologic agents causing Ludwig's angina

Staphylococcus sp.
Pneumococcus sp.
Haemophilus influenzae
Escherichia coli
Pseudomonas sp.
Neisseria sp.
Fusiform bacilli
Anaerobic streptococcus

Table 13.10 Etiology of myositis

Bacteria
Staphylococcus aureus
Group A β-hemolytic streptococci
Viruses
Influenza B
Coxsackie B
Herpes simplex
Parasites
Cysticercosis
Toxoplasmosis
Trichinosis

wrist, elbow, anterior axillary folds, female breasts, abdomen, penis and buttocks. In infants and young children atypical sites, such as the scalp, neck, palms, and soles, may be involved. Identification of the mite in skin scrapings is accomplished by placing a drop of mineral oil on a suspected lesion and scraping the lesion with a scalpel blade. The scrapings are examined under the light microscope.

The patient should shower and shampoo prior to treatment. Apply 5% permethrin (Elimite) cream to the entire body, sparing the face but including the scalp, temple and forehead; rub in gently. It should be left on for 8–14 h and then removed by washing (shower or bath). Repeat treatment is only needed should reinfection occur. Severe (Norwegian scabies) or refractory cases can be treated with a single oral dose of ivermectin (200 µg/kg). Bed linen and clothes need laundering at the start of treatment. All infected family members should be treated simultaneously.

SCROFULA

Tuberculosis of lymph nodes and overlying skin is called scrofula, cervical lymph nodes being most frequently involved. *Mycobacterium tuberculosis* or atypical mycobacteria (*M. kansasii* or *M. marinum*) are commonly identified agents. Scrofula may resolve spontaneously without therapy. The treatment of choice for persistent nodes is excisional biopsy. Specific chemotherapy depends upon the sensitivity of isolated agents. Often these micro-organisms are resistant to standard antituberculous therapy, but clarithromycin, rifampin and ethambutol have been used with some success.

WARTS (VERRUCAE)

Warts or verrucae are a common viral disease of the skin caused by a papovavirus. Transmission is thought to be by direct contact. Spontaneous resolution may occur. Topical application of podophyllin, 40% salicylic acid, 90% trichloroacetic acid, electrodesiccation, or liquid nitrogen freezing are usually effective treatments.

Central nervous system infections

14

BRAIN ABSCESS AND CEREBRITIS

The diagnosis and management of intracranial bacterial suppurative disease has evolved remarkably with the advent of computed tomography (CT), magnetic resonance imaging (MRI), and modern antibiotics. However, brain abscesses, subdural empyema and other suppurative intracranial disorders remain life-threatening and are frequently associated with significantly disabling neurologic deficits. Brain abscesses begin as focal bacterial encephalitis or cerebritis, characterized by neutrophilic infiltration and edema. Over several days fibroblastic proliferation and increased vascularity surround an increasingly necrotic core of liquified brain tissue forming the 'encapsulated' abscess. The source of infection of the abscesses varies, with 25% being hematogenous, 25% related to trauma, and 20% secondary to contiguous spread (otitis media, sinusitis, dental abscess, etc.). Approximately 20% have no apparent predisposing factor. Typically, brain abscesses arising from contiguous spread develop adjacent to the initiating site. Abscesses arising from hematogenous spread frequently occur in areas of middle cerebral artery distribution (namely at the cortical grey–white junction or within the basal ganglia). Factors which may contribute to brain abscess formation are given in Table 14.1.

Brain abscesses present initially with poorly localizable and vague neurologic complaints. Dull headache and low-grade fever associated with predisposing factors are sufficient to clinically raise the suspicion of an intracranial suppurative process. Typical signs and symptoms of brain abscess (Table 14.2) are variable and systemic signs of sepsis may be absent.

Table 14.1   Predisposing factors for brain abscess

Via contiguous spread
  Sinusitis
    Frontal
    Ethmoidal
  Mastoiditis and otitis media
  Trauma
    Cribriform plate fractures
    Middle cranial fossa/basilar skull fractures
      (across mastoid air cells, middle ear, etc.)
    Penetrating head injuries
  Postoperative (neurosurgical)
  Meningitis
  Infections of the face or scalp
  Dental infections
  Congenital anomalies of the skull (e.g.
    encephaloceles)

Via hematogenous spread
  Cyanotic heart disease
    Right-to-left shunts
    Valvular disease
    Septal defects
  Lung disease
    Bronchiectasis
    Lung abscess or empyema
    Rarely, cystic fibrosis
    Drug abuse (i.v.)
    Other distant focus of infection
Immunosuppression
  Steroids
  Antimetabolite therapy
  Congenital immunodeficiency disorders
  Acquired immunodeficiency syndrome
Neonates (particularly with *Citrobacter* meningitis)
Sickle cell disease
Congenital CNS malformations
  Dysraphic sites (myelomeningoceles, neurenteric
    cysts, etc.)
  Sinus tracts associated with dermoids, etc.

The current availability of CT and MRI has dramatically changed the timescale in which brain abscesses are diagnosed and

Table 14.2   Signs and symptoms of brain abscess

Headache
  Poorly localizable
  Dull
  Worsened by Valsalva maneuver or position
    change
Fever
  Prolonged course
  Absent in 30–50% of cases
Expanding mass and increased intracranial
    pressure
  Vomiting
  Somnolence, confusion
  Papilledema (late, and present in < 50% of
    cases)
  Focal signs; aphasia, hemiparesis, ataxia, lower
    cranial nerve findings, focal seizures with or
    without secondary generalization
  Presentations may be either insidious or
    'stroke-like'

treated. Initial confirmation of suspected cases as well as longitudinal follow-up can be achieved with serial CT scans. Ring enhancement does not necessarily correlate with surgical encapsulation. In the early stages of cerebritis (days 1 to 3), focal areas of cortical edema may appear on CT without evidence of contrast enhancement. As the lesion evolves into late cerebritis (days 4 to 9) and early encapsulated phases (days 10 to 13), contrast diffuses into the center of the lesion. After two weeks, CT imaging reveals an enhancing ring and a non-enhancing necrotic center. In all phases, periabscess edema may produce a significant mass effect. CT and MRI also allow accurate localization of abscesses for neurosurgical interventions, including open or guided needle drainage.

Lumbar puncture

Lumbar puncture may be significantly hazardous in patients with brain abscesses or other focal mass lesions. Increased intracranial pressure with focal masses may produce tangential forces which can herniate brain tissue across fixed structures, such as the tentorium cerebelli or other dural surfaces,

when lumbar puncture is performed and cerebrospinal fluid (CSF) removed. In most cases of unruptured brain abscesses, CSF examination does not contribute significantly to the diagnosis. Frequently, few or no inflammatory cells are present and often cultures of CSF do not reveal responsible micro-organisms. The opening pressure at the time of lumbar puncture may be significantly elevated, indicating a potential for subsequent brain herniation.

Radiographs of the skull

Radiographs of the skull contribute very little to the diagnosis of brain abscesses. Occasionally exudate may be detected in the frontal, ethmoid, or sphenoid sinuses. Evidence of mastoiditis may be present. The pineal gland is seldom calcified in children, thus mass shifts across the dura may not be detected.

Echoencephalography and electroencephalography

Echoencephalography and electroencephalography have very little or no current usefulness in the diagnosis and management of brain abscesses. Although electroencephalography may aid in the identification of abscesses, changes are generally non-specific. Localization is better achieved with CT or MRI.

Other studies to be considered for detecting potential predisposing factors or sources of infection in patients with brain abscesses should include echocardiography, which may indicate valvular defects or vegetations. Although a complete blood count (CBC) is routinely performed, it contributes little to the clinical differentiation of brain abscesses. Blood cultures, both for aerobic and anaerobic bacterial and fungal agents such as *Nocardia*, *Candida*, and *Cryptococcus* spp., should be obtained, particularly when valvular heart disease and right-to-left shunts are present. Bacteria responsible for brain abscesses are listed in Table 14.3.

Treatment

Early diagnosis and medical management of brain abscess and other intracranial suppurative lesions are now possible with CT. For this reason, the criteria for surgical intervention have changed. The size and stage of brain abscess encapsulation, amount of edema and mass effect on CT, and the general medical state of the patient often determine which general treatment option is followed (Tables 14.4 and 14.5).

FUNGAL INFECTIONS

Fungal infections of the central nervous system (CNS) may account for both acute and subacute deteriorations in neurologic function, particularly in children with factors predisposing them to opportunistic infections (Table 14.6). Even with a high index of clinical suspicion, the diagnosis of fungal infection is frequently delayed.

Insidious changes in neurologic function, such as unexplained lethargy, psychosis, or irritability, may be the earliest symptoms of fungal infection. More alarming features, including focal or generalized seizures, meningismus, single or multiple cranial neuropathies, hemiparesis and papilledema, occur as fungal diseases progress in the brain. It is crucial that patients be diagnosed early (Table 14.7), partly because of pre-existing and debilitating disorders and, in part, owing to the prolonged therapy with relatively toxic agents that is required following diagnosis. Emphasis must be placed on a high clinical index of suspicion. The typical pathological patterns of fungal CNS infections accounting for the evolution of signs and symptoms in these disorders are quite variable and usually subtle (Table 14.8).

Specific fungal organisms associated with CNS infections are numerous (Table 14.9). Only in unusual circumstances (e.g. mucormycosis), in which orbital and sinus complications are prominent, are characteristic features noted.

Table 14.3 Bacterial organisms causing brain abscess

Common causes
  Anaerobes*
  *Staphylococcus aureus**
  *Streptococcus pyogenes**
  *Streptococcus viridans**
  *Streptococcus pneumoniae**
  Citrobacter sp. (neonates)
  Mycobacterium tuberculosis
Less common causes
  Enterobacter sp.*
  Klebsiella sp.*
  Escherichia coli
  Proteus sp.
  *Staphylococcus epidermidis**
  Haemophilus sp.
  Nocardia sp.
  Listeria monocytogenes
  *Aspergillosis fumigatus**
  *Candida albicans**
  Crytpococcus spp.
Causes of barrier disruption
  Indwelling ventricular reservoir
  External ventriculostomy
  Cranial surgery
  Hyperalimentation
  Loss of cutaneous integrity

*Indicates those organisms more often seen in patients with barrier disruption

Table 14.4 General treatment options in brain abscess management

Broad-spectrum antibiotic therapy i.v. for several days to 2 weeks followed by surgical excision of the encapsulated brain abscess
Needle aspiration of the encapsulated abscess and appropriate i.v. antibiotic therapy determined by cultures of the exudate
Aspiration followed by complete excision and appropriate i.v. antibiotic therapy
Medical management alone with broad-spectrum i.v. antibiotic therapy without surgical intervention unless clinical or CT evidence of deterioration occurs

Table 14.5 Initial empiric antibiotic strategies for the treatment of brain abscess

Predisposing factor	Antibiotics
Uncertain, sinusitis, head trauma, or cyanotic heart disease	Vancomycin 60 mg/kg per day i.v. div. q.6h plus Ceftriaxone 100 mg/kg per day div. q.12h plus Metronidazole 30 mg/kg per day i.v. div. q.8h
Meningitis	Ceftriaxone 100 mg/kg per day div. q.12h or Cefotaxime 200 mg/kg per day i.v. div. q.6h or Guided by organism and sensitivities
Otitis/mastoiditis	Vancomycin plus metronidazole (as above) plus Ceftazidime 225 mg/kg per day i.v. div. q.8h Duration: 21 days minimum; thereafter guided by CT scan

Table 14.6 Factors predisposing children to fungal CNS infections

Primary immunodeficiency
Secondary immunodeficiency
   Corticosteroid therapy
   Antimetabolite therapy (e.g. azothioprine)
   Cytotoxic therapy (e.g. cyclophosphamide)
   AIDS
Chronic disease
   Diabetes mellitus
   Leukemia or lymphoma
   Chronic renal disease
   Cystic fibrosis
Organ transplantation
Intravenous therapy or drug abuse
Hematogenous spread from other foci
   Valvular heart disease
   Primary pulmonary fungal disease
   Primary cutaneous fungal disease
Contiguous spread
   Orbital, sinus, or cutaneous spread (e.g. mucormycosis)

Treatment of fungal infections of the CNS is crucially dependent on early recognition and alleviation of predisposing factors. The most widely used antifungal agents are fluconazole, amphotericin B, liposomal amphotericin B and flucytosine. Amphotericin B, when used intravenously, must be diluted with a 5% dextrose solution to a concentration no greater than 1 mg/10 ml and given as a 4–6 h infusion. Amphotericin B is highly nephrotoxic and has limited CNS penetration when used systemically. For that reason, intrathecally administered amphotericin B is often used, particularly in coccidioidal infections. Added CNS toxicity occurs with intrathecal administration.

When administered orally, flucytosine has excellent penetration into the CNS. The role

Table 14.7 Diagnostic approach to fungal CNS infections

Fungal cultures
    Cerebrospinal fluid (CSF)
    Blood
    Sputum
    Tissue aspirates
CSF analysis
    Cell count
    Glucose
    Protein
    Culture (a large volume of CSF is required)
    Serum and CSF cryptococcal antigen titers
    Special stains (e.g. India ink)
    Immunoglobulin electrophoresis or oligoclonal
      banding
Serum serologic assays
Tissue biopsy for histology and culture
    Meninges
    Brain
    Skin
    Lung

Table 14.8 Tissue reactions to fungal CNS infections

Meningitis; acute, subacute, or chronic
Meningoencephalitis
Abscess; solitary, multiple, or microabscesses
Granulomas
Arterial thrombosis

Table 14.9 Fungal organisms associated with CNS infection

Organism	Infection
Histoplasma capsulatum	Histoplasmosis
Coccidioides immitis	Coccidioidomycosis
Blastomyces dermatitidis	Blastomycosis, North American
Aspergillus fumigatus	Aspergillosis
Candida albicans	Candidiasis
Cryptococcus neoformans	Cryptococcosis (torulosis)
Rhizopus sp.	Mucormycosis
Allescheria boydii	Maduromycosis
Sporothrix schenckii	Sporotrichosis
Nocardia asteroides	Nocardiosis

of flucytosine remains controversial, however, and generally is used in combination with amphotericin B in patients with moderate to severe fungal CNS infections, and in neonates. Recent studies in adult patients with AIDS and cryptococcal meningitis have supported the use of higher dose amphotericin B (0.7 mg/kg/day) in conjunction with fluconazole or itraconazole for better CSF sterilization than with amphotericin B alone.

Fluconazole and itraconazole have selected indications in sensitive fungal invasive infections such as blastomycosis, coccidioidomycosis, histoplasmosis, cryptococcosis, and candidiasis. One may be the drug of choice in certain fungal infections poorly responsive to amphotericin B, including those caused by *Allescheria* sp. In CNS infections intrathecal administration may be required because antifungal agents have poor CNS penetration. Symptomatic care of children with CNS fungal infections includes clinical and laboratory evaluation for the syndrome of inappropriate secretion of antidiuretic hormone (SIADH), insidiously developing hydrocephalus and thrombotic infarctions. Seizures frequently occur and require therapy adapted to impaired renal and hepatic function.

VENTRICULITIS (SHUNT INFECTION)

Shunt obstruction and infection are the most frequent and serious complications following placement of ventriculoperitoneal shunts. As many as 20–40% of shunts ultimately become infected. In particular, shunts placed in neonates and young infants appear highly susceptible. There may also be an increased incidence of ventriculitis in children with hydrocephalus associated with myelomeningoceles (Arnold–Chiari malformation). The presence of intracranial infections or bacteremia are absolute contraindications to initial shunt placement, and frequently neurosurgeons consider any infection, including otitis media, a relative contraindication. In particular, prolonged operative time for shunt placement appears to correlate best with risk of infection. Immediately following shunt placement – and for the first 1–2 months postoperatively – the risk of infection is highest. Skin contamination is the probable source of colonization of the shunt. For this reason, by far the most common infective agent is *Staphylococcus epidermidis* or, less commonly, *Staphylococcus aureus*, diphtheroids and fungal organisms, in particular *Candida* sp. Occasionally Gram-negative bacilli including *Escherichia coli*, *Pseudomonas*, *Klebsiella*, and *Proteus* sp. may cause infection (Table 14.10).

Usually, clinical recognition of shunt infection is not difficult and occasionally the operative incision may appear frankly purulent, erythematous, and indurated. Fever, hypotension, or other clinical signs of sepsis may be present in these cases. Alternatively, shunt infection may occasionally present with abdominal distention and signs of bacterial peritonitis. On the other hand, infection with *S. epidermidis* may be more insidious, with local infection over the shunt incision site the only sign. In either case, shunt infections frequently present with signs and symptoms of shunt malfunction (decompensated hydrocephalus) with or without fever or other signs of infection. Findings of shunt malfunction/infection include lethargy or irritability, papilledema, cranial nerve palsies (especially 6th nerve palsies), impaired upgaze, and cortical spinal tract dysfunction. Pre-existing seizure disorders may worsen with the presence of shunt infection or obstruction.

The examination of CSF by shunt bulb aspiration is the most sensitive and safest procedure for documenting the etiology of shunt infection. Surgically preparing the site of the shunt bulb, and using a 26-gauge needle, permits aspiration of sufficient CSF for Gram stain, bacterial and fungal cultures, chemical analysis and cell count. Alternatively, a lumbar puncture may be performed in those instances where decompensated hydrocephalus is not clinically suspected. However, in the presence of complaints of an individual's typical decompensated hydrocephalus symptoms and physical findings of increased intracranial pressure on examination, lumbar puncture is usually contraindicated secondary to concerns of inducing brainstem herniation. Interval increased ventricle size on non-enhanced CT scans of the brain may aid in the diagnosis of decompensated hydrocephalus. However, the absence of increased ventricle size does not rule out shunt malfunction or infection as up to a third of surgically proven shunt malfunctions do not show interval changes on CT scan. Blood cultures should always be obtained as other abnormal laboratory findings may include prominent leukocytosis.

A difficult problem is the presence of positive cultures of shunt hardware removed electively at the time of surgery in the absence of evidence of CSF infection. At times, these shunt colonizations are considered asymptomatic and no antibiotic therapy may be warranted.

The approach to the treatment of ventriculitis depends somewhat on the causative organism. Traditionally, high-dose i.v. antibiotics combined with immediate shunt removal have been the treatment of choice. In about 15% of cases, high-dose i.v. antibiotics alone are sufficient. The combined approach of intrathecal and intraventricular antibiotics (Table 14.11) alone, or with high dose i.v. antibiotics (Table 14.12) and shunt removal, have also, occasionally, been reported to be successful with reduced neurologic morbidity and mortality.

Initial medical management of shunt infection includes vancomycin i.v. (40 mg/kg per day div. q.6h) pending the return of cultures.

Table 14.10 Bacterial organisms associated with shunt infections

Staphylococcus epidermidis
Staphylococcus aureus
Diphtheroids
Escherichia coli
Pseudomonas sp.
Klebsiella sp.
Proteus sp.
Haemophilus influenzae

Particularly in cases of staphylococcal infection, an adherent and sticky layer of mucus may be embedded on the shunt tubing, preventing total sterilization of the ventricle and shunt system by i.v. antibiotics alone. Where, after the first 48 h of treatment, clinical or bacteriologic improvement is not achieved, it is recommended that i.v. antibiotics be combined with shunt removal. Antibiotic therapy, at this point, should be tailored to the specific culture results and bacteriologic sensitivities (Tables 14.11 and 14.12).

Prophylactic therapy for shunt infections should be routinely used, particularly in those patients most susceptible to infection (e.g. neonates, those with Arnold–Chiari malformation, or debilitated patients). The most popular regimen is vancomycin, one preoperative and one or more postoperative dose(s) of 10 mg/kg. Other suggested prophylactic regimens include antistaphylococcal agents such as oxacillin or nafcillin in doses of 30–50 mg/kg given 2 h preoperatively and then repeated postoperatively. Vancomycin i.v. preoperatively, and rifampin i.v. preoperatively and postoperatively have also been used. No widespread consensus exists regarding recommendations for prophylactic antibiotic therapy. There is widespread agreement, however, that thorough skin preparation, reduced operative time and other aspects of meticulous surgical care minimize the chance of wound and shunt infection.

VIRAL DISEASE OF THE CENTRAL NERVOUS SYSTEM

Viral and postviral neurologic diseases are frequent in pediatric practice. Although the majority of these disorders are benign and self-limited, notable exceptions occur, including herpes encephalitis, some equine encephalitides, postinfectious encephalomyelitis, Guillain–Barré syndrome, and Reye syndrome.

Several viruses that cause meningoencephalitis (Table 14.13) appear clinically

Table 14.11 Intraventricular antibiotics for shunt infection

Antibiotic	Daily dose (mg)*
Amikacin	4–10
Ampicillin	10–25
Carbenicillin	25–40
Cephalothin	25–50
Chloramphenicol	25–50
Gentamicin	2–8
Kanamycin	4–10
Methicillin	25–100
Tobramycin	2–8
Vancomycin	5–20

*Higher dosages for large ventricles (hydrocephalus)

Table 14.12 Intravenous antibiotics for shunt infection*

Staphylococcus epidermidis or *Staphylococcus aureus*
    Nafcillin or oxacillin 200–400 mg/kg per day div. q.6h
    Vancomycin 60 mg/kg per day div. q.6h (for nafcillin-resistant organisms)
Gram-negative coliforms
    Ceftriaxone 100 mg/kg per day div. q.24h
    Cefotaxime 200 mg/kg per day div. q.6h

*Removal of the shunt may be necessary if prompt response to antimicrobial therapy is not obtained

similar. Seasonal occurrence and associated systemic signs and symptoms may suggest a specific viral cause. Endemic causes of encephalitis include Japanese B equine virus (the most common cause of encephalitis outside of the US) and the arboviruses. Sporadic encephalitis is usually caused by the enterovirus group. Equine encephalitis, a mosquito-borne viral disease, typically occurs in the warm months whereas herpes encephalitis is sporadic. The presence of gastrointestinal signs and symptoms may suggest an enteroviral agent whereas upper or lower respiratory tract infections may suggest adenovirus as a potential etiology. CNS infectious and postinfectious disorders may occur with common childhood disorders, such as varicella.

Table 14.13 Viruses associated with meningo-encephalitis

Arboviruses
  St Louis encephalitis
  Western equine encephalitis
  Eastern equine encephalitis
  California encephalitis
  Japanese B equine encephalitis
  Venezuelan equine encephalitis
Enteroviruses
  Polio types 1, 2 and 3
  Coxsackie groups A and B
  Enteric cytopathogenic human orphan
    (ECHO) virus
Herpes viruses
  Herpesvirus types 1 and 2
  Varicella-zoster
  Cytomegalovirus (CMV)
  Epstein–Barr
Miscellaneous viruses
  Mumps
  Measles
  Adenovirus
  Influenza A and B
  Lymphocytic choriomeningitis virus

The clinical signs and symptoms of viral meningoencephalitis are dependent upon the age of the child, severity of illness and, to a lesser extent, the specific viral agent. In general, mental-status changes ranging from coma to delirium, focal or generalized seizures, meningismus and fever, are typical presenting features. Diagnosis is usually confirmed by examination of CSF and exclusion of other bacterial, protozoan, or fungal organisms. Exceptions to this rule are chemical meningoencephalitis and Mollaret's meningitis, the latter being a disorder of recurrent aseptic meningitis of unknown etiology. Routine studies of CSF include measurement of the opening pressure, cell count and differential, protein and glucose determination (with comparison to the serum glucose level), and viral, bacterial and fungal cultures when appropriate. Polymerase chain reaction (PCR) diagnostic testing has been developed to detect a variety of pathogens including herpes simplex virus (HSV)-1,

HSV-2, varicella-zoster virus, JC virus, cytomegalovirus, enterovirus, tuberculosis, and Lyme disease. PCR analysis of the CSF for HSV-1 and -2 has a diagnostic sensitivity and specificity of well over 90%. While the diagnostic accuracy diminishes gradually after 24 h of acyclovir use, PCR may still be useful for up to 10 days of acyclovir use. The use of PCR has replaced the need for brain biopsy, viral culture, or serologic studies to confirm HSV encephalitis. Gram stain of the CSF should be carefully examined. The presence of gross or microscopic blood in CSF suggests the possibility of herpes or equine encephalitis.

Suspicion of herpes encephalitis is heightened by focal seizure activity, hemorrhagic CSF, and a fulminant course over several hours. Electroencephalography often reveals focal epileptiform activity and/or background slowing over the temporal lobes, ipsilaterally or bilaterally. The finding, when present, is not specific to HSV as other viruses and bacteria can affect the brain in a focal fashion. Despite strong clinical suspicion and focal epileptiform activity on EEG, CT findings may remain normal for several days into the clinical course. CT eventually reveals focal edema and possible hemorrhage in unilateral or bilateral temporal and orbitofrontal regions of the brain. T2-weighted MRI is more sensitive for picking up areas of focal edema in patients with encephalitis. MRI reveals edematous changes much sooner and with better delineation than does CT.

In general, treatment of viral meningoencephalitis involves supportive management, whether the patient is hospitalized or followed at home. Complications in treatment are summarized in Table 14.14. Analgesics in selected cases, and fluid and electrolyte therapy are usually sufficient. More fulminant cases of viral meningoencephalitis, in particular herpes encephalitis, may progress rapidly and leave the child with severe morbidity or death. The treatment for herpes encephalitis is acyclovir (30 mg/kg/day i.v. divided q.8h) for 14–21 days. The use of adenine arabinoside requires a significant

Table 14.14 Possible complications of viral meningoencephalitis

---

Acute development of the syndrome of inappropriate secretion of antidiuretic hormone (SIADH)
Vomiting and dehydration
Seizure disorder
Behavior disturbances; hyperactivity, delirium, attention deficits

---

amount of fluid to maintain drug solubility and may worsen some cases of focal cerebral edema associated with the viral encephalitis.

Postviral disorders of the CNS often occur in children recovering from seemingly mild, common viral illnesses. The presence of signs and symptoms of optic neuritis, focal seizure activity, myelitis, ataxia and other motor disturbances such as hemiparesis, monoparesis, or paraparesis suggests this neurologic disorder. The chronologic progression of postviral encephalitis may be insidious or fulminant. In addition to the studies used for the evaluation of acute meningoencephalitis, cerebrospinal immunoglobulin electrophoresis and oligoclonal banding are useful. CT scans, EEG, and the assessment of visual, auditory, and spinal pathways by evoked potentials permit adequate localization and documentation of multiple lesions in the neuraxis. High dose intravenous solumedrol (30 mg/kg/day divided q.6h up to 1 g per day for 3–5 days followed by an oral prednisone taper over 11 days), plasmapharesis and intravenous immune globulin have all been shown to be effective in acute demyelinating conditions (some of which are felt to be postviral), though controlled trials are lacking.

Surgical infections   15

INTRODUCTION

Infection, either endogenous or nosocomial, is a significant factor in the management of surgical care in children. Proper selection of preoperative management, intraoperative judgement and technique, and postoperative care of actual or potential infections can reduce the risk of complications.

A constant flux of new antibiotics may entice the physician into believing that their use alone provides a panacea for all surgical infections. Instead, use of percutaneous or open drainage in consort with antimicrobials should be preferred. Antibiotic choice demands a comprehensive knowledge of the signs and symptoms of common surgical infectious processes and their probable etiologies.

GENERAL PRINCIPLES

The development and progression of surgical infections require a colonizing organism, an appropriate nutritional milieu for that organism and lack of an appropriate host defense. The number of pathogens and their virulence affects the infectious potential of an inoculum although chronologic and species interactions will affect the gravity of a surgical infection, particularly in cases of aerobic–anaerobic synergism (e.g. *Escherichia coli* and *Bacteroides fragilis*). In addition, nutritional status, length of preoperative stay, perioperative cleansing and skin preparation, duration of the procedure, the immunologic status of the child and the use of cautery will significantly affect the incidence of infection.

Endogenous infections originate from altered skin or mucosal barriers. Bacterial translocation from the gut occurs following phagocytic ingestion of bacteria in the gut, lymphatic transport of these viable bacteria to extraintestinal tissue, and generation of sepsis from that locus. Although, historically, gut rest following accidental or operative trauma has been strongly advocated, clearly mucosal damage and subsequent microbial translocation can be prevented by early enteral diet. There is increased risk for translocation following prolonged shock, prolonged fast, protein malnutrition and total parenteral nutrition thus mandating an enhanced awareness of patient nutrition. Glutamine-supplemented diets decrease bacterial translocation and infection, while short-chain fatty acids from fermentable fiber decrease colonic mucosal atrophy and omega-6 polyunsaturated fatty acids promote survival of sepsis in animal models.

Preoperative hospital stay must be minimized. Preoperative shaving is deleterious and should be abandoned as a practice. Treating remote infections before operation reduces surgical infection risk. Personnel should wash their hands before and after taking care of a surgical wound. The surgeon should not directly touch a fresh wound or drainage without the use of sterile gloves. Any wound drainage should be cultured and examined with Gram's stain. Rigid aseptic technique and rapid but careful completion of the operation provide the greatest protection against postoperative infection. Despite these precautions, high rates of infection may occur without antimicrobial use. Seventy-five per cent of antibiotic orders on a surgical service, both appropriately and inappropriately, are for prophylaxis in an effort to improve outcome.

PROPHYLAXIS

Parenteral antimicrobial prophylaxis is recommended for operations associated with a high risk of infection or not frequently associated with infections but with severe or life-threatening consequences should they occur. Antimicrobials should be safe and effective for prophylaxis against organisms likely to contaminate the operative wound. Antimicrobial prophylaxis is initiated before the procedure – ideally 0–2 hours before – and promptly discontinued after the operation. Oral prophylactic antibiotics should not be used to supplement parenteral prophylaxis. Oral antibiotics are, however, used as prophylaxis for colorectal surgery to decrease the bacterial colony count in the gut flora for the purpose of minimizing potential exposure in the operating field. Their use should be limited to the 24 h period before operation.

Initial drug dosages should provide peak levels near to the maximum acceptable serum range. There are many suitable antibiotic choices but dosing, appropriate intervals, and maintaining appropriate blood levels are essential for maximum efficacy. The recommended dosages are detailed in Chapter 20. Recommendations must balance potential benefit againt the risk of complications, including allergy, toxicity, and creation of drug-resistant bacteria. Prophylactic antimicrobials are to be used only if the risk of infection outweighs the risk of complications. Risk of surgery can be quantitated by classification of operative procedures (Table 15.1).

A classification-specific wound infection rate should be surveyed for all operations. Clean procedures do not require prophylaxis unless the risk of infection during surgery is life-threatening. Prophylactic antibiotics are used in procedure classification clean/contaminated or higher.

Antibiotics given to patients whose wounds are classified as dirty and infected are strictly therapeutic, not prophylactic. Although guidelines are unclear, discontinuation of therapeutic antibiotics after the patient is clinically improved and afebrile for a minimum of 48 h is an acceptable use of these agents. Conversely, the child who remains ill and febrile is seldom likely to be helped by

Table 15.1 Classification of operative procedures

Clean
  Nontraumatic
  Noninflammatory
  No break in technique
  Respiratory, genitourinary, gastrointestinal
    tract not entered
Clean/contaminated
  Minor break in technique
  Oropharynx entered
  Respiratory or gastrointestinal tract entered
    without significant spillage, i.e.
    appendectomy, colorectal surgery with prior
    oral antibiotic therapy for gut flora
    prophylaxis
  Biliary tract entered (without infected bile) i.e.
    cholecystectomy for cholelithiasis or treated
    cholecystitis
  Vagina entered
  Genitourinary tract entered (without infected
    urine)
Contaminated
  Major break in technique
  Fresh traumatic wound
  Gross gastrointestinal spillage
  Biliary tract entered (infected bile) i.e.
    cholangitis
  Genitourinary tract entered (infected urine)
Dirty
  Bacterial inflammation encountered
  Transection of clean tissue for access to
    purulence
  Traumatic wound from 'dirty' source
  Traumatic wound with retained devitalized
    tissue, foreign body and/or fecal
    contamination
  Perforated viscus

unguided changes in antibiotics and there is no rationale for conversion to oral therapy to allow discharge.

WOUND INFECTION

Children have a lower incidence of wound infection than adults; however, a substantial number still occur. Surgical wounds are considered to be noninfected if there is no discharge during healing and infected if there is discharge of pus. Inflamed wounds or culture-positive serous fluid may signify infection. Criteria for infection generally exclude stitch abscess. Clean wound infection rates should be less than 1.5%. This rate may exceed 40% in contaminated or dirty cases. The lower incidence of wound infection in children is probably due to the fact that their delicate tissues require gentle handling, operations are brief, and postoperative stay is brief, reducing nosocomial infections. Wound infection rates are highest for abdominal operations and lowest for those on the extremities. Sutures themselves are foreign bodies; however, absorbable monofilament sutures without interstices provide the least nidus for bacteria. Although leaving the skin open in contaminated cases is advocated for adult patients, the technique need not be used in most pediatric wound infections. For example, most pediatric surgeons today primarily close all wounds in patients with perforated appendicitis.

Wound infection may occur as early as the first postoperative day up until many weeks after operation (Table 15.2). Group A streptococcus infection presents with rapidly advancing erythema and serous drainage. It is often unnecessary to immediately open the wound, but high dose intravenous penicillin or cefazolin should be given and if there is not the expected immediate improvement, the wound must be opened. Clostridia related cellulitis presents with pain, foul smelling exudate, and skin crepitus from subcutaneous emphysema and can rapidly progress to widespread necrotizing fasciitis. In addition to rapid institution of penicillin and clindamycin, a surgeon must open the wound and prepare for possible wide incision and debridement. Staphylococcal infection occurs 3–7 days after operation with gradual onset of fever, tenderness, induration, swelling and erythema. Palpation may elicit drainage but if not, the wound should be gently separated, all sutures removed, the wound irrigated with saline, and packed with saline damp to dry dressings. Use of iodoform-impregnated gauze for packing primary or secondary-infected wounds can cause wound-edge cytotoxicity and is thus far without definable benefit.

Infections caused by enteric bacteria occur from one to many weeks after operation. Erythema is limited, suppuration less prominent, and drainage watery-brown and foul smelling. Besides local signs, there is often systemic toxicity and an intra-abdominal source should be aggressively sought for where applicable.

SURGICAL WOUND INFECTION

The most common use of antibiotics in hospitals is surgical prophylaxis. Abundant

Table 15.2 Characteristics of wound infections

Organism	Onset (days)	Signs	Therapy
Streptococcus	< 1–2	Rapid spread of erythema and cellulitis	Penicillin G
Clostridia	< 1–2	Erythema, brown foul smelling drainage, skin crepitus	Penicillin G, clindamycin
Staphylococcus	4–7	Crepitus	Open, debride and pack wound
		Erythema, tenderness, cellulitis, purulent drainage	Oxacillin or nafcillin if cellulitis severe
Enteric Gram-negative	7–14	Induration, seropurulent drainage, systemic toxicity	Open, debride and pack wound
			Broad-spectrum antibiotics if cellulitis or toxicity severe

randomized clinical trials have well demonstrated their benefit. This includes clean, clean contaminated, contaminated, or infected surgical procedures. Major shortcomings are risk of drug toxicity, emergence of resistant organism, and superinfections. Chemoprophylaxis should be initiated before the surgical procedure for maximum efficacy so that peak serum levels are achieved during the operation and for a short time after. The duration of antibiotic administration should not exceed 48 h. Most surgical procedures require specific regimens directed at pathogens previously shown to cause postoperative infection (Table 15.3).

HIV, HEPATITIS B, AND SURGERY

Hepatitis B virus (HBV) and human immunodeficiency virus (HIV) remain threats to the operating surgeon's career and health. When healthcare workers follow recommended infection control procedures, the risks of acquiring disease from patients or transmitting these viruses to patients are quite small. Strict adherence to universal precautions, including the appropriate use of handwashing, protective barriers, and care in the use and disposal of needles and other sharp instruments, is essential. The recent mandatory use of needleless systems in many

Table 15.3   Recommended antimicrobial prophylaxis for certain surgical procedures

Surgical procedure	Prophylactic antibiotic
Tonsillectomy and adenoidectomy	No available data
Tympanostomy	Gentamicin eardrops
Cleft palate repair	p.o. TMP/SMX, sulfisoxazole, or ampicillin
Major head and neck surgery	i.v. cefazolin, ampicillin, or gentamicin plus clindamycin
Eye surgery	Gentamicin or tobramycin ophthalmic drops or cefazolin subconjunctival injection
Cardiovascular prosthetic implant	Cefazolin; vancomycin for methicillin resistant staphylococcus
Cardiothoracic and vascular surgery	i.v. cefazolin, oxacillin, or vancomycin
Inguinal hernia repair	No available data
Appendectomy	i.v. cefoxitin, cefazolin, or metronidazole
Colon surgery	Cefoxitin; gentamicin for ampicillin resistant enteric Gram-negative bacteria
Gastroduodenal surgery	i.v. cefazolin
Biliary tract surgery	i.v. cefoxitin; gentamicin for ampicillin resistant enteric Gram-negative bacteria
Elective splenectomy	Pneumococcal vaccine before the procedure
Penetrating abdominal trauma	i.v. cefoxitin
Urinary tract obstruction	p.o. TMP/SMX, ampicillin, or nitrofurantoin
Ruptured viscus	Aztreonam or mezlocillin or ampicillin/sulbactam plus metronidazole; aztreonam or gentamicin plus mitronidazole if penicillin resistant organisms identified
Abortion	
First trimester	i.v./i.m. penicillin G or p.o. doxycycline
Second trimester	i.v. cefazolin, i.v./i.m. penicillin G, or p.o. metronidazole
Orthopedic surgery	i.v. cefazolin or vancomycin
Cerebrospinal fluid shunting	i.v. cefazolin, oxacillin, or TMP/SMX procedures
Gastrostomy	i.v. cefazolin, vancomycin, or clindamycin
Burns	i.v. or p.o. penicillin plus 0.5% silver nitrate or 10% afenide acetate cream
Skin surgery	Cefazolin; penicillin; vancomycin if methicillin resistant *S. aureus* identified

hospitals has reduced the incidence of sharp instrument-related exposures. Open dermatitis should restrict the surgeon from patient care and handling of equipment and devices used in performing basic procedures until the condition resolves. Surgeons infected with HIV or HBV (HB$_S$Ag-positive) should not perform exposure-prone procedures without advice from an expert review panel.

BURNS

Infection in children with burns results from multiple systemic and local factors. Endogenous organisms grow easily in the burn eschar and invasion of viable tissue with subsequent systemic infection can follow. Fever is very common in the first three days following the burn and, therefore, only persistent hyperpyrexia (> 39.5°C) is considered abnormal. Observation of such children for changes in clinical behavior (e.g. increasing fever, poor appetite, or decreased sensorium) will optimize early recognition. Sepsis presents with hypothermia or hyperthermia, tachypnea, mental changes, oliguria, ileus, and hypotension. Crystalloid infusion, ventilatory support, and inotropes (along with antibiotic therapy against cultured organisms) are the cornerstones of sepsis management. Children with recurrent bacteremia should be examined for otitis media, urinary tract infections, tracheobronchitis, pneumonia, and cellulitis and treated accordingly.

Timely closure of the burn wound by excision and grafting with interim protection by topical antimicrobials are the essentials of burn wound treatment and will prevent most infections. The initial step is twice daily application of manfenide acetate owing to its increased eschar penetration. Tangential excision and perioperative vancomycin will minimize colonization by staphylococci. Gram-negative infections should be additionally treated with appropriate culture-guided antibiotics. *Pseudomonas* infection is best managed by subeschar injection of broad-spectrum β-lactam penicillin before operation (i.e. piperacillin sodium 200–300 mg/kg in 50 ml of saline).

Approximately two-thirds of burn wound infections are now of fungal origin (*Candida* sp. 25%, aspergillosis 15%, mucormycosis 8%, and other fungi 19%). Histologic biopsy examination is the most reliable means for diagnosis of fungal infections. Excision of involved tissue usually eliminates *Candida* and *Aspergillus*. Phycomycetes, however, cross tissue planes, have vascular invasion, and produce expanding necrosis. Systemic acidosis favors dissemination of fungi and must be treated to control fungal infection. Wounds should be widely excised and most patients treated with amphotericin B or fluconazole.

SOFT TISSUE INFECTION

Risk factors (other than burns) for soft tissue infection are listed in Table 15.4.

Table 15.4 Risk factors for soft tissue infection

Risk factor	Infection
Diabetes	All
Cancer, congenital agranulocytosis	*Clostridium septicum* gangrene
Omphalitis, urachal cyst, necrotizing enterocolitis, neonatal monitoring devices, varicella, circumcision, anorectal disease	Necrotizing fasciitis, Fournier's gangrene
Outdoor puncture wounds	Tetanus
Chronic immunosuppression i.e. transplant recipient, AIDS	All

SPECIAL INFECTIONS

Progressive bacterial synergistic gangrene

Progressive bacterial synergistic gangrene follows abdominal or thoracic wounds with contaminated foreign bodies or sutures. Necrotic ulcers with purple skin and erythema enlarge slowly, but progressively. Wide local excision usually cures the process.

Synergistic necrotizing cellulitis

Synergistic necrotizing cellulitis occurs in diabetics, particularly those with perineal infections. Tenderness and ulceration with vesicles containing so-called 'dishwater' pus in a toxic patient with diabetic ketoacidosis is the usual clinical setting. Skin may appear nearly normal and gas in underlying tissues occurs late in the disease. Anaerobic streptococcus and aerobic Gram-negative rods are causative. Fluid resuscitation, appropriate broad-spectrum antibiotic coverage, and radical debridement constitute optimal management.

Fournier's gangrene

Fournier's gangrene is necrotizing fasciitis of the genitalia. It frequently follows trauma or contaminated operations, initially presenting with decreased sensation, swelling, necrosis, and wound drainage. Polymicrobial etiology, particularly streptococci and enterobacteriaceae, is most likely. Dusky discoloration of the skin indicates impending gangrene. Diabetics are more prone to this infection. It may also follow circumcision, insect bites, or burns. Appropriate broad-spectrum antibiotics and radical debridement are necessary.

Clostridial cellulitis

Clostridial cellulitis presents with pain, swelling, foul-smelling exudate, and subcutaneous emphysema but with little systemic toxicity. Erythema and serosanguinous discharge progress to give bronzed skin with vesicles and crepitation. Underlying fascia and muscle have extensive necrosis. Wide debridement and high-dose penicillin are usually effective.

Clostridial myonecrosis

Clostridial myonecrosis (gas gangrene) is associated with diabetes, necrotic tissue, and arterial compromise. Infections of extremities have a better prognosis because of the option for amputation. Physical findings include tachycardia, severe local pain (disproportionate to the appearance of the wound), systemic toxicity, erythema and discharge. High-dose penicillin is the antibiotic of choice.

Clostridium septicum infection occurs in leukemia, chemotherapy, lymphoma, and congenital agranulocytosis. This organism is more aerotolerant than other clostridial pathogens. Its mode of invasion is translocation across the bowel wall in the absence of neutrophils. Treatment includes bone marrow-stimulating growth factors, aggressive resuscitation, and debridement with high-dose penicillin and clindamycin as the antibiotics of choice.

CARDIAC SURGERY

Patients undergoing open heart surgery, especially with placement of prosthetic heart valves or prosthetic intravascular or intracardiac materials, are at risk for bacterial endocarditis. Endocarditis associated with open heart surgery is most often due to *Staphylococcus aureus*, coagulase-negative staphylococci, or diphtheroids. Streptococci, Gram-negative bacteria, and fungi are less common. Penicillinase-resistant penicillins or 'first-generation' cephalosporins are most often selected, although the choice of antibiotic should be influenced by each hospital's antibiotic susceptibility data. Prophylaxis should be started immediately before the operative procedure and continued for more than 2 days postoperatively to minimize the emergence of resistant micro-organisms. The effects of cardiopulmonary bypass and compromised postoperative renal function on serum antibiotic levels should be considered and doses timed appropriately before and during the procedure.

CHEST INFECTION

Mediastinitis

The limits of the mediastinum are the medial pleura, the sternum, and the vertebral column. Contamination of the mediastinal space occurs by accidental or operative trauma or from spillage from adenopathy. Prompt surgical drainage is usually necessary to control serious infection, and continuous antibiotic irrigation can be used to supplement systemic broad-spectrum antibiotics which provides coverage for Gram-positive and Gram-negative bacteria. Granulomatous infections including tuberculosis and histoplasmosis can cause superior vena cava syndrome or obstruction of the trachea and esophagus secondary to direct compression or fibrosis. The features and management of mediastinitis are summarized in Table 15.5.

Empyema

The antibiotic era has gradually changed the causal factors, incidence, and seriousness of

Table 15.5 Features and management of mediastinitis

Symptoms
Pain
Dyspnea
Tachycardia
High fever
Radiographic signs
Mediastinal and/or subcutaneous emphysema
Mediastinal widening
Mediastinal air/fluid levels
Pericardial effusion on echocardiography
Organisms
Gram-positive cocci
Anaerobes
Treatment
Prompt drainage
Ticarcillin/clavulanate

empyema. Pleural fluid should be aspirated for culture and determination of character. Analysis for pH, white blood cell count, protein level, glucose, lactate dehydrogenase (LDH) and culture should be performed. Empyema must be regarded as an abscess and treated as such by complete evacuation of purulent material. Following thoracentesis or tube thoracotomy, the patient's clinical condition rather than radiography should guide therapy. The early use of thoracotomy, or preferably thoracoscopy with decortication should be considered if a patient with empyema has persistent difficulty in respiration, multiple loculations with pleural thickening, a febrile course, or persistent leukocytosis despite the use of drainage and antibiotics. In addition, empyemas in children with multiple organisms, immunocompromise, an infradiaphragmatic source, or those with empyema secondary to aspiration pneumonia can benefit from decortication if lesser measures are not rapidly effective. Antibiotic therapy for pneumonia-associated empyemas is outlined in Table 15.6.

Pulmonary abscess

Pulmonary abscess follows cavitation of suppurative lung infections. Very young, immunocompromised, or chronically ill children are most frequently affected. Precipitating factors may include aspiration, operation, or coma. *Staphylococcus* is the most frequently involved organism and α- and β-hemolytic streptococci, *Pseudomonas*, *Escherichia coli*, and *Klebsiella* are also seen. Careful bacteriologic examination for anaerobic organisms may yield *Peptostreptococcus*, *Peptococcus*, *Bacteroides melaninogenicus*, or *Bacteroides fragilis*. The empiric choice of antimicrobial therapy is penicillin G, or clindamycin for those with allergy. Antibiotics must be continued for six weeks. Bronchoscopic aspiration of contents will allow additional assessment of anatomic pathology, including retained foreign body examination. Lobectomy with thoracostomy drainage may be needed for chronic thick-walled abscesses which have

Table 15.6 Antibiotic therapy for pneumonia-associated empyemas

Organism	Age	Radiologic findings	Treatment
Staphylococcus	< 1 year	Patchy bronchopneumonia	Penicillinase-resistant penicillin
Streptococcus	3–5 years	Diffuse bronchopneumonia	Penicillin
			Ceftriaxone
Haemophilus influenzae	3 months to 3 years	Lobar pneumonia	Ceftriaxone
			Cefotaxime

not responded to 2 weeks of medical management.

ABDOMINAL INFECTION

Peritonitis

Following inflammation or perforation of the gastrointestinal tract, both a chemical and bacterial insult are introduced into the peritoneal cavity. Leukocyte and macrophage congregation into a fibrinopurulent serosal exudate and migration of the omentum usually convert generalized peritonitis into an abscess. Abdominal pain is the response to chemical irritation and cytokine release. This pain, although initially localized, soon spreads throughout the abdomen. A profound ileus with decreased bowel sounds and vomiting often occur. There is also abdominal guarding and rebound tenderness. The child with peritonitis usually appears toxic and third spacing causes vascular depletion. Fluid repletion and appropriate antibiotics with coverage for *Escherichia coli* and other coliform organisms, enterococcus, and *Bacteroides fragilis* should be provided (Chapter 20).

Appendicitis

Appendicitis is the most common surgical problem of the abdomen in children. At least 40% of cases in the pediatric age group have complicated forms of appendicitis. A typical presentation begins with a 'seasick' feeling followed by periumbilical pain, and subsequent right lower quadrant pain. Anorexia, nausea, vomiting, and fever may accompany the process. Persistent right lower quadrant tenderness is the most reliable indication of appendicitis. As simple appendicitis is impossible to differentiate from the more complex forms, intravenous fluid repletion and administration of antibiotics (i.e. cefoxitin) should precede operation (Table 15.7). A single preoperative dose is sufficient for negative exploration or simple acute appendicitis. If perforation has occurred, most authorities would recommend more generalized coverage consistent with gastrointestinal perforation elsewhere in the tract. The length of coverage in these cases is dependent on resolution of fever, leukocytosis, and symptoms.

Stomach and small bowel infection

The stomach and proximal small bowel have low concentrations of organisms and these are generally not pathogenic. However, hypo- or achlorhydria induced by prior operation, H_2 blockers or omeprazole, or intestinal obstruction permits polymicrobial bacterial overgrowth more characteristic of the terminal ileum and colon. Surgical intervention under these circumstances, as well as with associated obesity, malnutrition, high risk of contamination, immunocompromise, or presence of ventricular peritoneal shunt within the abdomen, requires prophylaxis with a first generation cephalosporin. Cefoxitin is the preferred choice for distal small bowel procedures.

Necrotizing enterocolitis

Although we are now approaching thirty years of management of necrotizing enterocolitis (NEC), the precise pathophysiology remains debatable. It occurs in 1 in 400 births and 2% of admissions to neonatal intensive care units (typically in stressed, prematurely born babies during the first two weeks of life). Initial findings include high gastric residuals, abdominal distention, vomiting, diarrhea, lethargy, apnea, bradycardia, poor perfusion, and blood per rectum. Pneumatosis cystoides intestinalis is the radiographic herald of NEC. There are multiple associated factors but nearly all neonates are found to have been fed. Many fecal organisms have been recovered but only enterotoxic *Escherichia coli* are associated with clusters. Clostridia-positive neonates have fulminant and highly lethal disease. The child culture-negative for *Clostridium* sp. can often be treated with medical therapy alone (nearly 90%). When diagnosis of NEC is entertained, the child is placed n.p.o., on gastric suction, and given ampicillin, an aminoglycoside, and metronidazole. Stool cultures may help identify abnormal flora. A summary of features of necrotizing enterocolitis and therapy is given in Table 15.8.

Elective colon surgery

The colon has 10^{11}–10^{13} bacteria/mm^3, with colonization occurring within hours of birth. A vigorous mechanical preparation with Go-Lytely® (30 ml/kg/h for 4 h) the day before operation can significantly reduce the bacterial count (to < 10^5/mm^3 ideally). Cefoxitin is used for elective prophylaxis. Combination broad-spectrum antibiotics should be used for fecal contamination.

Anorectal infection

The inherent resistance to infection of anorectal tissue means that special bowel preparations are not indicated for perianal

Table 15.7 Antibiotic use in appendicitis

Stage	Antibiotic	Duration
Normal or simple	Cefoxitin	1 dose preoperatively
Suppurative	Cefoxitin	1 dose preoperatively plus 2 doses postoperatively
Gangrene, perforation, or abscess	Mexlocillin, imipinem or aztreonam plus Metronidazole	Until afebrile, normalization of leukocytosis and resolution of symptoms; average 5 days

Table 15.8 Features of necrotizing enterocolitis and therapy

Signs
  Lethargy
  Thermolability
  Poor perfusion
  Increased gastric aspirate
Radiologic findings
  Pneumatosis cystoides intestinalis
Therapy
  Fluid and electrolyte repletion
  n.p.o.
  Gastric decompression
  Antibiotics (aminoglycoside, ampicillin, and metronidazole); average 10 days
  Nutritional support
  Operation for pneumoperitoneum, peritonitis, abdominal mass, fixed bowel loop on radiograph, uncorrectable acidosis, or positive findings on paracentesis

operations. However, cefoxitin should be used for prophylactic coverage. Perirectal infections occur with folliculitis in the very young infant and, in the slightly older infant, owing to malformation of the anal crypts with resulting persistent 'fistula-in-ano'. Recurrent perianal abscesses should be treated by fistulectomy or fistulotomy.

Biliary infection

Biliary atresia

Biliary atresia is the progressive obliteration of bile ducts in the newborn. Prompt diagnosis of infants presenting with direct hyperbilirubinemia beyond two weeks of age permits long-term survival after portoenterostomy. Prophylactic antibiotics for supressive therapy are continued indefinitely (Table 15.9). Cholangitis prompted by cholestasis and bacterial contamination from the intestinal conduit presents with fever, leukocytosis and jaundice. Bile quantity and concentration decrease if the conduit is external. Liver function deteriorates with each attack and cessation of bile flow can occur. Empiric, broad-spectrum, intravenous antibiotic therapy along with tapering dosages of methylprednisolone should be started when symptoms are first recognized. Imipenem/cilastatin or other drugs should be continued for a minimum of five days. Steroids act by increasing both bile acid-dependent bile flow and anti-inflammatory effect, thus reducing edema at the anastomosis. Failure of response to medical management within several days should prompt consideration for revision of the biliary conduit.

Gallbladder disease

Gallbladder disease in children consists of hydrops, acalculous cholecystitis, and cholelithiasis of hemolytic or cholesterol origin. Scarlet fever, Kawasaki disease, severe diarrhea, leptospirosis, familial Mediterranean fever, mesenteric adenitis, sepsis, typhoid fever, salmonellosis, a postoperative state, serious trauma, or extensive burns are

Table 15.9 Biliary atresia cholangitis

Signs
Fever
Leukocytosis
Decreased bile flow
Increased bilirubin
Suppression
Amoxicillin for first year of life;
Trimethoprim/sulfamethoxazole thereafter
Therapy
Imipenem/cilastatin
Steroids

associated processes causing hydrops of the gallbladder and acalculous cholecystitis. Cholecystectomy or cholecystostomy may be necessary and should be managed prophylactically with cefoxitin.

Hemolytic disorders cause bilirubinate stones, and cholecystectomy for symptomatic children requires cefoxitin coverage. Hemoglobin S levels must be below 30% before elective operation in children with sickle cell disease. Nonspecific abdominal pain is the herald for cholesterol cholelithiasis and ultrasonography defines the disease. Cholecystectomy requires cefoxitin prophylaxis.

Hepatic abscess

Hepatic abscess may be amebic or pyogenic. In the United States amebic abscess occurs most often in Hispanic males. *Entamoeba histolytica* titers of at least 1:512 are diagnostic. Treatment with metronidazole plus iodoquinol (Chapter 10) is appropriate. Antibiotics, percutaneous catheter drainage, open drainage, or a combination of these modalities are proper therapies for primary hepatic abscess or superinfection of an amebic abscess. Antibiotics are used to treat undrainable multiple microabscesses. Cefotaxime, metronidazole, and an extended penicillin (i.e. ticarcillin) are usually adequate therapy.

Trauma

Abdominal trauma

In cases of intestinal perforation following abdominal trauma, bacterial contamination is present at the time of antibiotic administration. However, lesser therapy is necessary than for patients with longer established peritonitis, as the interval before treatment is shorter than for other causes. Antibiotics must be given preoperatively and in proper dosage to cover aerobic cocci, especially enterococcus, anaerobic organisms and Gram-negative rods. Second or third generation cephalosporins are effective in preventing intra-abdominal abscesses and wound infection following abdominal exploration for penetrating abdominal wounds. Multiple studies show that there is no advantage in giving antibiotics for more than two days. Other drug combinations such as ticarcillin/clavulanate, mezlocillin, or ampicillin/sulbactam are also effective.

Splenic trauma

Splenectomy is associated with overwhelming operative post-splenectomy sepsis (OPSS) and is characterized by bacteremia with meningitis or pneumonia. The mortality is nearly 50% even in this day of multi-agent antibiotics. The usual causes are pneumococcus (50%), *Haemophilus influenzae* (30%), and meningococci (10%). There is no increased risk for viral, fungal, or mycobacterial infection. The greatest risk for bacterial infection following splenectomy is seen in the following cases: patients under 2 years of age, Wiskott–Aldrich syndrome, thalassemia, and during the first 2 years following splenectomy for trauma. Loss of the spleen causes loss of its dual function as a filter for bacteria and as a locus for antibody production. Nonoperative management, partial splenectomy, or splenorrhaphy can avoid the need for spleen removal in approximately 90% of instances of traumatic rupture of the spleen. Splenic function can then be most conveniently followed by looking for Howell–Jolly bodies, which are present in at least 50% of patients with functional asplenia.

Pneumococcal, *Haemophilus*, and meningococcal vaccination should precede elective splenectomy in children. Currently, recommendations for antibiotic prophylaxis reflect the experience gained with sickle cell disease. Prophylaxis with oral penicillin V is recommended for all asplenic children under 5 years of age (125 mg b.i.d.) and for older children (250 mg b.i.d.). Children under 2 years of age responded poorly to pneumococcal polysaccharide vaccine; therefore, it was not previously recommended. However, the newer conjugate pneumococcal vaccine is effective in children as young as 2 months of age and is now recommended not only for asplenic patients but routinely in all patients.

Antibiotic prophylaxis is most important in this high-risk group. If a patient presents with a high index of suspicion for overwhelming postsplenectomy sepsis, initial treatment should include antibiotics effective against streptococcus, *Neisseria meningitidis* and β-lactamase-producing *H. influenzae* type B.

POSTOPERATIVE FEVER

Fever is a common complication following operation. Identification of the pyrogenic source (Table 15.10) begins with physical examination. A pre-existing disease process can present in the postoperative period. If the patient has had an inflammatory process preoperatively, bacteremia from manipulation of the infected source can cause a vigorous postoperative fever. Continuation of preoperative and intra-operative antibiotics and antipyretics is the appropriate response.

Atelectasis is the usual cause of fever beginning in the 24 h following operation. Preoperative instruction in the use of incentive spirometry in older children can decrease the incidence. All children should be given analgesics sufficient to relieve postoperative pain. Diminished breath sounds are auscultated. Insufficient therapy may lead to more

Table 15.10   Causes of postoperative fever

Time of onset	Etiology
Immediate	Manipulation of infected focus
Day 1	Actelectasis, pre-existing illness, streptococcus, *Clostridium*
Day 2–3	Actelectasis, otitis media, phlebitis, urinary tract infection
Day 4	Staphylococcus
Day 5 (or later)	Enteric wound, otitis media, phlebitis, urinary tract infection, abdominal abscess

extensive segmental collapse requiring naso-tracheal suction or bronchoscopy for rein-flation. Invasive pulmonary infection may occur if this persists.

Pneumonia may also be respiration associated or result from aspiration in those who have altered sensorium while awakening from anesthesia. After the first day consider other causes, including otitis media induced from barotitis or irritation from nasogastric tubes, catheter-induced phlebitis, streptococcal wound infection, and catheter or instrument-induced urinary tract infections. Pyuria justifies urine culture, with a positive culture ($> 10^5$ bacteria/ml) requiring antibiotic therapy (Chapter 12).

Intra-abdominal infections are difficult to recognize because of the changes produced by the recent abdominal incision. Fever, leukocytosis, ileus, or diarrhea herald purulent collections, and ultrasound or computerized tomography can verify clinical suspicion. Occasionally operative exploration without verification of the locus is necessary for diagnosis. In children, other sources, although unusual, include parotitis, pancreatitis, and cholecystitis.

Sexually transmitted diseases and genital tract infections

16

CLINICAL PRESENTATIONS

Sexually transmitted diseases (STDs) can be broadly divided into those characterized by genital ulcers, with or without inguinal adenopathy, infections of epithelial surfaces, and specific well-defined syndromes (Table 16.1).

ETIOLOGIES

STDs can also be classified by specific pathogens (Table 16.2), although this is less practical than approaching etiologic diagnosis on the basis of clinical presentation. As an example, urethritis can be caused by bacteria, viruses, or even protozoa. A history of previous STD may also alter suspected pathogens. Repeat episodes of pelvic inflammatory disease (PID) are more likely to be produced by coliform bacteria than are initial infections. Selection of antimicrobial therapy may therefore vary for reinfection.

DISEASES ASSOCIATED WITH GENITAL ULCERS AND LYMPHADENITIS

Genital ulcers are most commonly associated with herpes simplex, syphilis or, less commonly, chancroid and can be differentiated by the presence or absence of pain. Syphilis is usually painless while herpes and chancroid are painful. Depending on this finding and other features such as adenopathy (syphilis, lymphogranuloma venereum

Table 16.1 Clinical presentations of STDs and genital tract infections

Syndrome	Etiology
Female and male	
Genital ulcers and lymphadenitis	Herpes, syphilis, chancroid, lymphogranuloma venereum
Urethritis	Gonococcus, chlamydia, *Ureaplasma* sp, herpes simplex virus, *Trichomonas* sp.
Arthritis-dermatitis syn.	*Neisseria gonorrhoeae*
Urethritis-arthritis-conjunctivitis syn.	Reiter's syndrome (uncertain etiology), possibly chlamydia
Warts	Human papilloma virus types 6 and 11
Hepatitis	Hepatitis B
Female	
Vaginitis	*Trichomonas, Gardnerella vaginalis, Candida* sp.
Cervicitis	Gonococcus, chlamydia, *Mycoplasma hominis*, herpes simplex virus, *Trichomonas* sp.
Pelvic inflammatory disease (PID)	Gonococcus, chlamydia, anaerobic bacteria, *M. hominis*, coliform bacteria
Postabortion postsalpingitis	Gonococcus, chlamydia, *M. hominis*
Male	
Epididymitis	Gonococcus, chlamydia
Balanitis	*Candida albicans, Trichomonas vaginalis, Gardnerella vaginalis*

(LGV), and chancroid), evaluation of genital ulcers would include the following: dark-field examination or direct immunofluor-escence test for *Treponema pallidum*; serologic tests for syphilis; culture, Tzanck test or fluorescence stains for herpes simplex virus (HSV); and culture for *Haemophilus ducreyi* (Table 16.3).

The appearance of skin lesions is often diagnostic. Genital warts (papilloma virus), ecchymoses of the arthritis–dermatitis syndrome (*Neisseria gonorrhoeae*), and the multiple painful ulcers of herpes simplex can easily be recognized.

Table 16.2 STDs classified by pathogen

Disease	Pathogen
Chancroid	*Haemophilus ducreyi*
Genital herpes	Herpes simplex virus type 2 (occasionally type 1)
Genital warts	Human papilloma virus type 6 and 11
Granuloma inguinale	*Calymmatobacterium granulomatis*
Lymphogranuloma venereum (LGV)	*Chlamydia trachomatis* (LGV serovars)
Pelvic inflammatory disease (PID)	Gonococcus, chlamydia, anaerobic bacteria, *Mycoplasma hominis*, coliform bacteria
Pubic lice	*Pthirus pubis*
Syphilis	*Treponema pallidum*
Vaginosis or nonspecific vaginitis	*Gardnerella vaginalis*, *Mobiluncus* sp., anaerobic bacteria

Table 16.3 Diagnostic studies for genital ulcers

Treponema pallidum	Specific treponemal serology
	Darkfield examination or direct immuno-fluorescence test
Herpes simplex virus	Antigen test (fluorescent or Tzanck prep) or culture
Haemophilus ducreyi	Culture
HIV	ELISA serology and/or PCR

Herpes simplex

Primary genital infection is characterized by painful ulcers which persist for 4–15 days until crusting (see Table 16.4 for treatment of HSV infection). Viral shedding occurs for an average of 12 days. There is then a 90% recurrence rate following HSV-2 genital infection, and 60% for HSV-1. The number of reactivation episodes varies considerably, averaging 5 episodes per year for the first 2 years but decreasing thereafter. Primary infection is associated with generalized signs and symptoms including fever, malaise, headache, myalgia and painful inguinal adenopathy. Aseptic meningitis with cerebrospinal fluid pleocytosis and positive viral cultures is seen in 1–3% of cases but is a benign disease which should not be confused with herpes encephalitis.

Syphilis

The four presentations of this disease commonly occurring in the pediatric population are: congenital syphilis, acquired disease in adolescents, asymptomatic adolescents with positive screening assays and sexual abuse. Each requires an understanding and interpretation of both screening and specific tests for syphilis. Those commonly available are as follows: nontreponemal – VDRL (Venereal Disease Research Laboratories test), RPR (rapid plasma reagin), ART (automated reagin test) – and treponemal – FTA-ABS (fluorescent treponemal antibody-absorption test) and MHA-TP (microhemagglutination-*Treponema pallidum* test). Screening assays are quite sensitive (95–100%) for secondary syphilis but positive in only 70–80% of primary, tertiary and latent disease and even lower for incubating and early primary infection (Table 16.5). Therefore, a history of possible recent exposure warrants retesting up to 90 days after initial negative results. Specific treponemal tests should be routinely ordered for patients in whom disease is strongly suspected.

Table 16.4   Oral antiviral therapy for genital herpes

First clinical episode; any of the following regimens given for 7–10 days:
Acyclovir: 400 mg t.i.d. or 200 mg 5 times per day
Famciclovir: 250 mg t.i.d.
Valacyclovir: 1 gm b.i.d.

Episodic recurrent infection; any of the following regimens given for 5 days:
Acyclovir: 800 mg b.i.d., 400 mg t.i.d. or 200 mg 5 times per day
Famciclovir: 125 mg b.i.d.
Valacyclovir: 500 mg b.i.d.

Daily suppressive therapy; duration generally one year but dependent on risk behavior and other personal issues:
Acyclovir: 400 mg b.i.d.
Famciclovir: 250 mg b.i.d.
Valacyclovir: 250 mg b.i.d., 500 mg q.d. or 1 g q.d.

Primary disease may be asymptomatic, particularly in women, since the chancre is usually not readily visible and is painless. Secondary syphilis is usually quite evident, characterized by a maculopapular rash, condyloma lata, mucous patches, lymphadenopathy, and fever. Disease tends to be remittent with variable intervals of asymptomatic latent infection. Half of untreated patients progress to a secondary phase, and half go directly into latency. Treatment depends on the stage of disease at diagnosis (Table 16.6).

Repeat quantitative nontreponemal tests are indicated until a 4-fold decrease in titer is seen (usually measured at 3, 6, and 12 months). Retreatment is recommended if clinical signs persist, a 4-fold increase in titer is documented, or the screening syphilis assay does not decrease 4-fold by 12 months.

Chancroid

Chancroid is distinguished by a painful genital ulcer accompanied, in about one-half of cases, by painful inguinal lymphadenopathy. Culture for *H. ducreyi* will confirm the etiology. Chancroid is highly associated with both HIV infection and syphilis, thereby necessitating serologic screens for these conditions. Following treatment of chancroid (Table 16.7), symptomatic improvement is expected within 3 days and improvement of lesions and reduction of exudate within 7 days. Adenitis may require needle aspiration.

Table 16.5   Sensitivity (%) of serology testing for syphilis

Assay	Test sensitivity (%) Stage of syphilis			
	Primary	Secondary	Latent	Tertiary
VDRL	72	100	73	77
FTA-ABS	91	100	97	100
MHA-TP	60	100	98	100

Table 16.6   Therapy for syphilis

Primary or secondary and early latent
  Benzathine penicillin G
  2.4 million units i.m., single dose
Late, latent or latent of unknown duration
  Benzathine penicillin G
  2.4 million units i.m., weekly for 3 weeks

Table 16.7   Therapy for chancroid

Azithromycin: 1 g p.o. single dose
Ceftriaxone: 250 mg i.m. single dose
Ciprofloxacin: 500 mg p.o. b.i.d. for 3 days
Erythromycin base 500 mg p.o. q.i.d. for 7 days

Lymphogranuloma venereum

Lymphogranuloma venereum (LGV) is caused by *Chlamydia trachomatis* (LGV serovars) and should be considered with the clinical presentation of persistent inguinal lymphadenopathy, although it is rare in the United States. Diagnosis is made by specific LGV serology. Treatment is with doxycycline (100 mg p.o. b.i.d. for 21 days). Alternative regimens are erythromycin (500 mg p.o. q.i.d. for 21 days) or sulfisoxazole (500 mg p.o. q.i.d. for 21 days).

DISEASES ASSOCIATED WITH URETHRITIS

Gonococcal infections

Neisseria gonorrhoeae are Gram-negative diplococci which cause infections only in humans and are transmitted by intimate sexual contact, parturition, and occasionally in prepubertal children from care-givers, following normal contact. Treatment decisions are influenced by changing sensitivity patterns of the organism, clinical manifestations, cost of therapy, and presence of other STDs. Uncomplicated gonococcal urethral, endocervical, or rectal infections can be treated with a single-dose regimen in conjunction with therapy for presumed chlamydial disease (Table 16.8). Ceftriaxone (125 mg) is adequate therapy for incubating syphilis. All patients with gonorrhea

Table 16.8 Therapy for gonococcal infection

Uncomplicated infections:
   ceftriaxone 125 mg i.m. single dose
   cefixime 400 mg p.o. single dose
   ciprofloxacin 500 mg p.o. single dose
   ofloxacin 400 mg p.o. single dose
Pharyngeal:
   ceftriaxone, ciprofloxacin or ofloxacin as above
Disseminated infection:
   ceftriaxone 1 g i.m. or i.v. q.d.

Note:
   Patients with gonococcal infection should also
   be treated for *Chlamydia trachomatis* with:
      azithromycin 1 g p.o. single dose or
      doxycycline 100 mg p.o. b.i.d. for 7 days

should be tested for syphilis (at the time of diagnosis and 1 month later) and, at least, counseled on HIV infection. Persons exposed to active gonorrhea cases within 30 days of diagnosis should be examined, cultured, and routinely treated. Follow-up cultures are not necessary since treatment failures with ceftriaxone are so rare.

Non-gonococcal urethritis

Painful urethritis, with an exudate containing abundant polymorphonuclear leukocytes but without Gram-negative intracellular diplococci, is caused by *C. trachomatis* in approximately 50% of cases and by *Ureuplasma urealyticum*, *Trichomonas vaginalis*, herpes simplex virus or other mycoplasmas in 10–20%. Specific etiologies are often difficult to confirm. Empiric treatment should be initiated in adolescents as soon as possible after diagnosis (Table 16.9), using either azithromycin (1 g p.o. single dose) or doxycycline (100 mg p.o. b.i.d. for 7 days). Children younger than 9 years of age can receive erythromycin (30–50 mg/kg per day p.o. div. q.i.d.) for 14 days. Failures should undergo a second treatment course.

Chlamydia trachomatis

Most treatment for chlamydia occurs as part of routine therapy in patients with gonorrhea, a recommendation based on the observation that one-third of patients with gonorrhea are concomitantly infected with *C. trachomatis*.

Diagnosis in infants with conjunctivitis and/or pneumonia also necessitates treatment of the mother and her sexual partner(s). Chlamydia is an STD transmitted to the newborn from the mother during childbirth, therefore clinical confirmation for infection in the mother already exists. Perinatal infection does not become clinically apparent until 2–20 weeks of life, when conjunctivitis and afebrile interstitial pneumonia are the most common manifestations. Failure to thrive is an occasional feature. Colonization rarely occurs after 20 weeks of age, and then

Table 16.9 Therapy for non-gonococcal urethritis

Recommended regimens
  Azithromycin 1 g orally in a single dose
  or
  Doxycycline 100 mg orally twice a day for 7 days

Alternative regimens
  Erythromycin base 500 mg orally four times a day for 7 days
  or
  Erythromycin ethylsuccinate 800 mg orally four times a day for 7 days
  or
  Ofloxacin 300 mg twice a day for 7 days
  If only erythromycin can be used and a patient cannot tolerate high-dose erythromycin schedules, one of the following regimens can be used:
  Erythromycin base 250 mg orally four times a day for 14 days
  or
  Erythromycin ethylsuccinate 400 mg orally four times a days for 14 days

Recommended treatment for recurrent/persistent urethritis
  Metronidazole 2 g orally in a single dose
  plus
  Erythromycin base 500 mg orally four times a day for 7 days
  or
  Erythromycin ethylsuccinate 800 mg orally four times a day for 7 days

Table 16.10 Therapy for *Chlamydia trachomatis* genital infections

Recommended regimens
  Azithromycin 1 g orally, single dose,
  or
  Doxycycline 100 mg orally b.i.d. for 7 days

Alternative regimens
  Erythromycin base 500 mg p.o. q.i.d. for 7 days
  or
  Erythromycin ethylsuccinate 800 mg p.o. q.i.d. for 7 days
  or
  Ofloxacin 300 mg p.o. b.i.d. for 7 days

only in asymptomatic infants or children. Sexually active male adolescents present with urethritis or epididymoorchitis while females may develop urethritis, cervicitis, or PID. Both culture and rapid antigen detection assays (ELISA, fluorescence, genetic probe) are available and should be obtained routinely for suspected infection in adolescents. Treatment of chlamydia is presented in Table 16.10.

Ureaplasma urealyticum

Approximately 25% of non-gonococcal, non-chlamydial urethritis in males is caused by *U. urealyticum*. Disease in women is usually asymptomatic. There is increasing evidence that this organism is associated with spontaneous abortion, sepsis, and bronchopulmonary dysplasia in neonates. This potential pathogen can be cultured in special broth medium containing urea, but since as many as half of sexually active adults are colonized, its presence is difficult to correlate with disease. Recommended treatment for adolescents and adults is doxycycline, 100 mg p.o. b.i.d. for 7 days. Children younger than 9 years of age, or those allergic to tetracycline, can be treated with erythromycin (30–50 mg/kg per day p.o. div. q.i.d.) for 7 days.

Trichomoniasis

Trichomonas vaginalis is a flagellated protozoan often identified as part of the vaginal flora in asymptomatic sexually active adolescent females. Moderate to heavy colonization produces a yellow-green discharge with a fishy odor associated with pruritic vaginitis, cervicitis, or urethritis. Their presence in postmenarchal girls strongly suggests sexual activity, while in premenarchal children their presence necessitates careful examination for sexual abuse. Males are more frequently symptomatic, with urethritis or prostatitis. Diagnosis is made by direct microscopic examination (wet preparation) of fresh vaginal discharge; treatment is by metronidazole 2 g p.o. single dose or 500 mg b.i.d. for 7 days.

DISEASES ASSOCIATED WITH VAGINAL DISCHARGE

Vaginosis

Bacterial vaginosis, also called nonspecific vaginitis, results from the overgrowth of *Gardnerella vaginalis* and/or anaerobes such as *Mobiluncus* sp. Diagnosis is suggested by the presence of a homogeneous discharge with a pH > 4.5, positive amine odor test and clue cells. Infection is of greatest concern during pregnancy, since bacterial vaginosis is associated with premature rupture of membranes and premature delivery. Only symptomatic infection should be treated. The recommended regimen is metronidazole (500 mg p.o. b.i.d.) for 7 days.

Alternatives are clindamycin cream 2%, one full applicator (5 g) intravaginally at bedtime for 7 days, metronidazole gel 0.75%, one full applicator (5 g) intravaginally b.i.d. for 5 days; metronidazole 2 g p.o. single dose or clindamycin 300 mg p.o. b.i.d. for 7 days.

Vulvovaginitis

Prepubertal vaginitis is usually secondary to *C. albicans, T vaginalis, N. gonorrhoeae*, foreign bodies, or irritation secondary to chemicals or pinworm; it may, however, be the only physical finding in sexual abuse. Gonococcal vaginitis in the prepubertal child is usually mild because it is localized to the superficial mucosa. Post pubertal vulvovaginitis is usually caused by *C. albicans*, and occasionally by other *Candida* sp., *Torulopsis* sp. or other yeasts. It may be the only physical finding in sexual abuse.

Major symptoms in vulvovaginitis include vaginal itching and a minor crusting discharge that discolors the underwear. Dysuria and pyuria are common. The character of the vaginal discharge in all patients, and the speculum examination in postpubertal (especially sexually active) females, are useful in establishing the diagnosis (Table 16.11). The treatment of vulvovaginitis is dependent on the etiologic agent (Table 16.12), while the numerous topical formulations for the treatment of vulvovaginal candidiasis in

Table 16.11 Clinical considerations in vulvovaginitis

Clinical examination	Vaginal discharge
Ectropion Oral contraceptives Pregnancy	Clear mucus
Cervicitis (gonococcal infection, *Chlamydia* sp., herpes simplex virus)	Purulent exudate, cervix friable
Vaginitis (*Candida albicans, Trichomonas vaginalis, Gardnerella vaginalis*)	Malodor, yellow to white, frothy discharge; cervicitis may be present

Table 16.12 Etiologic agents and treatment in vulvovaginitis

Candida albicans
    Discontinue antibiotics and oral contraceptives if possible. Topical antifungals: nystatin vaginal tablet b.i.d. for 7 days, or imidazole (clotrimazole or miconazole) intravaginally once daily for 7 days
Trichomonas vaginalis
    Metronidazole 10–30 mg/kg per day (maximum 2 g) p.o. single dose or 250 mg p.o. t.i.d. for 10 days
    Alternatives: tinidazole 2 g p.o. single dose. In pregnancy: clotrimazole 2–100 mg vaginal tablets h.s. for 7 days
    Neonatal trichomoniasis: symptomatic or persistent colonization; metronidazole 10–30 mg/kg per day p.o. for 5–8 days
Nonspecific vaginitis (*Gardnerella vaginalis*)
    Metronidazole 10–30 mg/kg per day (maximum 500 mg) p.o. b.i.d. for 7 days
    Alternatives: ampicillin 50 mg/kg per day (maximum 500 mg) p.o. q.i.d. for 7 days (pregnancy)
    Sexual partners: controversial; recommend treatment as in the female

Table 16.13 Treatment of vulvovaginal candidiasis

Intravaginal agents:

Butoconazole 2% cream 5 g intravaginally for 3 days

or

Clotrimazole 1% cream 5 g intravaginally for 7–14 days

or

Clotrimazole 100 mg vaginal tablet for 7 days

or

Clotrimazole 100 mg vaginal tablet, two tablets for 3 days

or

Clotrimazole 500 mg vaginal tablet, one tablet in a single application

or

Miconazole 2% cream 5 g intravaginally for 7 days

or

Miconazole 200 mg vaginal suppository, one suppository daily for 3 days

or

Miconazole 100 mg vaginal suppository, one suppository daily for 7 days

or

Nystatin 100 000-unit vaginal tablet, one tablet for 14 days

or

Tipconazole 6.5% ointment 5 g intravaginally in a single application

or

Terconazole 0.4% cream 5 g intravaginally for 7 days

or

Terconazole 0.8% cream 5 g intravaginally for 3 days

or

Terconazole 80 mg vaginal suppository, one suppository daily for 3 days

or

Oral agent:

Fluconazole 150 mg oral tablet, one tablet in single dose

---

postpubertal females are presented in Table 16.13. The oral antifungal agent fluconazole, one 150 mg tablet as a single dose, is also highly effective.

A thorough speculum examination is important to ascertain whether the discharge emanates from the vagina or the cervical os. The most common etiologies of vaginitis are: *Candida*, *Trichomonas* spp., and *G. vaginalis*. In *Candida* sp. vaginitis, the following are helpful in diagnosis: itching, dysuria, curds or plaques, 10% KOH test (no odor), yeast or pseudomycelia, pH < 4.5, and a positive culture for yeast. In vaginitis due to *Trichomonas* sp., the diagnosis is apparent with profuse, yellow-green discharge, 10% KOH test (amine odor), motile trichomonads (wet preparation, magnification × 400), and a vaginal pH 5.5–6.0. In nonspecific vaginitis due to *G. vaginalis*, the diagnosis is apparent with an adherent homogeneous discharge, also: 10% KOH test (amine odor), clue cells (secretions in a 1:1 dilution with normal saline), which are vaginal epithelial cells coated with coccobacillary forms of *G. vaginalis*, a pH > 4.5, and a positive culture. In some cases of vaginitis anaerobes have been isolated but no predominant organism has been demonstrated. For comparison, normal vaginal secretions have no odor with 10% KOH, and a pH < 4.5.

PELVIC INFLAMMATORY DISEASE

The spectrum of acute pelvic inflammatory disease (PID) includes endometritis, salpingitis, tubo-ovarian abscess, and pelvic peritonitis. Most infection is caused by *N. gonorrhoeae* and *C. trachomatis* although genital colonizing organisms (anaerobes, coliforms, streptococci, and mycoplasmas) are also potential pathogens, particularly for recurrent disease.

Diagnosis can be aided by pelvic ultrasonography or laparoscopy. Clinical findings are lower abdominal pain and tenderness, bilateral adnexal tenderness on motion of the cervix, recent-onset vaginal discharge, fever and abnormal menstrual bleeding. Even a low index of suspicion for infection necessitates early institution of antimicrobial therapy. Specific etiology is usually based on culture and rapid antigen detection assays of exudate from the lower genital tract.

Most adolescents should be hospitalized, not only for inpatient therapy (Table 16.14)

Table 16.14 Therapy for pelvic inflammatory disease (PID)

Parenteral regimen A
    Cefotetan 2 g i.v. every 12 h
    or
    Cefoxitin 2 g i.v. every 6 h
    plus
    Doxycycline 100 mg i.v. or orally every 12 h

Parenteral regimen B
    Clindamycin 900 mg i.v. every 8 h
    plus
    Gentamicin loading dose i.v. or i.m. (2 mg/kg
        of body weight), followed by a maintenance
        dose (1.5 mg/kg) i.v. every 8 hours. Single
        daily dosing may be substituted.

Alternative parenteral regimens
    Ofloxacin 400 mg i.v. every 12 h
    plus
    Metronidazole 500 mg i.v. every 8 h
    or
    Ampicillin/sulbactam 3 g i.v. every 6 h
    plus
    Doxycycline 100 mg i.v. or orally every 12 h
    or
    Ciprofloxacin 200 mg i.v. every 12 h
    plus
    Doxycycline 100 mg i.v. or orally every 12 h
    plus
    Metronidazole 500 mg i.v. every 8 hours

Regimen A
    Ofloxacin 400 mg orally twice a day for 14
        days
    plus
    Metronidazole 500 mg orally twice a day for
        14 days

Regimen B
    Ceftriaxone 250 mg i.m. once
    or
    Cefoxitin 2 g i.m. plus probenecid 1 g orally
        in a single dose concurrently once
    or
    Other parenteral third-generation
        cephalosporin (e.g. ceftizoxime or
        cefotaxime)
    plus
    Doxycycline 100 mg orally twice a day for 14
        days (include this regimen with one of the
        above regimens)

---

but to assure compliance in follow-up, to offer comprehensive counseling for sexual activity and other potential STDs, and to detect sequelae which are more severe in this age group. Complications are perihepatitis (Fitz-Hugh and Curtis syndrome), tubo-ovarian abscess, infertility, pelvic adhesions and ectopic pregnancy. PID is more severe in patients with intrauterine devices in place so these should be removed.

Follow-up of all patients is recommended at 3–5 days after beginning therapy and 7–10 days after completing antibiotics. Cultures should be obtained 21–28 days after completing therapy to document eradication of *C. trachomatis* and *N. gonorrhoeae*. Male sexual partners should be cultured and routinely treated for gonorrhea and chlamydia infection. Both patients and partner(s) should abstain from intercourse until therapy is complete.

MALE STD SYNDROMES

Balanitis

Cellulitis of the glans penis may occur as a consequence of poor hygiene in prepubertal uncircumcised children but is more commonly seen in sexually active males following intercourse with a partner who is colonized with *Candida albicans*, *Trichomonas vaginalis*, or *Gardnerella vaginalis*. Etiology can be determined by direct examination of the first aliquot of a voided urine and, if negative, examination of the female sexual contact. Inflammation may occasionally represent a hypersensitivity reaction from contact with *Candida albicans*; for these patients good hygiene and treatment of the sexual partner are curative. Balanitis may also be related to trauma or postcircumcision wound infections where streptococci and staphylococci are probable pathogens. Treatment of balanitis is summarized in Table 16.15.

Epididymitis

Epididymitis must be differentiated from testicular torsion, orchitis, or testicular cancer.

Table 16.15   Treatment of balanitis

Candida albicans
   Nystatin, butoconazole, or terconazole
      ointment applied q.i.d. for 3–7 days or until
      resolved, also treat sexual partner
Trichomonas vaginalis
   Children – metronidazole 10–30 mg/kg per day
      p.o. t.i.d. for 7 days
   Adults – metronidazole 2 g p.o. single dose or
      250 mg t.i.d. for 7 days
Gardnerella vaginalis
   Children – metronidazole 10–30 mg/kg per
      day p.o. t.i.d. for 7 days
   Adults – metronidazole 500 g p.o. b.i.d. for 7
      days
   or
   Ampicillin 500 mg p.o. q.i.d. for 7 days

Acute epididymitis in adolescents often occurs after trauma and/or heavy lifting but is occasionally a primary infection caused by *N. gonorrhoeae* or chlamydia. However, in most cases highly suspected of having infectious etiologies (scrotal edema and fever), no organism is recovered. There are, therefore, two distinct types of disease; nonspecific bacterial epididymitis and sexually transmitted epididymitis.

In acute epididymitis, ultrasonography shows the swollen epididymis as distinct parallel lines posterolateral to the discrete testicular echo and an enlarged, but separate, epididymal head. In torsion of the testis, the testicular echo is disrupted and the echogenic epididymis is inseparable from the testis. Urine culture may isolate the causative organism if this is an infectious process. Mumps orchitis is suspected by the lack of white blood cells in the urine of these patients, a negative culture, and an elevated serum amylase.

Scrotal elevation by an athletic supporter or towel across the thighs facilitates drainage and relief of pain. Sexual excitement may exacerbate pain and infection. Antibiotics active against gonococcus, chlamydia and coliform organisms (ceftriaxone and doxycycline) may be of benefit. Severe pain may be relieved by infiltrating the spermatic cord in the upper scrotum with xylocaine or other anesthetizing agents. Exploration and open biopsy are indicated to distinguish testicular tumors and to avoid spread of malignant cells.

Orchitis

Mumps and group B Coxsackieviruses are the most common causes of orchitis in children and adolescents, and orchitis is rarely considered an STD. The usual etiologies of orchitis can be differentiated clinically because mumps produces parotitis with elevated serum amylase. One-third to one-fourth of patients with mumps orchitis develop oligo- or aspermia in the involved testis. The other testis remains normal and potency is not affected. Treatment is symptomatic with analgesics and elevation of the scrotum.

OTHER SPECIFIC DISEASES

Genital warts

Exophytic genital and anal warts can be readily diagnosed clinically, only requiring biopsy to exclude dysplasia or carcinoma if lesions are atypical, pigmented, or persistent. Although human papilloma viruses (HPV) can cause laryngeal papillomatosis in infants, the method of transmission has not been defined and Cesarean section is not recommended to prevent disease in infants born to mothers with active genital warts. Treatment of HPV infection is summarized in Table 16.16.

Granuloma inguinale

Although rare in the United States, granuloma inguinale should be suspected with ulcerated cutaneous lesions, subcutaneous nodules, and granulomas (pseudobuboes) in the genital or anal regions. The demonstration of Donovan bodies on Wright's stain or Giemsa stain of a crush-preparation from a lesion confirms the diagnosis. Treatment alternatives include tetracycline, trimethoprim/sulfamethoxazole (TMP/SMX), ceftriaxone, gentamicin,

Table 16.16   Treatment of human papillomavirus (HPV) infection

External anogenital warts
  Patient applied:
    Podofilox 0.5% solution or gel or
    Imiquimod 5% cream
  Provider administered:
    Cryotherapy with liquid nitrogen or cryoprobe
    Alternatives: podophyllin, podophyllotoxin, trichloroacetic acid 80–90%, electrodesiccation/
      electrocautery, interferons, laser therapy
Vaginal warts
  Cryotherapy with liquid nitrogen
  Alternatives: trichloroacetic acid (80–90%), podophyllin (10–15%), 5-fluorouracil cream, laser therapy
Urethral meatus
  Cryotherapy with liquid nitrogen
  Alternatives: podophyllin (10–15%), 5-fluorouracil cream, laser therapy
Anal warts
  Cryotherapy with liquid nitrogen
  Alternatives: trichloroacetic acid, (80–90%), surgical removal (cold blade, laser therapy)
Oral warts
  Cryotherapy with liquid nitrogen
  Alternatives: electrodesiccation/electrocautery, surgical removal
Laryngeal papillomas
  Laser therapy
  Alternatives: photodynamic therapy, interferons

chloramphenicol and erythromycin – each given for 3 weeks, or until lesions have resolved. Response to therapy should occur within 7 days but failures are common.

Pediculosis pubis

Intense itching in the anogenital region is the most common manifestation of pubic lice but infestation may also involve other hairy areas such as eyelashes, eyebrows, beard, or axillae. A highly suggestive clinical finding is blue-gray macules on the chest, abdomen, or thighs. Numerous effective treatments are available (Table 16.17) but permethrin is preferred because it is available over-the-counter, has a high cure rate, and virtually no toxicity. Pediculosis of the eyelashes should be treated by smothering lice and nits with petrolatum ointment 3 or 4 times daily for 10 days.

Table 16.17   Treatment of pediculosis pubis

Permethrin 1% creme rinse: apply and wash off
  after 10 minutes
  or
Lindane 1% shampoo: apply and wash off after 4
  minutes
  or
Pyrethrin with piperonyl butoxide: apply and
  wash off after 10 minutes

SEXUAL ABUSE AND RAPE

Suspected sexual abuse requires a forensic as well as medical evaluation, which is in some ways different. As an example, rapid diagnostic tests, such as Gram stain, Tzanck test, ELISA, and direct fluorescence techniques are useful for early medical intervention but cannot be used as legal evidence. Routine tests carried out following suspected sexual abuse are listed in Table 16.18, while Table 16.19 shows a correlation between infection in children and the likelihood of the involvement of sexual abuse.

If the perpetrator is unknown or not available for testing, victims of recent abuse should usually be treated for gonorrhea, syphilis, chlamydia, and hepatitis B (Table 16.20).

Table 16.18 Routine testing following sexual abuse

	Organism/syndrome	*Specimens*
All children and adolescents	*Neisseria gonorrhoeae*	Rectal, throat, urethral, vaginal and/or endocervical culture(s)
	Chlamydia trachomatis	Throat, rectal, urethral, vulvovaginal, culture(s)
	Trichomonas vaginalis	Wet mount of vaginal discharge, culture of discharge
	Syphilis	Serologic tests at time of abuse repeated 6, 12 and 24 weeks later
	HIV	Serology of perpetrator (if possible), serology of patient at time of abuse and 6, 12 and 24 weeks later
	Hepatitis B	Serology of perpetrator and patient
Selected cases	Herpes simplex	Culture only if a lesion is present
	Bacterial vaginosis	Wet mount of vaginal discharge
	Human papilloma virus	Biopsy of lesion

Table 16.19 Infection and the likelihood of sexual abuse

Disease	*Likelihood of sexual abuse*
Neisseria gonorrhoeae	Almost certain
Chlamydia (child older than 2 years)	Probable
Syphilis	Almost certain
Herpes	Indeterminate
Genital warts (after 1 year)	Probable
Vaginosis	Possible
Mycoplasma hominis or *Ureaplasma urealyticum*	Indeterminate

Table 16.20 Empiric treatment for sexual abuse victim when the perpetrator cannot be examined

Potential disease	*Treatment*
Gonorrhea and incubating syphilis	Ceftriaxone 125 mg i.m. single dose
Chlamydia	Azithromycin 1 g p.o. single dose or doxycycline 100 mg p.o. b.i.d. for 7 days
Trichomoniasis and bacterial vaginosis	Metronidazole 2 g p.o. single dose
Hepatitis B	Hepatitis B immunoglobulin (HBIG) 0.5 ml i.m. Hepatitis B vaccine at 0, 1 and 6 months

AIDS

17

INTRODUCTION

The acquired immunodeficiency syndrome was first recognized in children in 1982, one year after the initial description in adults. Initially a large number of pediatric cases were transmitted through blood and blood products, but after 1985, when an antibody test for HIV became commercially available, blood bank screening essentially eliminated this as a route of transmission in the 'developed' world. Almost all infections in children in the US at the present time are the result of maternal disease. Without intervention, vertical transmission from HIV infected mothers to neonates is approximately 25%. With zidovudine treatment of the mother and neonate (Table 17.1), transmission is reduced to 6–8%. This is further decreased to 2–3% if the newborn is delivered by Cesarean section.

Additional general principles have been developed by the US Public Health Service to further define appropriate interventions for pregnant HIV infected mothers (Table 17.2), modified according to the gestational age of the fetus, maternal CD4 lymphocyte count, clinical disease stage, and previous antiretroviral therapy.

DIAGNOSIS

Differentiating infected from noninfected infants has been greatly simplified with the development of highly sensitive and specific polymerase chain reaction (PCR) assays. HIV infection can be identified in many infected infants by age 1 month and in virtually all infected infants by age 4 months using viral diagnostic assays (Table 17.3). A positive virologic test result at birth (i.e. detection of HIV by culture, DNA, or RNA PCR) indicates probable HIV infection and should be

confirmed by a repeat virologic test on a second specimen at 1 to 2 months of age. It is recommended for all infants born to HIV positive mothers to obtain a DNA-PCR determination before the infant is 48 hours of age, at 1 to 2 months, and at 4 months. These HIV-exposed infants should be evaluated by or in consultation with a specialist in HIV infection in pediatric patients.

HIV DNA-PCR is the preferred virologic method for diagnosing HIV infection during infancy. Of infected children, 38% have positive PCR test results by 48 hours of age. No substantial change in sensitivity during the first week of life occurs, but sensitivity increases rapidly during the second week, with over 90% of infected children testing PCR-positive by age 14 days. Some experts therefore recommend repeat testing of PCR-negative neonates at two weeks of age. Data are more limited regarding the sensitivity and specificity of HIV RNA assays compared with HIV DNA-PCR for early diagnosis.

For infants born to HIV infected mothers who are not identified until some time after delivery, diagnosis in the infant is usually made by the subsequent clinical course or persistence of antibody beyond 15 months of

Table 17.1 Prevention of pediatric AIDS

Routine testing of pregnant women
HIV-infected pregnant women
    Zidovudine (AZT) 100 mg p.o. 5 times per day
      beginning in the second trimester
During labor
    Zidovudine 2 mg/kg loading dose, 1 mg/kg
      per h continuous infusion
Newborn
    Zidovudine syrup 2 mg/kg per dose q.i.d. for 6
      weeks

Table 17.2 US Public Health Service recommendations for use of zidovudine to reduce perinatal HIV transmission

Clinical scenario	Recommendations

CD4 ≥ 200/mm³
  14–34 weeks of gestation
  No maternal clinical indication for zidovudine
	Risk vs benefit discussion
	Recommend full protocol (Table 17.1) zidovudine regimen

CD4 ≥ 200/mm³
  >34 weeks of gestation
  No maternal clinical indication for zidovudine
  No extensive history (> 6 months) of prior zidovudine
	Risk vs benefit discussion
	Recommend full protocol (Table 17.1) zidovudine regimen
	May be less effective because therapy is initiated late

CD4 < 200/mm³
  14–34 weeks of gestation
  No extensive history (> 6 months) of prior zidovudine
	Risk vs benefit discussion
	Recommend antenatal zidovudine therapy for woman's health
	Recommend intrapartum and neonatal components of zidovudine regimen (Table 17.1)

Significant prior administration of zidovudine or other antiretroviral therapy (> 6 months)	Risk vs benefit discussion
	Recommend zidovudine therapy on a case-by-case basis
	Issues to consider
	  Likelihood of resistance to therapy
	  Duration of prior zidovudine therapy
	  Reason alternative therapy was given, if received (intolerance vs progression of disease despite therapy)

Woman is in labor and has not had antepartum zidovudine therapy	Risk vs benefit discussion Discuss and offer intrapartum and neonatal ZDV if clinical situation permits

Infant is born to a woman who has not received intrapartum zidovudine	Risk vs benefit discussion
	If ≤ 24 h old and clinical situation permits:
	  Discuss and offer neonatal zidovudine
	  Start zidovudine as soon as possible after birth
	If > 24 h old: no data support offering zidovudine therapy

age. The classification system of the Centers for Disease Control (CDC), outlined in Table 17.4, was designed both to identify the variable clinical characteristics of AIDS and to categorize patients for future treatment protocols.

HUMAN IMMUNODEFICIENCY VIRUS (HIV) THERAPY

Decisions for HIV-specific antiviral therapy must take into consideration clinical and immunologic parameters as well as quality-of-life issues (Tables 17.6 and 17.7). It should also be remembered that although early intervention is theoretically advantageous, most current medications have significant potential adverse effects and the risk of development of resistance.

Recommendations for antiretroviral therapy (beyond 6 weeks postnatally when used prophylactically) in HIV-infected children have been based on viral load, CD4 lympho-cyte count and percentage, and clinical

Table 17.3 Laboratory tests for HIV

Test	Advantages and disadvantages
PCR (polymerase chain reaction)	Rapid, sensitive, and specific Requires only 1–3 ml of blood
Viral culture	Highly specific Not routinely available Requires 7–28 days Labor intensive
p24 Antigen assay	Highly specific when positive Lacks sensitivity particularly with high titers of antibody Improved with immune complex dissociation (ICD)
Antibody assays ELISA and Western blot	 Standard screening assays for older patients; not diagnostic at <15 months of age
Latex agglutination	Lacks sensitivity
HIV-IgM, HIV-IgA	Not routinely available

Immune function assays
    CD4 quantitation
    CD8 quantitation
    CD4:CD8 ratio
    Mitogen-induced lymphocyte stimulation
    Quantitative immunoglobulins
    Specific antibody responses
	Surrogate tests (non-specific) – meet CDC criteria in symptomatic infant for starting antiretroviral therapy

conditions. Owing to rapidly expanding knowledge concerning the dynamic interaction of the HI virus with the host's immune system and owing to the availability of multiple new antiretroviral drugs, recommendations for antiretroviral therapy are being revised. Thus, decisions regarding antiretroviral therapy in HIV-infected children should be made in conjunction with a physician with expertise in pediatric HIV infection.

The CD4+ T-lymphocyte count or percentage value is used in conjunction with other measurements to guide antiretroviral treatment decisions and primary prophylaxis of PCP after age 1 year (Table 17.5). However, measurement of CD4+ cell values can be associated with considerable intrapatient variation. Even mild concomitant illness or undergoing vaccination can produce a transient decrease in CD4+ cell number and percentage; thus, CD4+ values are best measured when patients are clinically stable. No modification in therapy should be made in response to a change in CD4+ cell values until the change has been substantiated by at least a second determination, with at least one week between measurements.

There are a number of antiretroviral agents approved for use in HIV-infected adults in the United States, but many of these are not approved at the present time for pediatric patients (Table 17.7). The agents available fall into three major classes: (1) nucleoside analog reverse transcriptase inhibitor (NRTI) agents (zidovudine, didanosine, stavudine, lamivudine and zalcitabine); (2) non-nucleoside analog reverse transcriptase inhibitor (NNRTI) agents (nevirapine and delavirdine); and (3) protease inhibitor (PI) agents (saquinavir hard and soft gel capsules, indinavir, ritonavir and nelfinavir).

Table 17.4 1994 revised HIV pediatric classification system: clinical categories

Category N: not symptomatic
Children who have no signs or symptoms considered to be the result of HIV infection or who have only one of the conditions listed in category A

Category A: mildly symptomatic
Children with two or more of the conditions listed below but none of the conditions listed in categories B and C
  Lymphadenopathy ($\geq$ 0.5 cm at more than two sites; bilateral = one site)
  Hepatomegaly
  Splenomegaly
  Dermatitis
  Parotitis
  Recurrent or persistent upper respiratory infection, sinusitis or otitis media

Category B: moderately symptomatic
Children who have symptomatic conditions other than those listed for category A or C that are attributed to HIV infection. Examples of conditions in clinical category B include but are not limited to:
  Anemia (< 8 gm/dl), neutropenia (< 1000/mm^3) or thrombocytopenia (< 100 000/mm^3) persisting $\geq$ 30 d
  Bacterial meningitis, pneumonia, or sepsis (single episode)
  Candidiasis, oropharyngeal (thrush) persisting (> 2 months) in children > 6 months old
  Cardiomyopathy
  Cytomegalovirus infection, with onset before 1 month of age
  Diarrhea, recurrent or chronic
  Hepatitis
  Herpes simplex virus stomatitis, recurrent (more than two episodes within 1 year)
  Herpes simplex virus bronchitis, pneumonitis, or esophagitis with onset before 1 month of age
  Herpes zoster (shingles) involving at least two distinct episodes or more than one dermatome
  Leiomyosarcoma
  Lymphoid interstitial pneumonitis (LIP) or pulmonary lymphoid hyperplasia complex
  Nephropathy
  Nocardiosis
  Persistent fever (lasting > 1 month)
  Toxoplasmosis, onset before 1 month of age
  Varicella, disseminated (complicated chickenpox)

Category C: severely symptomatic
Children who have any condition listed in the 1987 surveillance case definition for AIDS, with the exception of LIP (which is a category B condition)
  Serious bacterial infections, multiple or recurrent (i.e. any combination of at least two culture-confirmed infections within a 2-year period) of the following types: septicemia, pneumonia, meningitis, bone or joint infection, or abscess of an internal organ or body cavity (excluding otitis media, superficial skin or mucosal abscesses, and in-dwelling catheter-related infections)
  Candidiasis, esophageal or pulmonary (bronchi, trachea, lungs)
  Coccidioidomycosis, disseminated (at site other than or in addition to lungs or cervical or hilar lymph nodes)
  Cryptococcosis, extrapulmonary
  Cryptosporidiosis or isosporiasis with diarrhea persisting > 1 month
  Cytomegalovirus disease with onset of symptoms at age > 1 month (at a site other than liver, spleen, or lymph nodes)

Continued

Table 17.4 Continued

Encephalopathy (at least one of the following progressive findings present for at least 2 months in the absence of a concurrent illness other than HIV infection that could explain the findings): 1) failure to attain or loss of developmental milestones or loss of intellectual ability, verified by standard developmental scale or neuropsychological tests; 2) impaired brain growth or acquired microcephaly demonstrated by head circumference measurements or brain atrophy demonstrated by CT or MRI (serial imaging is required for children < 2 years of age); 3) acquired symmetric motor deficit manifested by two or more of the following: paresis, pathologic reflexes, ataxia, or gait disturbance

Herpes simplex virus infection causing a mucutaneous ulcer that persists for > 1 month, or bronchitis, pneumonitis, or esophagitis for any duration affecting a child > 1 month of age

Histoplasmosis, disseminated (at a site other than or in addition to lungs or cervical or hilar lymph nodes)

Kaposi's sarcoma

Lymphoma, primary, in brain

Lymphoma, small, noncleaved cell (Burkitt's), or immunoblastic or large cell lymphoma of B-cell or unknown immunologic abnormality

Modified from Centers for Disease Control 1994 revised classification system for human immunodeficiency virus infection in children less than 13 years of age. MMWR 1994;43 (No. RR-12):1-10

Table 17.5 1994 revised pediatric HIV classification system: immunologic categories based on age-specific CD4 lymphocyte count per μl and percentage

| | Age of child | | | | | |
| | <12 months | | 1–5 years | | 6–12 years | |
Immune category	n	%	n	%	n	%
Category 1: no suppression	≥ 1500	≥ 25	≥ 1000	≥ 25	≥ 500	≥ 25
Category 2: moderate suppression	750–1499	15–24	500–999	15–24	200–499	15–24
Category 3: severe suppression	< 750	< 15	< 500	< 15	< 200	< 15

Modified from Centers for Disease Control 1994 revised classification system for human immunodeficiency virus infection in children less than 13 years of age. MMWR 1994;43(No. RR-12): 1-10; values are CD4 lymphocytes per μl, and percentages are per cent of normal for age

INFECTIOUS COMPLICATIONS

Many children initially exhibit HIV-induced changes in immune function by developing unusual infections. Unfortunately, once established, infectious diseases are often difficult to treat because immunosuppression is so severe. Therefore, early recognition and therapy are essential. Some of these opportunistic pathogens are predictable enough to offer prophylaxis.

Prophylaxis

There are four potential secondary infections in pediatric acquired immunodeficiency syndrome (AIDS) that warrant prophylaxis: bacteremia/sepsis, *Pneumocystis carinii* infection,

Table 17.6 Clinical manifestations warranting HIV antiviral therapy

AIDS-definitive infection (see Table 17.4)
Wasting or failure to thrive (or lower than the 5th percentile)
HIV encephalopathy
AIDS-associated malignancy (see Table 17.4)
Two episodes of sepsis or meningitis

tuberculosis, and *Mycobacterium avium–M. intracellulare* infection. Table 17.8 summarizes criteria for these indications and currently recommended treatment.

Intravenous immunoglobulin has been used in infants and children infected with human immunodeficeincy virus (HIV), with

Table 17.7   Drugs used in pediatric HIV infection

Drug	Dosage
Nucleoside analog reverse transcriptase inhibitor (NRTI) agents	

Didanosine (ddI) (dideoxyinosine)
   VIDEX
 Preparations:
 Pediatric powder for oral solution (when
   reconstituted as solution containing antacid
   10 mg/ml)
 Chewable tablets with buffers, 50, 100 and 150 mg
 Buffered powder for oral solution, 100, 167,
   and 250 mg
	Neonatal dose (infants < 90 days):
	   50 mg/m^2 q.12 h
	 Pediatric usual dose: in combination with other anti-
	   retrovirals, 90 mg/m^2 q.12 h
	 Pediatric dosage range: 90 to 150 mg/m^2 q.12 h
	   (Note: may need higher dose in patients with
	   CNS disease)
	 Adolescent/adult dose:
	   >60 kg, 200 mg b.i.d.
	   <60 kg, 125 mg b.i.d.

Lamivudine (3TC)
   EPIVIR
 Preparations:
 Solution, 10 mg/ml
 Tablets, 150 mg
 Tablets: COMBIVIR (150 mg lamivudine in
   combination with 300 mg zidovudine)
	Neonatal dose (infants < 30 days):
	   2 mg/kg b.i.d.
	 Pediatric dose: 4 mg/kg b.i.d.
	 Adolescent/adult dose:
	   > 50 kg, 150 mg b.i.d.
	   < 50 kg: 2 mg/kg b.i.d.

Stavudine (d4T)
   ZERIT
 Preparations:
 Solution, 1 mg/ml
 Capsules, 15, 20, 30 and 40 mg
	Neonatal dose: under evaluation
	 Pediatric dose: 1 mg/kg q.12h (up to body weight
	   of 30 kg)
	 Adolescent/adult dose:
	   ≥ 60 kg, 40 mg b.i.d.
	   < 60 kg, 30 mg b.i.d.

Zalcitabine (ddC)
   HIVID
 Preparations:
 Syrup, 0.1 mg/ml
 (investigational; available through
   compassionate use program)
 Tablets, 0.375 mg and 0.75 mg
	Neonatal dose: unknown
	 Pediatric usual dose: 0.01 mg/kg q.8h
	 Pediatric dosage range: 0.005 to 0.01 mg/kg q.8h
	 Adolescent/adult dose: 0.75 mg t.i.d.

Zidovudine (ZDV, AZT)
   RETROVIR
 Preparations:
 Syrup, 10 mg/ml
 Capsules, 100 mg
 Tablets, 300 mg
 Tablets: COMBIVIR (300 mg zidovudine
   in combination with 150 mg lamivudine)
 Concentrate for injection, for intravenous
   infusion: 10 mg/ml
	Dose in premature infants: (standard neonatal
	   dose may be excessive in premature infants)
	     Under study: oral or i.v. 1.5 mg/kg q.12h from
	     birth to 2 weeks of age; then increase to
	     2 mg/kg q.8h after 2 weeks of age
	 Neonatal dose: oral, 2 mg/kg q.6h
	   Intravenous 1.5 mg/kg q.6h
	 Pediatric usual dose: oral, 160 mg/m^2 q.6h
	 Intravenous (intermittent infusion), 120 mg/m^2 q.6h
	 Intravenous (continuous infusion), 20 mg/m^2/h
	 Pediatric dosage range: 90 mg/m^2 to 180 mg/m^2 q.6–8h
	 Adolescent/adult dose: 200 mg t.i.d. or 300 mg b.i.d.

Continued

Table 17.7 Continued

Non-nucleoside analog reverse transcriptase inhibitor (NNRTI) agents

Delavirdine (DLV)
  RESCRIPTOR
Preparations:
  Tablets, 100 mg

Neonatal dose: unknown
Pediatric dose: unknown
Adolescent/adult dose: 400 mg t.i.d.

Nevirapine (NVP)
  VIRAMUNE
Preparations:
Suspension, 10 mg/ml
  (investigational; available through compassionate
  use program)
Tablets, 200 mg, scored

Neonatal dose (through 3 months): under study
  5 mg/kg once daily for 14 days, followed by
  120 mg/m^2 q.12 h for 14 days, followed by
  200 mg/m^2 q.12h
Pediatric dose: 120 to 200 mg/m^2 q.12h
Initiate therapy with 120 mg/m^2 given once daily for
  14 days. Increase to full dose administered q.12 h
  if no rash or other untoward effects
Adolescent/adult dose: 200 mg q.12h
Initiate therapy at half dose for the first 14 days.
  Increase to full dose if no rash or other untoward
  effects.

Protease inhibitor (PI) agents

Indinavir (IDV)
  CRIXIVAN
Preparations:
Capsules, 200 and 400 mg

Neonatal dose: unknown; because of side effect of
  hyperbilirubinemia, should not be given to
  neonates until additional information available
Pediatric dose: under study in clinical trials, 500 mg/m^2
  q.8h
Adolescent/adult dose: 800 mg q.8h

Nelfinavir (NFV)
  VIRACEPT
Preparations:
Powder for oral suspensions,
  50 mg per 1 level scoop
  (200 mg per 1 level teaspoon)
Tablets, 250 mg

Neonatal dose: under study: 10 mg/kg t.i.d.
  (note: no preliminary data available,
  investigational)
Pediatric dose: 25 to 30 mg/kg q.8h
Adolescent/adult dose: 750 mg t.i.d.

Ritonavir (RTV)
  NORVIR
Preparations:
Oral solution, 80 mg/ml
Capsules, 100 mg

Neonatal dose: under study
Pediatric dose: 400 mg/m^2 q.12h
To minimize nausea/vomiting, initiate therapy at
  250 mg/m^2 q.12h and increase stepwise to full
  dose over 5 days as tolerated
Pediatric dosage range: 350 to 400 mg/m^2 q.12h
Adolescent/adult dose: 600 mg q.12h (single PI
  therapy)
  400 mg q.12h (in combination with SQV)
  To minimize nausea/vomiting, initiate therapy at
  300 mg q.12h and increase stepwise to full dose
  over 5 days as tolerated

Continued over

Table 17.7 Continued

Saquinavir (SQV)
    INVIRASE (hard gel capsule)
    FORTOVASE (soft gel capsule)
Preparations:
Hard gel capsules (HGC) 200 mg
Soft gel capsules (SGC) 200 mg
	Neonatal dose: unknown
	Pediatric dose: SGC: under study:
	    50 mg/kg t.i.d.
	
	Adolescent/adult dose: HGC, 600 mg t.i.d.
	    SGC, 1200 mg t.i.d. (single PI therapy)
	    400 mg b.i.d. (in combination with RTV)

Table 17.8 Routine prophylaxis for children infected with human immunodeficiency virus

Clinical syndrome	Indications	Prophylaxis and dosage

Bacterial sepsis	Hypogammaglobulinemia
	    Abnormal antibody formation
	Serious bacterial infection
	or
	Presumed bacterial
	    pneumonia × 2
		IVIG, *400 mg/kg/month

Pneumocystis carinii
    pneumonia (PCP)
	Age (yr) CD4$^+$ cells/mm^3
	  < 1 <1500 (20% of total lymphocytes)
	  1–2 < 750 (20%)
	  2–6 < 500 (20%)
	  > 6 < 200 (20%)
		TMP/SMX
		150 mg/m^2/day
		    TMP p.o. divided
		    b.i.d. on 3 consecutive days
		    (M, T, W) each week
		or
		Dapsone, 1 mg/kg/day
		    p.o. (max. 100 mg)
		or
		Aerosolized pentamidine

Tuberculosis (TB)	At birth (when immune function is near
	    normal) for neonates born to HIV-positive
	    mothers if high risk for TB
		BCG vaccine

MAI/MAC	Same as in PCP	Rifabutin 5 mg/kg/day p.o. (max. 300 mg, once daily)

encouraging reports of its efficacy in preventing bacterial sepsis and decreasing the number of hospitalizations.

Pneumocystis carinii pneumonia (PCP), the most common infection in pediatric AIDS and often the first manifestation of disease, warrants an early primary prevention strategy. Trimethoprim–sulfamethoxazole is currently the drug of choice for prophylaxis, with dapsone or aerosolized pentamidine reserved as alternatives for patients intolerant of TMP/SMX.

Although the incidence of *Mycobacterium tuberculosis* infection in pediatric patients with AIDS is considerably lower than in adults, a prevention strategy should be considered for children living in an environment of high tuberculosis (TB) prevalence. The World

Health Organization (WHO) currently recommends the administration of bacilli Calmette-Guerin (BCG) vaccine for HIV-infected patients in high TB-prevalence areas. However, disseminated BCG infection has been reported in children with symptomatic HIV infection who have received this vaccine. *Mycobacterium avium–M. intracellulare* complex (MAC) infection has been recognized with increased frequency and is associated with high morbidity and short survival. Prophylaxis is recommended for adult patients with AIDS, and many experts also recommend treatment for children seen in centers where MAC is commonly encountered. Rifabutin has been approved for prophylaxis. Additional options currently under investigation include azithromycin, clarithromycin and biological-response modifiers. Other clinical syndromes and opportunistic infections in patients with HIV may require suppressive or secondary prevention since recurrence of these diseases is common (Table 17.9).

Bacteremia and sepsis

In contrast to adults with AIDS, children are uniquely susceptible to serious bacterial infections early in the course of HIV disease. Pathogens are those that are also the more common etiologies of infection in normal children (Table 17.10). Infection is sufficiently common that IVIG prophylaxis is recommended as described previously (Table 17.8).

Empiric therapy for a toxic febrile child can be provided with a broad-spectrum cephalosporin (ceftriaxone, cefotaxime or ceftazidime) as a single agent if there is no central intravenous access line in place. For patients with a central line, it would be prudent to offer additional coverage for staphylococci by adding vancomycin, nafcillin, or oxacillin. Antimicrobial therapy can be adjusted as soon as culture results are available. As with any immunocompromised patient, bactericidal antibiotics are preferred to bacteristatic agents, using synergistic combinations when available. Antimicrobial agents should be given in maximum dosages and for maximum durations.

Respiratory infections

Although pneumonia is the most commonly reported bacterial respiratory tract disease in childhood AIDS, upper respiratory tract infections, particularly otitis media and sinusitis, are far more frequent, and both tend to be recurrent. Oral candidiasis is also quite common, occurring early in the course of HIV disease. Mucocutaneous herpes simplex can be severe and may produce recurrent or chronic gingivostomatitis. Therefore intravenous antiviral therapy is sometimes necessary. Pathogens causing otitis media and sinusitis in childhood AIDS are somewhat different from those causing disease in otherwise normal children in that staphylococci (both *S. aureus* and *S. epidermidis*), enterococcus and Gram-negative coliform organisms are relatively more common. However, antibiotics routinely recommended for infection in all children are still appropriate for childhood AIDS patients (Table 17.11).

Table 17.9 Suggested antimicrobial therapy for suppressive or secondary prevention of opportunistic infections in patients infected with human immunodeficiency virus

Clinical syndrome for which initial therapy has been completed	Prophylaxis
Oral and esophageal candidiasis	Clotrimazole, fluconazole, or ketoconazole
Toxoplasma cerebritis	TMP/SMX or pyrimethamine plus sulfadiazine
Cytomegalovirus	High-dose acyclovir, ganciclovir, or foscarnet
Herpes simplex	Acyclovir or vidarabine
Cryptococcosis	Fluconazole or ketoconazole

The differential diagnosis of lower respiratory tract disease (Table 17.12) is unusual, often requiring open lung biopsy for final resolution. One difference as contrasted with adult AIDS is that fungal pneumonias such as histoplasmosis and coccidioidomycosis are extremely rare.

Gastrointestinal infections

In patients with AIDS, normally non-pathogenic gastrointestinal colonizing parasites may produce prolonged symptomatic disease. For this reason, available treatment should be offered if the clinical course suggests an etiologic relationship (Table 17.13). Usual stool pathogens such as rotavirus, *Salmonella, Shigella, Campylobacter, Yersinia* spp., and *Giardia lamblia* can be diagnosed and treated in the usual fashion (see Chapter 10). Additional stool and gastrointestinal studies might include a modified acid-fast or monoclonal antibody stain of stool or duodenal aspirate (*Cryptosporidium* sp. and *Isospora belli*), small bowel biopsy (*Cryptosporidium* and *Microsporidium* spp.), duodenal biopsy (*Isospora belli, G. lamblia*, and *Strongyloides stercoralis*), and ELISA of stool for *G. lamblia*.

Tuberculosis

Propensity to mycobacterial disease results both from immunodeficiency and increased exposure to adults with tuberculosis. By definition, all children born to HIV-positive mothers may be at risk because of the high incidence of tuberculosis among their mothers and other family members. Therefore, any child born into this setting would be a candidate for BCG vaccination. Once disease develops, therapy must be continued for a prolonged period of time (Table 17.14). Atypical mycobacteria are extremely difficult to treat and ideal regimens have really not been determined.

Varicella-zoster

Primary infection (i.e. chickenpox), can be severe and prolonged in children with AIDS. Therefore, exposure to disease warrants the use of varicella-zoster hyperimmune immuno-globulin (VZIG) within 96 h of initial contact (see Chapter 3). Once disease has developed, most AIDS patients should be hospitalized and begun on intravenous acyclovir (30 mg/kg per day or 1500 mg/m^2 per day div. t.i.d.) for 6–14 days, depending on the clinical course. If vesicles continue to erupt but there is no visceral involvement, and cutaneous disease is mild, oral acyclovir (20 mg/kg per dose 5 times per day div. q.4h) can be offered. Response to oral therapy is quite variable so duration of treatment should be individualized.

Table 17.10 Bacterial pathogens causing serious infection in children with AIDS

Streptococcus pneumoniae
Haemophilus influenzae
Salmonella spp.
Staphylococcus aureus
Staphylococcus epidermidis
Pseudomonas spp.
Klebsiella sp.
Streptococci, Group A and B
Enterococcus
Escherichia coli

Table 17.11 Treatment of common upper respiratory infections

Disease	Therapy
Otitis media	Macrolide or cephalosporin
Sinusitis	Macrolide or cephalosporin
Oral candidiasis	Nystatin, clotrimazole, ketoconazole, or fluconazole
Herpes gingivostomatitis	Acyclovir p.o. or i.v.

Table 17.12 Differential diagnosis and treatment of lower respiratory tract infections in childhood AIDS

Etiology	Treatment
Lymphoid interstitial pneumonitis	Prednisone 2 mg/kg per day p.o. div. q.d. for 4–12 weeks; taper dose to lowest maintenance level
Pneumocystis carinii	TMP/SMX 20 mg TMP/100 mg SMX/kg per day p.o. or i.v. div. q.6h for 21 days plus Prednisone 2 mg/kg per day p.o. div. b.i.d. for 5 days, then 1 mg/kg per day div. q.d. for 5 days, then 0.5 mg/kg per day div. q.d. for 11 days Alternative: pentamidine isethionate 4 mg/kg per day i.m. div. q.d. for 12–14 days
Bacterial: *Streptococcus pneumoniae, Pseudomonas aeruginosa, Staphylococcus aureus, Klebsiella* sp., *Haemophilus influenzae,* enterococcus, *Salmonella* sp., *Nocardia* sp., *Listeria* sp., *Pertussis, Legionella* sp., *Moraxella catarrhalis*	See individual pathogen
Tuberculosis and atypical mycobacteria (MAI)	See Tuberculosis section; Chapter 17
Viral: Respiratory syncytial virus (RSV)	Aerosolized ribavirin (20 mg/ml in the reservoir) 18 h per day for 5–10 days
Influenza A	Amantadine 5–8 mg/kg per day (max. 200 mg) p.o. div. b.i.d. for 7–14 days Rimantadine 5 mg/kg per day p.o. div. q.12–24h
Influenza A and B, parainfluenza, measles	Aerosolized ribavirin (as above)
Cytomegalovirus (CMV)	Ganciclovir 7.5 mg/kg per day i.v. div. t.i.d. for 14–21 days then 10 mg/kg per day div. b.i.d.; only treat if biopsy is positive for interstitial inflammation with CMV inclusions and no other pathogens

Table 17.13 Treatment of gastrointestinal protozoa in childhood AIDS

Pathogen	Treatment
Cryptosporidium sp.	Paromomycin 30 mg/kg per day p.o. div. t.i.d.
Isospora belli	TMP/SMX 40 mg TMP/200 mg SMX/kg per day p.o. div. q.i.d. for 10 days (maximum 640 mg TMP, 3200 mg SMX per day) then 20 mg TMP 100 mg SMX/kg per day (mximum 320 mg TMP, 1600 mg SMX per day) for 3 weeks
Microsporidium sp.	None Albendazole investigational
Strongyloides stercoralis	Thiabendazole 50 mg/kg per day div. b.i.d. for 2 days
Blastocystis hominis	Metronidazole 35–50 mg/kg per day p.o. div. t.i.d. for 10 days
Dientamoeba fragilis	Metronidazole 35–50 mg/kg per day p.o. div. t.i.d. for 10 days or Iodoquinol 40 mg/kg per day (maximum 2 g) p.o. div. t.i.d. for 20 days
Balantidium coli	Metronidazole 35–50 mg/kg per day p.o. div. t.i.d. for 7 days
Entamoeba coli	Treatment rarely necessary Metronidazole 35–50 mg/kg per day p.o. div. t.i.d. for 10 days

Table 17.14 Treatment of tuberculosis and atypical mycobacterial disease

Mycobacterium tuberculosis	Isoniazid, rifampin, and pyrazinamide for 2 months followed by Isoniazid and rifampin for 10 months (for dosages see Table 9.13)
Mycobacterium avium –M. intracellulare complex (MAI, MAC)	Clarithromycin 15 mg/kg per day p.o. div. b.i.d. plus Rifampin 20 mg/kg per day i.v. or p.o. div. b.i.d. plus Amikacin 22.5 mg/kg per day i.v. div. t.i.d. plus Ciprofloxacin 30 mg/kg per day i.v. or p.o. div. b.i.d.

Measles

Wild measles is a life-threatening infection in childhood AIDS patients and, unfortunately, there is no antiviral therapy of proven benefit. Early in the course of infection, all cases should be treated with a single oral dose of vitamin A; 200 000 U for children over 1 year and 100 000 U for infants 6 months to 1 year of age. In addition, the antiviral agent ribavirin has been shown *in vitro* to exhibit virucidal activity against measles and, in limited clinical trials, both the aerosolized and intravenous preparations have been used.

Fungal infections

Systemic mycoses are relatively rare in childhood AIDS but, when present, are managed as for other immunosuppressed pediatric patients (see Chapter 18 and Tables 20.19 and 20.20). Oral candidiasis is quite common, often requiring continual suppressive therapy for recurrent or chronic disease. If disease remains uncontrolled with nystatin oral suspension (200 000 U (2 ml) p.o. q.i.d.) for 6–12 days, either fluconazole (1–2 mg/kg per day p.o. div. q.d.) or ketoconazole (3–5 mg/kg per day p.o. div. b.i.d.) may be substituted.

HIV EXPOSURE IN HOSPITAL PERSONNEL

Primary prophylaxis against HIV following exposure to contaminated needles remains controversial. The risk for HIV-1 transmission associated with a single parenteral exposure to a contaminated needle is 0.37%. Zidovudine (AZT) alone or in combination with other antiretroviral agents is currently recommended but efficacy for prophylactic use has not been established.

The immunocompromised host 18

NEONATES

The largest group of patients with immuno-deficiency are newborn infants, who have been shown to exhibit a variety of immune defects that predispose these otherwise healthy neonates to life-threatening illness (Table 18.1). It is unclear which defects might be relatively more important and which may be related to specific disease processes. The absence of IgM is considered one of the more important deficiencies, and one that at least partially accounts for propensity to Gram-negative bacterial meningitis and sepsis (see Chapter 2).

The newborn is particularly vulnerable to treatment modalities that may further depress immune function; splenectomy is associated with a much higher long-term morbidity in the neonate as compared to older children and adults, and steroid therapy, similarly, is

Table 18.1 Maturational defects of immunity in neonates

Humoral: absent IgM and IgA
Complement levels: 50% adult concentrations
Specific antibody production: poor response to polysaccharide antigens
Cell-mediated immunity: increased CD8 suppressor cells; decreased killer cell function
Skin test responses: decreased reaction to recall antigens
Phagocytosis: particularly with low concentrations of opsonizing antibody
Inflammatory response
Intracellular killing of bacteria
Viral killing by monocytes
Polymorphonuclear leukocyte and monocyte chemotaxis
Random migration of phagocytes
Polymorphonuclear leukocyte deformability
Generation of serum chemotactic factors

fraught with more complications in this age group. The trauma of both surgery and thermal burns suppresses immune function in patients of all ages but, in neonates, it may have a more potent influence on immune capabilities with resulting fatal infection. Most of the basic principles that apply to the management of immunocompromised patients are relevant to neonates. Maximum doses of bactericidal antibiotics should be given, with duration of therapy often being longer than for similar diseases in infants and children.

IATROGENIC FACTORS

Secondary immunodeficiency is often iatrogenically introduced (Table 18.2). Chemotherapeutic regimens for cancer patients, directed at inhibiting tumor replication are, at the same time, toxic to all elements in bone marrow, including immunologically competent white blood cells. In addition, patients with a variety of diseases are kept alive for longer periods of time using extra-ordinary supportive measures that offer a much greater chance for eventual coloni-zation with multiresistant or unusual micro-organisms, and eventual overt infectious disease. The infectious agents which cause such disease are often opportunistic organ-isms. For each medical intervention in these fragile patients, the physician must calculate risk factors and anticipate complications. Some common complications involve local factors related to diagnostic or therapeutic proce-dures, and to the placement of indwelling catheters, cannulae, or other foreign bodies. This sets the stage for colonization by oppor-tunistic pathogens, which may then account for significant morbidity and mortality.

Table 18.2 Iatrogenic predisposition to infection

Local factors; mucosal and skin lesions
   Drugs (e.g. cyclophosphamide)
   Procedures (i.v. administration, cutdown, bone
     marrow biopsy)
   Surgical wounds
Urinary catheters
Intravascular devices (intravenous, intra-arterial,
   central venous pressure, Swan-Ganz catheters,
   etc.)
Respiratory support (ventilator, intermittent
   positive pressure breathing, etc.)
Transfusion transmitted disease
Splenectomy
Hospital-acquired resistant bacteria (owing to
   inadequate handwashing)

Table 18.3 Infections transmitted by blood transfusions

Bacterial
   Bacterial sepsis
   Endotoxemia
   Brucellosis
   Syphilis
   Salmonellosis
Viral
   Hepatitis A, B and C viruses (now rare)
   Cytomegalovirus (CMV)
   Epstein–Barr virus
   Measles virus
   Rubella virus
   Colorado tick fever virus
   Human immunodeficiency virus
Other
   Toxoplasmosis
   Babesiosis
   Malaria
   Leptospirosis
   Filariasis
   Trypanosomiasis
   Chagas' Disease
   Creutzfeldt–Jakob variant (not established)

Most patients with diseases that result in secondary immunodeficiency receive blood or blood products during the course of their therapy. The transmission of infectious diseases to these patients represents a significant risk, particularly if multiple transfusions are given (Table 18.3). It should be noted that many of these agents are not routinely screened for in potential blood donors. Hepatitis is the best understood and most carefully monitored disease, but recent literature incriminates cytomegalovirus as an agent that is increasingly likely to cause severe illness. Blood donors are often asymptomatic for infectious agents at the time of phlebotomy. In the compromised host additional care should be taken in screening donors and in providing follow-up medical examination of donors as a routine aspect of the recipient's care. Additional problems of transfusion therapy are pulmonary edema from volume overload, hemolytic reactions, and other incompletely understood febrile reactions.

PRIMARY IMMUNODEFICIENCY

It is difficult to determine the incidence of primary immunodeficiency syndromes because many of the more severe forms may result in early infant death before diagnosis is made. In one British study it was estimated that 1 in 50 child deaths was a result of immune dysfunction. Realistically, the more severe defects are only occasionally encountered by primary care physicians. The more common deficiencies, such as transient hypogammaglobulinemia of infancy and selective IgA deficiency, are familiar to clinicians.

Most primary immunodeficiency syndromes present during infancy or early childhood with the most notable exceptions being common variable hypogammaglobulinemia, cyclic neutropenia, and complement deficiencies which may not become clinically apparent until later in life. The deficiencies of the latter components of complement (C5–8) are not seen until adolescence or early adulthood, with the presentation of recurrent meningococcal and gonococcal disease. Immunodeficiency syndromes and their usual age at diagnosis are summarized in Table 18.4.

The approach to therapy varies according to the specific defects demonstrated (Table

Table 18.4 Primary immunodeficiency syndromes in order of their frequency

Syndrome	Usual age at diagnosis	Gender
Transient hypogammaglobulinemia of infancy	6–12 months	Both
Selective IgA deficiency	4–16 years	Both
Common variable hypogammaglobulinemia	All ages	Both
Chronic mucocutaneous candidiasis	1–2 years	Both
Cyclic neutropenia	All ages	Both
X-linked hypogammaglobulinemia (Bruton type)	6–12 months	Male
Ataxia telangiectasia	3–5 years	Both
Chronic granulomatous disease	2 years	Male
Severe combined immunodeficiency (SCID)	9 months	Both
Wiskott–Aldrich syndrome	1–2 years	Male
Thymic hypoplasia (Di George syndrome)	3 months	Both
Complement deficiencies	All ages	Both

Table 18.5 Therapeutic approaches to immunodeficiency syndromes

Syndrome	Therapy
T cell deficiency	
Di George syndrome (thymic aplasia)	Bone marrow transplantation
Nezelof syndrome (thymic hypoplasia)	Antimicrobial therapy, bone marrow transplantation
Wiskott–Aldrich syndrome	Bone marrow transplantation
Ataxia telangiectasia	Fresh plasma, antibiotics
Chronic mucocutaneous candidiasis	Ketoconazole, fluconazole suppressive therapy
B cell deficiency	
Hypogammaglobulinemia	i.v. Immunoglobulin replacement
Selective IgA deficiency	Antibiotics
Complement deficiencies	Antibiotics, fresh plasma, meningococcal vaccine
T and B cell deficiency	
Severe combined immunodeficiency (SCID)	Bone marrow transplantation
Phagocytosis	
Chronic granulomatous disease	Antibiotics, interferon, bone marrow transplantation
Neutropenia	Antibiotics, granulocyte colony stimulating factor (GCSF); granulocyte transfusions

18.5). The most difficult deficiencies to manage are those with T lymphocyte or combined T and B lymphocyte abnormality where bone marrow transplantation usually represents definitive therapy. Selective B lymphocyte deficiencies with hypogammaglobulinemia are treated with immunoglobulin replacement, and this is best managed by the primary care physician. Intravenous preparations of human serum immunoglobulin are readily available for therapy and are generally given at a dosage of 400 mg/kg monthly. These should be used only for patients with documented hypogammaglobulinemia accompanied by recurrent clinical infection, or with demonstrated inability to produce specific antibody following antigenic challenge (e.g. tetanus). The 'physiologic' hypogammaglobulinemia, apparent at 3–6 months of age, does not require supplemental immunoglobulin and must be distinguished from transient hypogammaglobulinemia of infancy. The latter deficiency represents a delay in normal antibody synthesis after maternal IgG is no longer at protective levels; these infants occasionally require immunoglobulin supplementation until approximately 18 months of age.

Defects in neutrophil function are characteristically followed closely and treated aggressively with antibiotics especially during acute infectious episodes. Thus, good communication between patient and physician becomes the most important aspect of management.

SECONDARY IMMUNODEFICIENCY

Suppression of immunologic function with resulting increased susceptibility to infection may occur as a result of a number of primary diseases (Table 18.6). This circumstance is more common in adults than in children because of the higher incidence of malignancy and greater use of immunosuppressive chemotherapy for a variety of diseases. AIDS is the most common predisposing factor in children and its management is covered in detail in Chapter 17. More than 2% of all hospitalized children demonstrate secondary immunodeficiency. Recognition and treatment of these host defense abnormalities have therefore become a very important aspect of hospital practice. Secondary deficiency is actually much more common than primary immunologic disorders, even in infants and children, and is usually managed by primary care physicians with consultative support.

Recognition of associations between specific infectious processes and primary disease offers important guidance to diagnosis and treatment (Table 18.7). All these should be well understood by the physician caring for pediatric patients.

Neutropenia

The congenital neutropenias may present either in childhood or during the adult years and include benign neutropenia with variants thereof, cyclic neutropenia, and what

Table 18.6 The most common causes of secondary immunodeficiency in children

AIDS	Splenectomy
Sickle cell disease	Poor nutrition
Leukemia	Other malignancies
Nephrotic syndrome	Autoimmune disease
Down syndrome	Immunosuppressive chemotherapy

Table 18.7 Unusual pathogens and disease entities associated with secondary immunodeficiency

Leukemia	Disseminated chickenpox
	Pneumocystis carinii pneumonia
	Herpes simplex
	Candida sp. sepsis
	Ecthyma gangrenosum (*Pseudomonas*, *Aeromonas* spp.)
	Aspergillus sp. pneumonia
Sickle cell disease	Pneumococcal meningitis, bacteremia and pneumonia
	Salmonella sp. osteomyelitis
Nephrotic syndrome	Pneumococcal peritonitis
	Disseminated chickenpox
Down syndrome	Pneumococcal pneumonia
	Hepatitis
Splenectomy	Pneumococcal sepsis
Diabetes	Malignant otitis externa (*Pseudomonas* sp.)
	Phycomycosis (mucormycosis)
	Listeriosis

is termed infantile genetic agranulocytosis. These syndromes are secondary to inadequate production of granulocytes and, although a large spectrum of clinical consequences has been described, most patients do not experience a significantly increased propensity to infection. Inadequate production of neutrophil precursors may also be the consequence of nutritional deficiencies, including vitamin B_{12} and folate, or may be secondary to infectious processes such as typhoid fever, infectious mononucleosis, and viral hepatitis. More common are neutropenic states secondary to cytotoxic drugs used in cancer therapy, autoimmune disease, and excessive destruction of granulocytes (either as inherited disorders, hypersplenism, or as a result of artificial heart valves or hemodialysis).

More recently described is an autoimmune process where antibodies directed at neutrophils produce profound neutropenia. These autoantibodies are often seen in conjunction with autoimmune states such as lupus erythematosus and Felty's syndrome. In such cases, infectious diseases are difficult to manage and account for the observed high mortality. Granulocyte transfusions are of no benefit because antineutrophil antibodies destroy donor cells. The clinical approach for patients with neutropenia secondary to immunosuppressive chemotherapy is careful monitoring for infectious episodes and early institution of antimicrobial therapy. Once acute infection is documented, these patients must be treated for much longer periods as it is extremely difficult to eradicate bacteria without the help of the host's granulocyte killing capacity.

Normal neutrophil counts are generally in the range of 2000–5000/mm³, with variations accounted for by age, gender, and race. Although neutropenia is defined as an absolute neutrophil count of < 1500/mm³, increased infection is not observed until a neutrophil count of < 1000/mm³. The absolute neutrophil count is an important objective parameter for making clinical decisions for patients with fever in the face of neutropenia (Table 18.8). It has become a fairly standard protocol to offer antibiotics, pending results of culture, to febrile patients who have a neutrophil count of < 500/mm³.

Table 18.8 Susceptibility staging for neutropenia secondary to immunosuppressive chemotherapy

Absolute neutrophil count/mm³	Predisposition to bacterial infection
> 1000	Little
500–1000	Mild
< 500	Moderate (50%)
< 100	Severe (100%)

During periods of anticipated transient neutropenia, such as during induction therapy for cancer, patients may benefit from granulocyte transfusions. This is impractical unless the period of neutropenia is 6 weeks or less but, under these defined conditions, benefits from such transfusions have been demonstrated.

Neutropenia and fever

The most common clinical circumstance in which the physician must make decisions for the immunocompromised host is fever in the neutropenic patient. In pediatrics this individual is most likely to be a child with leukemia who is neutropenic secondary to chemotherapy administered during treatment of the oncologic process. Such patients are not only neutropenic, but their remaining granulocytes function poorly in phagocytosis and bacteria killing, unlike other neutropenic states (e.g. congenital neutropenia) where remaining neutrophils function normally. This accounts for the increased susceptibility of neutropenic cancer patients over those with neutropenia of other etiology. The etiology of infection in childhood leukemia is summarized in Table 18.9.

The best indicator of susceptibility to systemic bacterial disease is the absolute neutrophil count (see Table 18.8). A count of < 500/mm³ in a febrile patient dictates empiric antimicrobial therapy (Table 18.10). If therapy is not instituted and blood cultures are obtained daily for 5 days, 50–80% will eventually demonstrate bacteremia. If antibiotics are not started until a positive culture is obtained, mortality under these circumstances is over 80%.

Diagnostic evaluation should include cultures of blood, urine, stool, throat and any other suspicious focus, with chest X-ray and lumbar puncture if CNS infection cannot be ruled out clinically. Baseline liver enzymes, renal function studies, and serum electrolytes should also be obtained before beginning antimicrobial therapy. Selection of antibiotics must obviously provide coverage for the most probable pathogens yet be particularly directed at the most difficult-to-treat organisms; in most settings, *Pseudomonas aeruginosa* represents the most resistant organism.

There is at present no clinical evidence that one particular combination from the list in Table 18.10 is more efficacious than another. Monotherapy is preferred unless *Staphylococcus aureus* is a major consideration, or absolute neutrophil counts are < 200/mm^3.

The final general comment is that the duration of recommended therapy is different from that for routine infections; treatment courses are dependent on the duration of fever and granulocytopenia. If a patient shows return of peripheral neutrophils after three days of therapy (Table 18.11), then intravenous antibiotics could be discontinued and the patient changed to oral therapy, particularly if cultures are negative and the patient is afebrile. On the other hand, if fever and granulocytopenia persist, antibiotics are usually continued even after what would normally be considered adequate therapy (Table 18.12).

Candidemia

Recovery of *Candida* sp. from the blood of immunosuppressed patients has become

Table 18.9 Documented etiology of infection in childhood leukemia

Bacteria	(75%)
Staphylococcus epidermis	50%
Staphylococcus aureus	15%
Escherichia coli	3%
Pseudomonas aeruginosa	2%
Klebsiella/Enterobacter sp.	1%
Others	4%
Viral	(20%)
Varicella-zoster virus	7%
Herpes simplex virus	5%
Cytomegalovirus	5%
Fungal	(5%)
Candida albicans	4%

Table 18.10 Initial management of the febrile neutropenic patient

Monotherapy (preferred)
    cefepime
    ceftazidime
    meropenem
    imipenem cilastatin
Staphylococcus aureus or *S. epidermidis* highly suspected
    add vancomycin
Gram (–) highly suspected
    add aminoglycoside
    other combinations with aminoglycoside
        ticarillin
        ticarcillin/clavulanic acid
        azlocillin
        mezlocillin
        piperacillin
Reassess after 3 days (Tables 18.11 and 18.12)

Table 18.11 Continued management of the neutropenic patient after 3 days of i.v. antibiotics

Afebrile and etiology identified
    Adjust to most appropriate management
Afebrile and etiology not identified
    Low risk
        Oral antibiotics: cefprozil, cefpodoxime, cefixime
        ANC > 500/mm^3 at day 7: stop
    Intermediate risk (ANC < 500/mm^3 at day 7)
        Clinically well: stop antibiotics when afebrile 5 days
    High risk (unstable or ANC < 100/mm^3)
        Continue same i.v. antibiotic(s)

ANC, absolute neutrophil count

Table 18.12 Management of patients with persistent fever (5–7 days)

Options for management
    Continue initial antibiotics, stop vancomycin if stable;
    Change antibiotics for progressive disease; or
    Add i.v. fluconazole or amphotericin B
Duration of therapy
    Day 7: afebrile and ANC > 500/mm^3 stop antibiotics
    Day 7: afebrile and ANC < 500/mm^3 continue oral or i.v. antibiotics for 14 days; reassess
    Day 7: febrile continue i.v. antibiotics until afebrile 5 days

commonplace, and is usually the result of two predisposing factors: the use of long-term, broad-spectrum antibiotics and the presence of intravascular access lines. In almost all cases medically placed catheters or other offending foreign bodies should be removed to allow eradication of this fungus. Consideration must also be given to limiting the number of broad-spectrum antimicrobial agents used. Table 18.13 summarizes the management of candidemia. Amphotericin

Table 18.13 Treatment of candidemia in neutropenic patients

Stable patients
    Fluconazole 12 mg/kg/day i.v. div. b.i.d.
Unstable patients
    Amphotericin B 0.8–1.0 mg/kg/day i.v. div. q.24h
    plus
    5-Flurocytosine 100 mg/kg/day p.o.. div. q.6h
    or
    Fluconazole 12 mg/kg/day i.v. div. b.i.d.
    When stable: fluconazole
Empirical therapy (including other fungi)
    Fungus unlikely: fluconazole
    Fungus likely: amphotericin B

B, in relatively low doses and short duration, is usually effective in the treatment of this infection. In the immunologically normal host with candidemia, removal of the intravascular line is often the only step necessary.

PROPHYLAXIS

Some infections in a well-defined group of immunosuppressed hosts are frequent enough to warrant prophylactic therapy (Table 18.14). Circumstances indicating prophylaxis in the immunologically normal host are reviewed in Chapter 5.

CUTANEOUS ANERGY

Transient defects in cell-mediated immunity are commonly encountered during the course of acute or chronic illnesses (Table 18.15). For a variable period of time patients may fail to demonstrate positive delayed hypersensitivity to intradermal skin testing. This presents an enigma to the clinician using a skin test to diagnose a patient's primary illness. To differentiate global cutaneous anergy, a

Table 18.14 Prophylaxis for the immunocompromised host

Underlying disease	Infectious agent	Prophylactic regimen
Leukemia	*Pneumocystis carinii*	Trimethoprim/sulfamethoxazole
Primary immunodeficiency		(TMP/SMX) 4 mg
SCID		TMP/20 mg SMX/kg per day
Di George syndrome		p.o. div. q.12h
Nezelof syndrome		
Asplenia	*Streptococcus pneumoniae*	Pneumococcal vaccine at age
Splenectomy		2 years and 5 years later
Sickle cell disease		plus
Congenital complement		Benzathine
deficiencies (C2, C3, C3b		Penicillin G 1.2×10^6 U i.m.
inhibitor, C5)		q.3 wk [> 27 kg (60 lb)]; 600 000 U
		[< 27 kg (60 lb)]
		or
		Penicillin V 250 mg p.o. b.i.d.
		[> 27 kg (60 lb)];
		125 mg [< 27 kg (60 lb)]
Chronic granulomatous disease	*Staphylococcus aureus*	TMP/SMX
		4 mg TMP/20 mg SMX/kg
		per day p.o. div. q.12h

SCID, severe combined immunodeficiency

battery of skin tests might be applied along with the test antigen. A positive skin test to a recall antigen such as tetanus or candida along with a negative skin test to the pathogen in question would reassure the physician that this patient can respond to specific antigens, and she/he would then interpret the negative specific skin test as evidence against disease. However this reactivity is not absolute, particularly when skin testing for tuberculosis, since antigen-specific non-reactivity has been observed.

The PHA (phytohemagglutination) skin test is probably most sensitive for evaluating anergy; therefore a more rapid resolution of the question would be achieved with this mitogen in the initial skin test battery. Placing other skin tests first would create a delay of 2 days while reading these tests before the PHA skin test could be applied as a second step in the diagnostic work-up.

It is always better to monitor patients with diseases known to be associated with cellular immunodeficiency to alert the physician that a patient is highly predisposed to viral and fungal infectious processes. The degree of cellular immunosuppression can be roughly determined by quantitating T lymphocyte CD4 subpopulations. This testing for clinical management helps to direct early and aggressive use of antifungal or antituberculous medication for the severely immunosuppressed individual, often before receiving final culture results. Using a staging system (Table 18.16), patients can be categorized into those who have mild suppression of cellular immunity and those severely immunosuppressed. The latter group of patients is at extremely high risk for infection with opportunistic pathogens, particularly fungi and herpes group viruses.

TRANSPLANT RECIPIENTS

Patients who have recently undergone transplantation, either bone marrow or solid organs, represent a population with moderate to severe immunodeficiency and with a high risk for opportunistic infections, many of which are caused by reactivated pathogens present in the host or donor organs at the time of transplant. Etiology varies with

Table 18.15 Causes of cutaneous anergy

Primary immunodeficiency
Secondary immunodeficiency
  AIDS
  Malignancy
  Immunosuppressive therapy
  Autoimmune disease
  Surgery (recent)
  Trauma
  Burns
  Poor nutritional status
  Advanced age
  Acugte disease process
Infectious diseases
  Bacterial
  Viral
  Fungal
  Rickettsial
Chronic diseases
  Sarcoidosis
  Rheumatoid
  Renal
  Alcoholism
  Cirrhosis
  Diabetes

Table 18.16 Cellular immunosuppression and susceptibility staging of patients

Degree of immunosuppression		CD4 cells/mm^3
Severe		
Age (years)	< 1	< 700
	1–2	< 500
	2–6	< 250
	> 6	< 100
Moderate		
Age (years)	< 1	700–1200
	1–2	500–750
	2–6	250–500
	> 6	100–250
Mild		
Age (years)	< 1	1200–1750
	1–2	750–1000
	2–6	500–750
	> 6	250–500

timing pre- or post-transplant and is consistent enough to use this parameter in the initial approach to a differential diagnosis (Figure 18.1). Reactivation of herpes group viruses, particularly cytomegalovirus, is so common in these patients that it is critical to obtain serologic data before transplant to determine previous infection with these potential pathogens for both recipient and donor. Prophylactic antiviral and antibacterial therapy is often warranted (Chapter 5).

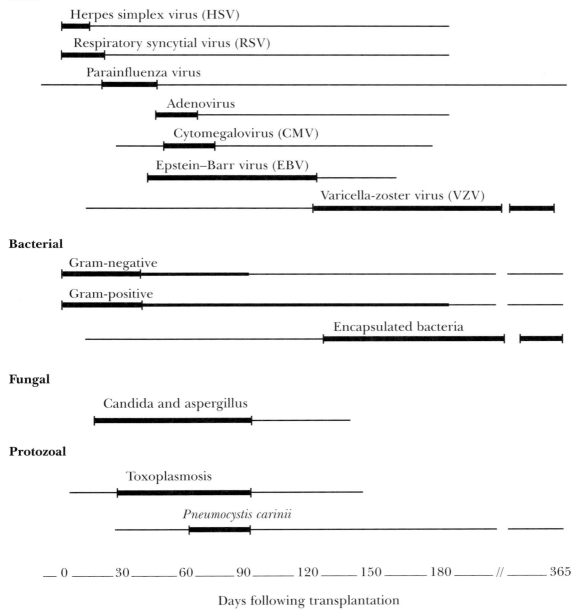

Figure 18.1 Timetable for infection following transplantation

Infection control 19

INFECTIONS IN PEDIATRIC HOSPITAL PERSONNEL

The hospital provides an environment that contains unique, antibiotic-resistant micro-organisms and susceptible, immunosuppressed individuals. In such a setting hospital personnel are exposed to multiple agents and many patients, and may serve as vectors for disease transmission. The infections for which pediatric hospital personnel are at particular risk are given in Table 19.1.

MECHANISMS OF DISEASE TRANSMISSION

Hospital infections are transmitted by airborne dissemination, exposure to a contaminated common vehicle, and person-to-person contact. Because the pediatric patient is usually an ineffective aerosolizer, the hands of hospital personnel become the primary vehicle for carrying micro-organisms from one patient to another.

CONTROL MEASURES

Prevention of infection acquired during hospitalization is a goal of all physicians. A firm understanding of the mechanisms of disease transmission is foremost in infection control; control measures include hand washing, recognition of infectious processes, appropriate treatment of infection, proper handling of patient and body secretions and isolation (when necessary).

ISOLATION POLICIES

Isolation policies must be modified to meet the needs of individual hospitals. For the purposes of this book, representative diseases, as outlined in the Centers for Disease Control manual *Guidelines for Prevention and Control of Nosocomial Infections*, have been selected to illustrate disease-specific isolation techniques.

All infection control groups now recommend standard – blood and body fluid – precautions since medical history and examination cannot identify all patients infected with HIV. These precautions are especially relevant to blood and blood-containing fluids; see list below.

Hand washing: after touching blood, body fluids, secretions, excretions, and

Table 19.1 Infections for which pediatric personnel are at special risk

Bacteria	Viruses	Parasites
Meningococcus	Cytomegalovirus	Pediculosis
Pertussis	Enteroviruses	Scabies
Staphylococcus (methicillin resistant – MRSA)	(e.g. hand-foot-mouth disease)	Tinea capitis and corporis
Tuberculosis	Hepatitis A, B and C	
	HIV	
	Influenza A and B	
	Parvovirus B19	
	Rotavirus	
	Rubella	
	Varicella-zoster	

contaminated items, whether or not gloves are worn. Hands should be washed immediately after removing gloves, between patient contacts, and when otherwise indicated to avoid transfer of micro-organisms to other patients or environments;

Gloves: worn when touching blood, body fluids, secretions, excretions and items contaminated with these fluids. Clean gloves should be used before touching mucous membranes and non-intact skin. Gloves should be promptly removed after use, before touching noncontaminated items and environmental surfaces, and before going to another patient;

Masks, eye protection, and face shields should be worn to protect mucous membranes of the eyes, nose, and mouth during procedures and patient care activities that may generate splashes or sprays of blood, body fluids, secretions, or excretions;

Nonsterile gowns will protect skin and prevent the soiling of clothing during procedures and patient care activities likely to generate splashes or sprays of blood, body fluids, secretions, or excretions. Soiled gowns should be promptly removed;

Patient care equipment that has been used should be handled in a manner that prevents skin and mucous membrane exposures and contamination of clothing.

Linen soiled with blood and body fluids, secretions, and excretions should be handled, transported, and processed in a manner that prevents skin and mucous membrane exposure and contamination of clothing;

Blood-borne pathogen exposure should be avoided by taking all precautions to prevent injuries when using, cleaning, and disposing of needles, scalpels and other sharp instruments and devices; and

Mouthpieces, resuscitation bags, and other ventilation devices should be readily available in all patient care areas and used instead of mouth-to-mouth resuscitation.

General isolation categories are summarized in Table 19.2 and disease-specific recommendations are listed in Table 19.3. Many hospitals use color-coded cards that list requirements for each category and post these on doors of patient rooms. Standard precaution cards are unnecessary since they apply to all patients.

Table 19.2 Infection control categories for hospitalized children

Category of precaution	Hand washing before and after contact	Negative pressure room	Private room	Masks	Gowns	Gloves
Standard	Yes	No	No	During procedures	During procedures	When touching blood and body fluids
Airborne	Yes	Yes	Preferred	At all times	No	No
Droplet	Yes	No	Preferred	If within 3 feet of patient	No	No
Contact	Yes	No	Preferred	No	At all times	At all times

Table 19.3 Disease specific isolation precautions

Agent	Category	Duration of precautions
Adenovirus	Both droplet and contact	Duration of illness
Abscess, etiology unknown (major draining)	Contact	Duration of illness

Comments: major – no dressing or dressing does not adequately contain the pus

Continued

Table 19.3 Continued

Agent	Category	Duration of precautions
(minor or limited draining)	Contact	Duration of illness

Comments: minor or limited-dressing covers and adequately contains pus, or infected area is small (e.g. stitch abscess)

Agent	Category	Duration of precautions
Bronchiolitis, usual etiology, respiratory syncytial virus	Contact	Duration of illness

Comments: various etiologic agents (e.g. respiratory syncytial virus, parainfluenza viruses, adenoviruses, influenza viruses) have been associated with this syndrome

Agent	Category	Duration of precautions
Bronchitis, infective etiology unknown		
Infants and young children	Contact	Duration of illness
Other	Standard	Duration of illness
Chickenpox (varicella)	Both airborne and contact	Minimum 5 days after onset of rash in the nomal host; in immunocompromised patients, as long as the rash is vesicular

Comments: persons who are not susceptible need not wear a mask. Susceptible persons should, if possible, stay out of the room. Special ventilation for the room, if available, may be advantageous, especially for outbreak control. Neonates of mothers with active varicella should be placed on isolation precautions at birth. Exposed susceptible patients should be placed on isolation precautions beginning 10 days after exposure and continuing until 21 days after last exposure. (see *CDC Guideline for Infection Control in Hospital Personnel* for recommendations for exposed susceptible personnel)

Agent	Category	Duration of precautions
Common cold		
Infants and young children	Contact	Duration of illness

Comments: although rhinoviruses are most frequently associated with the common cold, which is mild in adults, severe infections may occur in infants and young children. Other etiologic agents (e.g. respiratory syncytial viruses) may also cause this syndrome

Agent	Category	Duration of precautions
Croup	Contact	Duration of illness

Comments: viral agents (e.g. parainfluenza A virus) have been associated with this syndrome.

Agent	Category	Duration of precautions
Cytomegalovirus	Standard	Hospital stay

Comments: pregnant personnel may need special counseling (see *CDC Guideline for Infection Control in Hospital Personnel*)

Agent	Category	Duration of precautions
Diphtheria	Droplet	Until 2 cultures are negative
Enterovirus	Contact	Duration of hospitalization
Epiglottitis	Droplet	24 h after start of effective therapy
Gastroenteritis		
Campylobacter sp.; *Clostridium difficile*; *Escherichia coli* (enteropathogenic, enterotoxic, or enteroinvasive); *Giardia lamblia*; *Salmonella* sp; *Vibrio parahaemolyticus*; viral; *Yersinia enterocolitica*; unknown etiology	Contact for diapered or incontinent children	Duration of illness

Continued over

Table 19.3   Continued

Agent	Category	Duration of precautions
Rotavirus	Contact	Duration of illness
Shigella sp.	Contact in diapered or incontinent children	Duration of illness
Haemophilus influenzae	Droplet	24 h after start of effective therapy
Hepatitis A	Contact for diapered or incontinent children	Duration of illness
Herpes simplex	Contact for primary neonatal disease	Duration of illness
Influenza	Droplet	Duration of illness
Lice	Contact	24 h after effective therapy
Measles	Airborne	Duration of illness
Meningitis		
Aseptic nonbacterial or viral meningitis (see also specific etiologies)	Contact	Duration of hospitalization

Comments: enteroviruses are the most common cause of aseptic meningitis

Bacterial, Gram-negative enteric in neonates	Standard	Duration of hospitalization

Comments: during a nursery outbreak, cohort ill and colonized infants, and use gowns if soiling likely and gloves when touching feces

Haemophilus influenzae	Droplet	24 h after start of effective therapy
Meningococcus	Droplet	24 h after start of effective therapy
Meningococcemia	Droplet	24 h after start of effective therapy

Comments: see Chapter 5 for recommendation for prophylaxis after exposure

Mumps	Droplet	9 days after onset of disease
Mycoplasma pneumoniae	Droplet	Duration of illness
Parainfluenza	Contact	Duration of illness
Parvovirus B19	Droplet	7 days after onset of disease
Pertussis	Droplet	5 days after start of effective therapy
Respiratory syncytial virus	Contact	Duration of illness
Rubella	Droplet	7 days after onset of rash
Scabies	Contact	24 h after effective therapy
Staphylococcal disease	Contact	Duration of illness
Streptococcal disease	Contact	24 h after start of effective therapy
Tuberculosis, only pulmonary with cavitation	Airborne	Individually based
Zoster (in immunocompromised host)	Both airborne and contact	Duration of illness

Comments: see Chapter 5 for recommendations for prophylaxis after exposure

Antimicrobial therapy 20

EMPIRIC THERAPY

Initial selection of antimicrobial agents is usually made before definitive cultures and sensitivities are available. The physician must, therefore, first have an understanding of the pathogens that commonly cause the specific infectious process under consideration. Other chapters in this book discuss in greater detail anticipated etiologic agents. This understanding must then be translated into initial empiric therapy (Tables 20.1 and 20.2). With the increasing number of new pharmaceutical products entering the market, there are now many alternatives for this selection.

It is, of course, essential to obtain all necessary Gram stain and culture specimens before beginning treatment. In many cases, Gram stains of body fluids (buffy coat, joint aspiration, cerebrospinal fluid, urine, pleural effusion, etc.) will guide selection of antimicrobial agents.

ADVERSE REACTIONS

An appreciation of untoward side-effects is as important as a knowledge of the therapeutic potential of antibiotics. Many antibiotics are of equal efficacy, therefore selection is often determined on the basis of relative toxicity (Tables 20.3 and 20.4). Third generation cephalosporins (ceftriaxone, cefotaxime, etc.)

Table 20.1 Initial empiric therapy for serious neonatal infections (birth to 2 months)

Disease	Antibiotics
Sepsis or meningitis (Chapters 1 & 2)	Ampicillin plus Gentamicin, cefotaxime, or ceftriaxone
Necrotizing enterocolitis (Chapter 15)	Clindamycin or Metronidazole plus Ampicillin plus Cefotaxime, ceftriaxone, gentamicin or amikacin
Osteomyelitis (Chapter 11)	Oxacillin or nafcillin
Peritonitis (Chapter 15)	Ampicillin plus Clindamycin plus Cefotaxime, ceftriaxone or gentamicin
Pneumonia	Oxacillin or nafcillin plus Cefotaxime, ceftriaxone or gentamicin
Septic arthritis (Chapter 11)	Nafcillin or oxacillin plus Ceftriaxone
Urinary tract infections (Chapter 12)	Ceftriaxone, cefotaxime or gentamicin

Table 20.2 Initial empiric therapy for infants and children (> 2 months old)

Disease	Antibiotics
Sepsis or meningitis (Chapters 1 & 2)	Ceftriaxone or cefotaxime plus Vancomycin (add clindamycin if Group A streptococcus is considered)
Cellulitis (Chapter 6)	
Facial, orbital, preseptal	Ceftriaxone or cefotaxime
Facial (following trauma)	Nafcillin or oxacillin
Trunk or extremities	Ceftriaxone or cefotaxime
Osteomyelitis (Chapter 11)	Nafcillin or oxacillin
Foot (following trauma)	Ticarcillin plus Gentamicin plus Nafcillin or oxacillin
Otitis media (Chapter 6)	Macrolide or cephalosporin
Pneumonia (Chapter 9)	
< 5 years	Amoxicillin
> 5 years	Macrolide
Severe or with empyema	Nafcillin or oxacillin plus Ceftriaxone, cefotaxime or cefuroxime
Septic arthritis (Chapter 11)	Cefazolin, nafcillin or oxacillin
Shunt infections (ventriculoperitoneal) (Chapter 14)	Vancomycin plus Ceftriaxone or cefotaxime
Sinusitis (Chapter 9)	Macrolide or cephalosporin
Urinary tract infections (Chapter 12)	
Cystitis	Amoxicillin, TMP/SMX, sulfisoxazole, or cephalosporins

Pyelonephritis	Gentamicin, 3rd gen. cephalosporins,
	  or TMP/SMX; add ampicillin for
	  adolescents

TMP/SMX, trimethoprim/sulfamethoxasole

are desirable because they circumvent the potential toxicity of chloramphenicol and aminoglycosides when treating *Haemophilus influenzae* or Gram-negative coliform infection, respectively. Similarly, oxacillin is preferred over nafcillin, because phlebitis is relatively less common. Oxacillin should be used in neonates because nafcillin serum and tissue levels are erratic in this age group. Tetracyclines should be avoided in children under 8 years of age, as this drug is deposited in teeth and bones.

There is a narrow margin between therapeutic and toxic levels of chloramphenicol

Table 20.3 Relative frequency of allergic reactions to commonly used antibiotics

Highest frequency
  Tetracyclines
  Sulfonamides
  Penicillins
  Cephalosporins
  Aminoglycosides
  Quinolones
  Chloramphenicol
Lowest frequency
  Erythromycin

Table 20.4 Important adverse reactions associated with antibiotics

All antibiotics
  Gastrointestinal symptoms most common
  Overgrowth of resistant bacteria and fungi
    (*Candida albicans*)
  Hypersensitivity skin rashes
  Serum sickness
  Anaphylaxis
  Bone marrow toxicity
  Nephrotoxicity
  Pseudomembranous colitis
  Drug fever
Aminoglycosides
  Nephrotoxicity (reversible)
  Ototoxicity (permanent)
Cephalosporins
  Nephrotoxicity
  Direct Coomb's reaction (probably of no
    clinical significance)
  Phlebitis and phlebothrombosis
    Cefaclor
      Serum sickness-like reaction
    Cefamandole
      Antabuse (disulfiram) effect
Chloramphenicol
  Aplastic anemia
  Circulatory collapse (gray syndrome)
  Hypoplastic bone marrow
Erythromycin
  Nausea
  Abdominal pain
  Cholestatic hepatitis
  Phlebitis
Penicillins
  Ampicillin
    Diarrhea
  Tircarcillin, piperacillin
    Platelet dysfunction
Quinolones
  Destruction of developing cartilage (only seen
    in animals)
Rifampin
  Gastrointestinal distress
  Thrombocytopenia
Sulfonamides
  Stevens–Johnson syndrome
Tetracycline
  Decreased bone growth and staining of teeth
    in children under 8 years of age
  Photosensitivity
  Abdominal pain

Continued

Table 20.4   Continued

  Diarrhea
  Pseudotumor cerebri
  Angioedema
  Brown tongue
  Glossitis
  Anal pruritis
  Fanconi's syndrome
Minocycline
  Vestibular toxicity
Trimethoprim/sulfamethoxazole
  Hypersensitivity skin rashes
  Stevens–Johnson syndrome

and aminoglycosides. Therefore, monitoring of peak and trough levels is essential for individual dosage adjustment. For most other antibiotics, toxic levels far exceed the usual therapeutic ranges.

HOST FACTORS RELATED TO ANTIBIOTIC SELECTION

The compromised host

The selection of antibiotics for the compromised host, particularly the granulocytopenic patient, requires three major alterations in prescribing practice. First, two agents rather than one should be given and these should be chosen for their potential synergism against the presumed or identified pathogen (Table 20.5). Second, maximum dosages and duration of therapy should be employed. Finally, where alternatives are available, bactericidal rather than bacteriostatic agents should be given (Table 20.6). This is necessary because bacteriostatic agents primarily inhibit bacterial growth while relying on host factors for complete killing of the organisms. Following therapy with these agents in the compromised host relapse is frequent. Bactericidal agents are much more effective in totally eliminating pathogens in the absence of adequate mechanisms of host defense.

Table 20.5   Antibiotic synergism for the immunocompromised patient

Pathogens	Synergistic combinations
Pseudomonas aeruginosa	Aminoglycoside plus A broad-spectrum penicillin or a broad-spectrum cephalosporin
Staphylococcus aureus	Gentamicin plus Nafcillin, oxacillin or vancomycin
Enterococci	Gentamicin plus Ampicillin, penicillin or vancomycin
Klebsiella pneumoniae	Aminoglycoside plus Cephalosporin
Coliforms (*Escherichia coli, Enterobacter proteus*, and *Providencia*)	Gentamicin plus Ampicillin, broad-spectrum penicillins or cephalosporins
Mycobacterium tuberculosis	Isoniazid plus Rifampin

Table 20.6   *In vitro* classification of antibiotics

Bactericidal
  Aminoglycosides
  Carbapenems (imipenem, meropenem)
  Cephalosporins
  Monobactams (aztreonam)
  Penicillins
  Quinolones
  Vancomycin
Bacteriostatic
  Chloramphenicol
  Clindamycin
  Erythromycin
  Tetracyclines

Table 20.7   Antibiotics not requiring dosage adjustments for renal impairment

Amphotericin B
Azithromycin
Ceftriaxone
Chloramphenicol
Clindamycin
Doxycycline
Minocycline
Nafcillin
Oxacillin
Pyrimethamine
Rifabutin

Renal failure

In patients with abnormal renal function, dosages of many antibiotics must be altered relative to the degree of renal impairment. In some circumstances an antibiotic can be chosen that is excreted by extrarenal mechanisms – avoiding potential increased toxicity (Table 20.7).

However, most antibiotics require some adjustment calculated on the basis of creatinine clearance and its percentage of normal (Table 20.8); if such a selection is made, it becomes more important to monitor drug serum levels when this can be done.

Creatine clearance (CrC1) in ml/min/1.73 m² for renal impairment is calculated from the formula

$$CrC1 = kL/Pcr$$

where L is the height of the patient in cm, Pcr is plasma creatinine (mg/dl) and k is a

Table 20.8 Normal glomerular filtration rate (GFR) by age

Age	GFR – mean ml/min/1.73 m²
Neonates < 34 weeks gestational age	
2–8 days	11
8–28 days	20
30–90 days	50
Neonates > 34 weeks gestational age	
2–8 days	39
8–28 days	47
30–90 days	58
1–6 months	77
6–12 months	103
12–19 months	127
2–12 years	127

'constant' which, in fact, varies according to the patient; for LBW during the first year of life k = 0.33, for term AGA during the first year of life k = 0.45, for children and adolescent girls k = 0.55, and for adolescent boys k = 0.70.

After estimating creatinine clearance for patients with renal impairment and determining the percent of CrCl compared to normal values as given in Table 20.8, adjustments in antibiotic dosing can be determined using Table 20.9.

There are two basic approaches to dosage modification: increasing the dosing interval or decreasing the individual dosage. For severe infections, particularly with bacteremia, many experts recommend the latter approach, which best assures longer intervals with high serum levels of antibiotic. This approach, however, is more likely to result in higher trough levels, which may increase the risk of nephrotoxicity for aminoglycosides. For most other infections, it is more prudent to increase the dosing interval and obtain peak and trough levels to further guide therapy.

Hepatic failure

For patients with severe hepatic disease the following antibiotics, that are metabolized by the liver, or excreted through the biliary tract, should be avoided: cefoperazone; chloramphenicol; clindamycin; isoniazid; macrolides; nitrofurantoin; rifampin; tetracyclines. Adequate guidelines for dosage modification are simply not available. The only approach which might assure safe administration is frequent measurement of serum drug levels.

Penicillin allergy and desensitization

In patients with documented allergic reactions to penicillins, one of this class of antibiotics may still have to be given for certain life-threatening infections. The most common clinical circumstance is streptococcal or staphylococcal endocarditis. For most other severe infections (meningitis, pneumonia, etc.) cephalosporins represent adequate alternatives.

Penicillin allergy skin testing may be undertaken to confirm hypersensitivity in a patient with a questionable history. Such testing is time consuming and, with currently available reagents, yields a 5% false-negative and 80% false-positive reaction rate. Limitations of this testing are primarily attributable to the absence of a reliable minor determinant mixture (MDM). Major determinant, benzylpenicilloyl/polylysine (PPL), can be obtained through commercial sources (Pre-pen; Kremers-Urban, Milwaukee, WI). Some studies have used a fresh solution of crystalline penicillin G as the source of MDM. If the antibiotic to be given is a derivative of penicillin, skin testing should include this derivative in addition to testing with PPL and penicillin G. With each product scratch testing should be followed by intradermal injection (0.01–0.02 ml). For scratch testing, a drop of the test solution is placed on the forearm and a 3–5 mm scratch made at this site with a 20-gauge needle. For penicillin G or penicillin derivative testing, serial scratch tests followed by serial intradermal injections with solutions of 0.25 mg/ml, 2.5 mg/ml, and 25 mg/ml are recommended. Each test should be observed for 15 min before proceeding to

Table 20.9 Dosages of antimicrobial agents for patients with renal impairment

Antibiotic	Adjustment for creatinine clearance (% of normal)		
	50–90	*10–50*	*10*
Aminoglycosides (except streptomycin)	75% q.12h*	50% q.12h	20% q.24h
Streptomycin	50% q.24h	50% q.48h	50% q.72h
Carbapenems			
Imipenem	75% q.8h	50% q.8h	25% q.12h
Meropenem	100% q.8h	75% q.12h	25% q.24h
Cephalosporins	100%	100%	100%
Cefazolin	q.8h	q.12h	q.24h
Cefepime	q.12h	q.16h	q.24h
Cefotaxime	q.8h	q.12h	q.24h
Cefoxitin	q.8h	q.12h	q.24h
Ceftazidime	q.12h	q.24h	q.48h
Ceftriaxone	–	no adjustment	–
Cefuroxime	q.8h	q.12h	q.24h
Fluconazole	100% q.24h	100% q.24h	100% q.48h
Macrolides			
Azithromycin	–	no adjustment	–
Clarithromycin	100% q.12h	75% q.12h	50% q.12h
Erythromycin	100% q.6h	100% q.6h	75% q.6h
Metronidazole	100% q.6h	100% q.6h	50% q.6h
Monobactams			
Aztreonam	100% q.8h	50% q.8h	25% q.8h
Penicillins			
Amoxicillin	100% q.8h	100% q.8h	100% q.24h
Ampicillin	100% q.6h	100% q.6h	100% q.12h
Mezlocillin	100% q.6h	100% q.6h	100% q.8h
Penicillin G	100% q.6h	75% q.6h	50% q.6h
Piperacillin	100% q.6h	100% q.6h	100% q.8h
Ticarcillin	50% q.6h	50% q.8h	50% q.12h
Ticarcillin/clavulanate	100% q.6h	75% q.6h	75% q.12h
Tetracycline	100% q.8h	100% q.12h	100% q.24h
Trimethoprim/ sulfamethoxazole	100% q.12h	100% q.18h	100% q.24h
Vancomycin	50% q.12h	25% q.24h	25% q.48h

*% of dosage for children with normal renal function (with dosing interval)

the next. A positive reaction is a wheal greater than 5 mm. Normal saline and histamine (1 mg/ml) should be included as negative and positive controls.

When a penicillin must be given to an allergic patient, desensitization, beginning with oral administration, should be accomplished – this can be done with penicillin G or any derivative (Table 20.10). Desensitization should be undertaken in the hospital where careful monitoring and treatment for allergic reactions are available.

Table 20.10 Penicillin desensitization

Time	Dose (mg)	Units	Route
0	0.05	100	p.o.
15 min	0.10	200	p.o.
30 min	0.25	400	p.o.
45 min	0.5	800	p.o.
1 h	1	1600	p.o.
1 h 15 min	2	3200	p.o.
1 h 30 min	4	6400	p.o.
1 h 45 min	8	12 500	p.o.
2 h	15	25 000	p.o.
2 h 15 min	30	50 000	p.o.
2 h 30 min	60	100 000	p.o.
2 h 45 min	125	200 000	p.o.
3 h	250	400 000	p.o.
3 h 15 min	125	200 000	s.c.
3 h 30 min	250	400 000	s.c.
3 h 45 min	500	800 000	s.c.
4 h	625	1 000 000	i.m.
4 h 15 min	Begin full dose i.v.		

DOSAGES OF ANTIBIOTICS

Neonates

There are actually very few antibiotics commonly used for the treatment of neonatal infection. Pharmacokinetics, however, change rapidly during the first weeks of life and differ between prematurely born and full term neonates. Dosages and intervals of administration (Tables 20.11 and 20.12) must therefore be adjusted frequently during the course of treatment, and this requirement represents the most unique feature of therapy in the neonatal patient. Selection of an aminoglycoside in a particular institution is more predicated on resistance patterns of coliforms for that institution than on pharmacokinetic differences. It is always necessary to monitor peak and trough levels of aminoglycosides, so laboratory capabilities may influence choices among these agents.

Infants and children

After 28 days of age pharmacokinetic patterns are quite constant, although different from adult patterns which have a relatively smaller volume of distribution. This simply means that relatively higher amounts of antibiotics must be given to children to achieve the same serum concentrations. Dosages can be calculated according to weight for most children (Tables 20.13 amd 20.14), exceptions being those with excessive obesity or malnutrition (cystic fibrosis and cancer patients). In these cases dosages should be calculated by body surface area (see Table 20.16). For children over 12 years of age or weighing more than 40 kg, maximum dosage limitations should be reviewed (see Table 20.15).

Monitoring of drug levels for aminoglycosides, vancomycin, and chloramphenicol should be undertaken for patients who will be on these antimicrobial agents for more than 48 h (after initial culture information is available). Other antibiotic concentrations may be indirectly measured by performing serum bactericidal assays with the recovered pathogen. These assays should be considered for any patient with serious infection who demonstrates a poor clinical response to apparently appropriate therapy.

For the three most common minor infections requiring antibiotic therapy, otitis media, streptococcal pharyngitis and skin infections, a maximum dosage of 1 g of a penicillin, cephalosporin, or erythromycin is recommended. In the case of ampicillin, this maximum dosage is reached as early as 1 year of age or in children weighing at least 10 kg.

Dosage calculations need not be exact but should be calculated so that a convenient individual dose is prescribed (½ teaspoon, 1 teaspoon, etc.). Whenever possible q.d. or b.i.d. rather than t.i.d. or q.i.d. dosing intervals should be used as these are more realistic for patients' and parents' night-time compliance.

Maximum (adult) dosages

For many antibiotics, maximum dosage limitations (Table 20.15) are reached by approximately 12 years of age (40–50 kg). In these older children the volume of distribution is decreased, thereby increasing the possibility of overdosing, with accompanying

Table 20.11 Daily dosages of intravenous antibiotics for neonates with serious infections

Antibiotic	Gestational age in weeks	Dose in mg/kg/dose	Interval in hours (postnatal age)
Acyclovir	> 34	10	8
	< 34	10–15	12
Amikacin	≤ 29	15	48
	30–33	14	48
	34–37	12	36
	≥ 38	12	24
Amphotericin B	All	0.25–0.5	Initial dose
		0.5–1	24–48
Amphotericin B liposome	All	1 (increase daily 1mg)	Initial dose
		1–5	24
Ampicillin	≤ 29	25 to 100	12 (0–28 days)
			8 (> 28 days)
	30–36		12 (0–14 days)
			8 (> 14 days)
	37–44		12 (0–7 days)
			8 (> 7 days)
	> 45		6
Aztreonam	≤ 29	30	12 (0–28 days)
			8 (> 28 days)
	30–36		12 (0–14 days)
			8 (> 14 days)
	37–44		12 (0–7 days)
			8 (> 7 days)
	≥ 45		6
Cefazolin	< 29	25	12 (0–28 days)
			8 (> 28 days)
	30–36		12 (0–14 days)
			8 (> 14 days)
	37–44		12 (0–7 days)
			8 (> 7 days)
	> 45		6
Cefotaxime	≤ 29	50	12 (0–28 days)
			8 (> 28 days)
	30–36		12 (0–14 days)
			8 (> 14 days)
	37–44		12 (0–7 days)
			8 (> 7 days)
	≥ 45		6
Ceftazidime	≤ 29	30	12 (0–28 days)
			8 (> 28 days)
	30–36		12 (0–14 days)
			8 (> 14 days)
	37–44		12 (0–7 days)
			8 (> 7 days)
	≥ 45		8
Ceftriaxone	All	100 (loading)	
		80	24

Continued

Table 20.11 Continued

Antibiotic	Gestational age in weeks	Dose in mg/kg/dose	Interval in hours (postnatal age)
Chloramphenicol	All	20 (loading)	
	< 37	2.5 (< 1 month)	6
		5.0 (> 1 month)	
	> 37	5.0 (< 7 days)	6
		12.5 (> 7 days)	
Clindamycin	< 29	5–7.5	12 (0–28 days)
			8 (> 28 days)
	30–36		12 (0–14 days)
			8 (> 14 days)
	37–44		8 (0–7 days)
			6 (> 7 days)
	> 45		6
Erythromycin	All	5–10	6
Fluconazole	All	12 (loading)	
	≤ 29	6	72 (0–14 days)
			48 (> 14 days)
	30–36		48 (0–14 days)
			24 (> 14 days)
	37–44		48 (0–7 days)
			24 (> 7 days)
	≥ 45		24
Gentamicin	≤ 29	5	48
	30–33	4.5	48
	34–37	4	36
	≥ 38	4	24
Imipenem/cilastatin	All	20–25	12
Meropenem	All	20 (sepsis)	12
		40 (meningitis)	8
		40 (*Pseudomonas* sp.)	8
Methicillin	≤ 29	25–50	12 (0–28 days)
			8 (> 28 days)
	30–36		12 (0–14 days)
			8 (> 14 days)
	37–44		12 (0–7 days)
			8 (> 7 days)
	≥ 45		6
Metronidazole	All	15 (loading)	
	≤ 29	7.5 (maintenance)	48 (0–28 days)
			24 (> 28 days)
	30–36		24 (0–14 days)
			12 (> 14 days)
	37–44		24 (0–7 days)
			12 (> 7 days)
	≥ 45		8
Mezlocillin	≤ 29	50–100	12 (0–28 days)
			8 (> 28 days)
	30–36		12 (0–14 days)
			8 (> 14 days)

Continued over

Table 20.11 Continued

Antibiotic	Gestational age in weeks	Dose in mg/kg/dose	Interval in hours (postnatal age)
Mezlocillin (cont'd)	37–44		12 (0–7 days)
			8 (> 7 days)
	≥ 45		6
Nafcillin	≤ 29	25–50	12 (0–28 days)
			8 (> 28 days)
	30–36		12 (0–14 days)
			8 (> 14 days)
	37–44		12 (0–7 days)
			8 (> 7 days)
	≥ 45		6
Oxacillin	≤ 29	25–50	12 (0–28 days)
			8 (> 28 days)
	30–36		12 (0–14 days)
			8 (> 14 days)
	37–44		12 (0–7 days)
			8 (> 7 days)
	≥ 45		6
Penicillin G	All	75–100 000 IU per dose (meningitis)	
		25–50 000 IU per dose (bacteremia)	
		200–400 000 IU per day (Group B strep)	
	≤ 29		12 (0–28 days)
			8 (> 28 days)
	30–36		12 (0–14 days)
			8 (> 14 days)
	37–44		12 (0–7 days)
			8 (> 7 days)
	≥ 45		6
Piperacillin	≤ 29	50–100	12 (0–28 days)
			8 (> 28 days)
	30–36		12 (0–14 days)
			8 (> 14 days)
	37–44		12 (0–7 days)
			8 (> 7 days)
	≥ 45		6
Rifampin	All	5–10	12–24
Tobramycin	≤ 29	5	48
	30–33	4.5	48
	34–37	4	36
	≥ 38	4	24
Vancomycin	≤ 29	20	24
	30–33	20	18
	34–37	20	12
	38–44	15	8
	≥ 45	10	6
Zidovudine	All	1.5	
	< 37		12 (0–14 days)
			6 (> 14 days)
	> 37		6

Table 20.12 Dosages of oral antibiotics for neonates

Antibiotic (trade name)	Daily dosage (mg/kg except where otherwise stated)
Amoxicillin (numerous trade names)	20–40 div. q.8h
Ampicillin (numerous trade names)	50–100 div. q.8h
Cefaclor (Ceclor)	40 div. q.8h
Cephalexin (Keflex)	50 div. q.6h
Chloramphenicol (Chloromycetin)	< 14 days; 25 div. q.8h
	> 14 days; 50 div. q.6h
Clindamycin (Cleocin)	20 div. q.6h
Cloxacillin (Tegopen)	> 2.5 kg; 50–100 div. q.6h
	< 2.5 kg; 50 div. q.8h
Dicloxacillin (Dycill, Dynapen, Pathocil)	> 2.5 kg; 50–100 div. q.6h
	< 2.5 kg; 50 div. q.8h
Erythromycin (numerous trade names)	30–40 div. q.6–8h
Flucytosine (Ancobon)	50–150 div. q.6h
Metronidazole (numerous trade names)	25 div. q.12h
Nystatin (Mycostatin)	800 000 U div. q.6h
	Premature 400 000 U div. q.6h
Oxacillin (Bactocill, Prostaphlin)	> 2.5 kg; 50–100 div. q.6h
	< 2.5 kg; 50 div. q.8h
Penicillin V (numerous trade names)	50 000 U/kg div. q.8h
Rifampin (Rifadin, Rimactane)	10–20 div. q.24h
Zidovudine (Retrovir)	8 div. q.6h
	Premature infants < 14 days 4 div. q.12h
	Premature infants > 14 days 8 div. q.6h

Table 20.13 Intravenous and intramuscular antibiotic dosages for serious infections in infants and children

Antibiotic (trade name)	Daily dosage (mg/kg unless otherwise stated)
Aminoglycosides	
Amikacin (Amikin)	22 div. q.8h
Gentamicin (numerous trade names)	7.5 div. q.8h
Kanamycin (Kantrex, Klebcil)	30 div. q.8h
Netilmicin (Netromycin)	7.5 div. q.8h
Streptomycin	20 div. q.12h
Tobramycin	7.5 div. q.8h
Aztreonam (Azactam)	100 div. q.6h
Cephalosporins	
Cefamandole (Mandol)	150 div. q.6h
Cefazolin (Ancef, Kefzol)	100 div. q.8h
Cefepime (Maxipime)	150 div. q.8h
Cefoperazone (Cefobid)	> 12 years; 150 div. q.8h
Cefotaxime (Claforan)	200 div. q.6h (300 mg/kg for CNS)
Cefoxitin (Mefoxin)	100 div. q.6h
Ceftazidime (Fortax, Taxicef, Tazidime)	150 div. q.8h
Ceftizoxime (Cefizox)	> 6 months; 200 div. q.6h
Ceftriaxone (Rocephin)	50 div. q.24h (80 mg/kg for CNS)
Cefuroxime (Zinacef)	150 div. q.8h
Cephalothin (Keflin)	100 div. q.6h
Cephradine (Anspor, Velosef)	100 div. q.6h

Continued over

Table 20.13   Continued

Antibiotic (trade name)	Daily dosage (mg/kg unless otherwise stated)
Chloramphenicol (Chloromycetin)	50 div. q.6h (100 mg/kg for CNS)
Ciprofloxacin (Cipro)	20–30 div. q.12h
Clindamycin (Cleocin)	40 div. q.6h
Erythromycin (numerous trade names)	40 div. q.6h
Fluconazole (Diflucan)	12 div. q.12h
Imipenem/Cilastatin (Primaxin)	40–60 div. q.6h
Meropenem (Merem)	60 div. q.8h (120 mg/kg for CNS)
Metronidazole (Flagyl)	30 div. q.6h
Penicillins	
Ampicillin (numerous trade names)	200 div. q.6h (400 mg/kg for CNS)
Mezlocillin (Mezlin)	200 div. q.6h
Nafcillin (Nafcil, Unipen)	150 div. q.6h
Oxacillin (Bactocill, Prostaphlin)	200 div. q.6h
Penicillin G	400 000 U/kg div. q.6h
Penicillin G benzathine i.m.	50 000 U/kg single dose i.m.
Penicillin G procaine i.m.	50 000 U/kg div. q.12h i.m.
Piperacillin (Pipracil)	200–300 div. q.6h
Ticarcillin (Ticar)	300 div. q.6h
Ticarcillin/clavulanate (Timentin)	200–300 div. q.6h
Rifampin (Rifadin, Rimactane)	10–20 div. q.12h
Streptomycin i.m.	30 div. q.12h i.m.
Tetracyclines	
Doxycycline (numerous trade names)	4 div. q.24h
Minocycline (Minocin)	4 div. q.12h
Trimethoprim/sulfamethoxazole (TMP/SMX) (Bactrim, Septra)	20 TMP/100 SMX/kg div. q.6h
Vancomycin (Vancocin)	40 div. q.6h

Table 20.14   Dosages of oral antibiotics for infants and children

Antibiotic (trade name)	Daily dosage (mg/kg unless otherwise stated)
Azithromycin (Zithromax)	10 mg/kg loading dose then 5 mg/kg; strep throat 12 mg/kg
Cephalosporins	
Cefaclor (Ceclor)	50 div. q.8h
Cefadroxil (Duricef, Ultracef)	30 div. q.12h
Cefdinir (Omnicef)	14 div. q.24h
Cefixime (Suprax)	8 single daily dose
Cefpodoxime (Vantin)	10 div. q.12h
Cefprozil (Cefzil)	30 div. q.12h
Ceftibuten (Cedax)	9 single daily dose
Cefuroxime (Ceftin)	30 div. q.12h
Cephalexin (Keflex)	25–50 div. q.6h
Cephradine (Velosef)	25–50 div. q.6h
Chloramphenicol	50–100 div. q.6h
Ciprofloxacin (Cipro)	20–30 div. q.12h

Continued

Table 20.14   Continued

Antibiotic (trade name)	Daily dosage (mg/kg unless otherwise stated)
Clarithromycin (Biaxin)	15 div. q.12h
Clindamycin (Cleocin)	10–20 div. q.6h
Clostin (Coly-Mycin)	5–15 div. q.8h
Dapsone	1 single daily dose
Erythromycin (numerous trade names)	25–50 div. q.6h
Erythromycin and sulfisoxazole (Pediazole)	25–50 of erythromycin div. q.6h
Ethambutol (Myambutol)	15 div. q.24h
Ethionamide (Trecator-SC)	10–20 div. q.12h
Isoniazid (INH, Nydrazid)	10–20 div. q.12–24h
Loracarbef (Lorabid)	15–30 div. q.12h
Methenamine mandelate (Mandelamine, Thiacide, Uroquid)	50 div. q.6h
Metronidazole (Flagyl, Metric, Protostat)	35 div. q.8h
Nalidixic acid (NegGram)	50 div. q.6h
Neomycin (Mycifradin, Neobiotic)	50–100 div. q.6h
Nitrofurantoin (Furadantin, Macrodantin)	7 div. q.6h
	2 div. q.24h (for urinary tract suppressive therapy)
Penicillins	
Penicillin V (numerous trade names)	< 10 kg; 375 div. q.8h
	> 10 kg; 750 div. q.8h
Amoxicillin (numerous trade names)	20–40 div. q.8h
Amoxicillin/clavulanate (Augmentin)	20–40 div. q.8h
Ampicillin (numerous trade names)	50–100 div. q.6h
Bacampicillin	25–50 div. q.12h
Carbenicillin (Geocillin)	25–50 div. q.6h
Cloxacillin (Tegopen)	50–100 div. q.8h
Cyclacillin (Cyclapen-W)	50–100 div. q.8h
Dicloxacillin (Dycill, Dynapen, Pathocil)	25 div. q.6h
Hetacillin (Versapen)	50–100 div. q.6h
Nafcillin (Nafcil, Unipen)	50–100 div. q.6h
Oxacillin (Bactocil, Prostaphlin)	50–100 div. q.6h
Pyrazinamide	30 div. q.12h
Rifampin (Rifadin, Rimactane)	20 div. q.24h
Sulfonamides	
Sulfadiazine	150 div. q.6h
Sulfamethoxazole (Gantanol)	50 div. q.12h
Sulfisoxazole (Gantrisin, SK-Soxazole)	100–150 div. q.6h
Tetracyclines	
Tetracycline (numerous trade names)	50 div. q.6h
Demeclocycline (Declomycin)	8–12 div. q.6h
Doxycycline (Vibramycin)	4 div. q.12h
Methacycline (Rondomycin)	10 div. q.6h
Minocycline (Minocin)	4 div. q.12h
Oxytetracycline (Terramycin)	25 div. q.6h
Trimethoprim/sulfamethoxazole (TMP/SMX)	6–20 TMP/30–100 SMX/kg div. q.12h
(Bactrim, Septra, Cotrim, Sulfatrim)	4 TMP/20 SMX/kg div. q.12h for *Pneumocystis* prophylaxis
Vancomycin (Vancocin)*	50 div. q.6h

*Vancomycin is not absorbed

Table 20.15 Maximum (adult) dosages for parenteral antibiotics

Antibiotic	Maximum daily dosage
Aminoglycosides	
Amikacin	1 g
Gentamicin	300 mg
Kanamycin	1 g
Netilmicin	300 mg
Streptomycin	2 g
Tobramycin	300 mg
Aztreonam	
Cephalosporins	
Cefamandole	6 g
Cefeprime	4 g
Cefazolin	6 g
Cefonicid	2 g
Ceforanide	2 g
Cefotaxime	12 g
Cefoxitin	12 g
Ceftazidime	8 g
Ceftizoxime	12 g
Ceftriaxone	4 g
Cefuroxime	6 g
Cephalothin	12 g
Meropenem	6 g
Chloramphenicol	4 g
Clindamycin	4 g
Erythromycin	4 g
Metronidazole	4 g
Penicillins	
Penicillin G	24×10^6 U
Penicillin G benzathine	2.4×10^6 U
Penicillin G procaine	4.8×10^6 U
Ampicillin	12 g
Azlocillin	24 g
Mezlocillin	24 g
Nafcillin	12 g
Oxacillin	12 g
Piperacillin	24 g
Ticarcillin	24 g
Spectinomycin	4 g
Tetracycline	2 g
Vancomycin	4 g

toxicity, if calculations are made by body weight as with younger patients. Maximum dosages of oral antibiotics are reached even earlier in life, and amounts of antibiotic in tablets and capsules (commonly 250 mg and 500 mg) reflect this limitation.

Body surface area

Patients who are excessively obese or malnourished will be overdosed or underdosed, respectively, if antibiotic dosages are calculated by body weight. For these patients body surface area may be determined using scales or by equation (Figure 20.1). Table 20.16 lists antibiotic dosages calculated by body surface area.

ANTIBIOTICS FOR SPECIFIC PATHOGENS

For many patients a clinical syndrome is apparent at presentation. Pending results of cultures and their antibiotic sensitivities, therapy should be instituted based on reported susceptibility or efficacy data. Table 20.17 summarizes recommended initial antimicrobial therapy. Antibiotic therapy should be re-evaluated once culture information is available.

ANTIVIRAL AGENTS

Antiviral therapy of proven efficacy is currently available for the treatment of the following viruses: cytomegalovirus, hepatitis B, hepatitis C, herpes simplex types 1 and 2, HIV, influenza A, respiratory syncytial virus and varicella-zoster. For herpes-group virus infections therapy is initiated only for certain well-defined infections. Many other antiviral agents are currently under investigation. Table 20.18 offers a summary of therapy for viral infections.

ANTIFUNGAL AGENTS

Systemic fungal infections are being seen with increased frequency as a result of longer survival for patients with severe disease and compromised immune function. Broad-spectrum antibiotics and indwelling foreign bodies (central i.v. lines, urinary catheters, and arterial monitoring devices) are the most significant predisposing factors, particularly for infection with *Candida albicans*. Therefore,

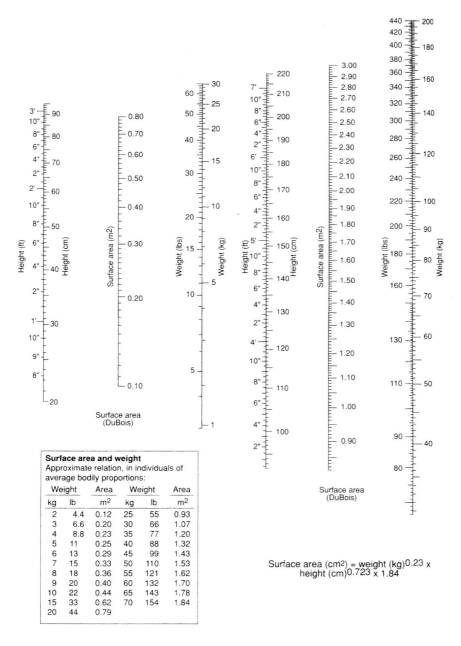

Surface area and weight
Approximate relation, in individuals of average bodily proportions:

Weight		Area	Weight		Area
kg	lb	m²	kg	lb	m²
2	4.4	0.12	25	55	0.93
3	6.6	0.20	30	66	1.07
4	8.8	0.23	35	77	1.20
5	11	0.25	40	88	1.32
6	13	0.29	45	99	1.43
7	15	0.33	50	110	1.53
8	18	0.36	55	121	1.62
9	20	0.40	60	132	1.70
10	22	0.44	65	143	1.78
15	33	0.62	70	154	1.84
20	44	0.79			

Surface area (cm²) = weight (kg)$^{0.23}$ x height (cm)$^{0.723}$ x 1.84

Figure 20.1   Scales for determination of body surface area

241

Table 20.16 Dosages of antibiotics by body surface area

Antibiotic	Daily dosage/m²
Aminoglycosides	
Amikacin	600 mg div. q.8h
Gentamicin	180 mg div. q.8h
Kanamycin	600 mg div. q.8h
Netilmicin	180 mg div. q.8h
Tobramycin	180 mg div. q.8h
Aztreonam	3.2 g div. q.6h
Cephalosporins	
Cefamandole	4.2 g div. q.8h
Cefazolin	2.4 g div. q.8h
Cefonicid	1.1 g div. q.12h
Ceforanide	1.1 g div. q.12h
Cefotaxime	4.2 g div. q.8h
Ceftazidime	4.2 g div. q.8h
Ceftizoxime	4.2 g div. q.8h
Ceftriaxone	2.8 g div. q.24h
Cefuroxime	2.4 g div. q.8h
Cephalothin	5.6 g div. q.6h
Chloramphenicol	2.8 g div. q.6h (CNS)
	1.8 g div. q.6h
Imipenem	2.2 g div. q.6h
Metronidazole	840 mg div. q.8h
Penicillins	
Penicillin G	10.5×10^6 U div. q.6h (CNS)
	2.7×10^6 U div. q.6h
Ampicillin	5.6 g div. q.6h
Azlocillin	10 g div. q.6h
Methicillin	5.6 div. q.6h
Mezlocillin	10 g div. q.6h
Nafcillin	4.2 g div. q.6h
Oxacillin	5.6 g div. q.6h
Piperacillin	10 g div. q.6h
Ticarcillin	10 g div. q.6h
Trimethoprim/ sulfamethoxazole (TMP/SMX)	300 mg TMP/1.5 g SMX div. q.8h
Vancomycin	1.7 g div. q.6h (CNS)
	1.1 g div. q.6h
Zidovudine	640 mg div. q.6h

strong consideration must be given to discontinuing these antibiotics and removing any indwelling source of fungal colonization. Amphotericin B was previously the most commonly recommended agent for invasive *Candida albicans* infection but because of its toxicity has been largely replaced by fluconazole (Chapter 18, Table 18.13). Therapy for fungal infections is summarized in Tables 20.19 and 20.20. Renal function must be carefully monitored and, whenever possible, both dosage and duration of therapy should be minimized.

ANTIPARASITIC AGENTS

Parasitic infections are much less commonly encountered in medical practice in the USA today as contrasted with just one generation ago. This change is attributed primarily to improved urban sanitation. Moreover, few cities have retained soil conditions necessary for maintenance of the life cycle of most parasites. Pinworm remains the most common parasitic infestation in the United States and therapy is indicated only when symptoms are of clinical significance or the worm burden is excessive, since recurrence is almost universal. Giardiasis is being seen with greater frequency as a result of increased use of day care centers, where disease is readily transmitted. Therapy for parasitic infections is shown in Table 20.21. For unusual parasitic infections telephone consultation should be obtained from the Centers for Disease Control, Atlanta, GA, where many of the preferred therapeutic agents are available. The telephone number is (770) 488-7760.

Table 20.17 Therapy for defined clinical syndromes or specific micro-organisms

Infection	Drug of choice	Alternatives
Actinomycosis	Penicillin G	Tetracycline, clindamycin
Adenitis (Chapter 6)	Cloxacillin, dicloxacillin, oxacillin, cephalexin or erythromycin	
Aeromonas spp.	Trimethoprim/sulfamethoxazole (TMP/SMX)	Aminoglycoside; imipenem
Anthrax	Penicillin	Erythromycin
Arcanobacterium hemolyticum	A macrolide	Penicillin
Bacillary angiomatosis	A macrolide	TMP/SMX
Bacillus spp.	Vancomycin	Clindamycin
Bartonellosis	Chloramphenicol	Penicillin or tetracycline
Botulism (Chapter 1)	Penicillin	Tetracycline
Brucellosis	Gentamicin plus Tetracycline	TMP/SMX, rifampin
Burkholderia cepacia	TMP/SMX	Cefazidime
Campylobacter enteritis (Chapter 10)	Erythromycin	Tetracycline
Capnocytophagacanimorsus	Penicillin	A macrolide
Cat-scratch disease	Azithromycin	Gentamicin, TMP/SMX, rifampin
Chancroid (Chapter 16)	Ceftriaxone, a macrolide	Ciprofloxacin
Chlamydia trachomatis (Chapter 16)	A macrolide	Sulfisoxazole
Chlamydia pneumoniae	Azithromycin, clarithromycin	Tetracycline
Cholera	Tetracycline	TMP/SMX
Clostridium difficle	Metronidazole	Vancomycin
Diphtheria (Chapter 1)	A macrolide	Penicillin
Ehrlichiosis	Tetracycline	Chloramphenicol
Endocarditis (Chapter 1)	Ampicillin plus Vancomycin	
Erysipelas (Chapter 6)	Penicillin	A macrolide
Erysipeloid	Ampicillin	Gentamicin, tetracycline
Erythrasma	Topical miconazole or clindamycin	A macrolide
Gas gangrene	Penicillin	Tetracycline
Glanders	Gentamicin plus Tetracycline	Chloramphenicol
Gonorrhea (Chapter 16)	Ceftriaxone	Cefixime, ofloxacin, ciprofloxacin, tetracycline, spectinomycin, cefoxitin, or cefotaxime
Granuloma inguinale (Chapter 16)	Tetracycline	Erythromycin
Helicobacter pylori	Amoxicillin plus Metronidazole plus Pepto-Bismol	Clarithromycin plus Omeprazole
Impetigo (Chapter 13)	Erythromycin	Mupirocin (topical)
Kingella kingae	Ampicillin	Ceftriaxone
Legionnaires' disease (Chapter 9)	A macrolide and rifampin	TMP/SMX; ciprofloxacin

Continued over

Table 20.17 Continued

Infection	Drug of choice	Alternatives
Leprosy	Clofazimine plus Dapsone plus Rifampin	Clarithromycin, sparfloxacin; minocycline
Leptospirosis	Penicillin	Tetracycline
Listeriosis	Ampicillin plus Gentamicin	TMP/SMX; vancomycin
Ludwig's angina (Chapter 13)	Ceftazidime plus Clindamycin	
Lyme disease (early) (severe)	Tetracycline Ceftriaxone	Amoxicillin
Melioidosis	Ceftrazidime plus Sulfisoxazole plus Gentamicin	TMP/SMX; tetracycline
Meningococcemia (Chapter 11)	Ceftriaxone or penicillin	Chloramphenicol
Mycoplasma pneumoniae	Azithromycin or clarithromycin	Tetracycline
Necrotizing fasciitis	Clindamycin plus Penicillin or ceftriaxone	
Nocardiosis	Sulfisoxazole or TMP/SMX plus Amikacin (for first 7 days)	Amikacin
Otitis externa (Chapter 6)	Antibiotic–steroid ear drops	
Otitis media (Chapter 6)	Macrolide, cephalosporin or amoxicillin	
Parotitis, suppurative	Nafcillin or oxacillin plus Gentamicin	
Pertussis (Chapter 9)	A macrolide	TMP/SMX
Plague	Gentamicin plus Tetracycline	Chloramphenicol
Pneumocystis carinii (Chapters 17 & 18)	TMP/SMX	Pentamidine
Pseudomembranous colitis (Chapter 10)	Metronidazole p.o.	Vancomycin p.o.
Psittacosis	Tetracycline	Chloramphenicol
Q fever	Tetracycline	Chloramphenicol
Rat-bite fever	Penicillin	Tetracycline
Relapsing fever	Tetracycline	Penicillin
Rickettsial	Tetracycline	Chloramphenicol
Salmonellosis (Chapter 10)	Ceftriaxone	TMP/SMX; ampicillin (if susceptible)
Scarlet fever	Pencillin	Erythromycin

Continued

Table 20.17   Continued

Infection	Drug of choice	Alternatives
Shigellosis (Chapter 10)	TMP/SMX	Ceftriaxone, ciprofloxacin
Sinusitis (Chapter 9)	A macrolide or cephalosporin	Amoxicillin/clavulanate, or erythromycin–sulfa combination
Staphylococcal scalded skin syndrome	Nafcillin/oxacillin	Vancomycin
Syphilis (Chapter 16)	Penicillin	Tetracycline, ceftriaxone
Tetanus (Chapter 1)	Penicillin	Tetracycline
Toxoplasmosis (Chapter 2)	Pyrimethamine plus Sulfadiazine	Spiramycin
Traveler's diarrhea (Chapter 4)	TMP/SMX	Doxycycline or ciprofloxacin (over 18 years)
Tuberculosis (Chapter 9)	Isoniazid plus Rifampin plus Pyrizinamide plus Streptomycin or ethambutol (older child)	
Tularemia	Gentamicin	Tetracycline
Typhoid fever	Ceftriaxone	TMP/SMX, or chloramphenicol
Typhus	Tetracycline	Chloramphenicol
Ureaplasma urealyticum	A macrolide	Tetracycline
Vaginosis (bacterial)	Metronidazole	Clindamycin
Vincent's angina	Penicillin	Erythromycin
Yersiniosis	TMP/SMX	A macrolide, tetracycline or an aminoglycoside

Table 20.18   Therapy for viral infections

Viral infection	Drug of choice	Dosage
Cytomegalovirus pneumonia	Ganciclovir plus IVIG	2.5 mg/kg q.8h i.v. for 20 days 500 mg/kg q.o.d. for 10 doses then ganciclovir 5 mg/kg/day 3–5 times/week for 20 doses plus IVIG 500 mg/kg 2 times/week for 8 doses
retinitis	Ganciclovir or foscarnet	5 mg/kg i.v. b.i.d. for 14–21 days 60 mg/kg i.v. q.8h for 14–21 days
Hepatitis B virus chronic hepatitis	Interferon α-2b	5×10^6 U/day s.c. for 4 months
Hepatitis C virus chronic hepatitis	Interferon α-2b plus ribavirin	3×10^6 U s.c. or i.m. 3 times per week for 24 weeks

Continued over

Table 20.18 Continued

Viral infection	Drug of choice	Dosage
Herpes simplex virus		
Bell's palsy	Acyclovir plus	20 mg/kg p.o. q.i.d. for 10 days
	prednisone	0.5–1 mg/kg/day d.i.v. q.12h for 10 days
conjunctivitis	Trifluridine	1 drop of 1% solution topically q.2h, up to 9 times per day
encephalitis	Acyclovir	30 mg/kg/day i.v. d.i.v. q.8h for 14–21 days
genital herpes (see Chapter 16)	Acyclovir	
mucocutaneous disease in immunocompromised host	Acyclovir	5 mg/kg i.v. q.8h or 400 mg p.o. 5 times per day for 7–14 days
neonatal	Acyclovir	30 mg/kg/day i.v. div. q.8h for 14–21 days
acyclovir-resistant	Foscarnet	40 mg/kg i.v. q.8h
HIV (see Chapter 17)		
Influenza A virus	Rimantadine	5 mg/kg per day p.o. d.i.v. q.12–24h (maximum 200 mg/day)
	Amantadine	5–8 mg/kg per day p.o. div. q.12h (maximum 200 mg/day)
Respiratory syncytial virus	Ribavirin	Aerosol treatment 12–18 h per day for 3–7 days (20 mg/ml in the reservoir)
Rotavirus – gastroenteritis in immunocompromised host	Immunoglobulin p.o.	
Varicella-zoster virus		
chickenpox	Acyclovir	20 mg/kg p.o. q.i.d. for 5 days (800 mg maximum)
varicella zoster	Acyclovir	
varicella or zoster in immunocompromised host	Acyclovir	1500 mg/m^2/day i.v. div. q.8h until improved then p.o. as above
acyclovir-resistant	Foscarnet	40 mg/kg i.v. q.8h

Table 20.19 Therapy for systemic fungal infections

Infection	Drug of choice
Aspergillosis	Amphotericin B × 30 days
	Alternative: itraconazole
	For patients with decreased renal function:
	amphotericin B lipid complex (Abelcet, ABLC)
	liposomal amphotericin B (AmBisome)
	amphotericin B cholesteryl complex (Amphotec)
	amphotericin B colloidal dispersion (ABCD)
Blastomycosis	Moderate infection: itraconazole p.o. for 3–6 months
	Severe infection: amphotericin B i.v. for 2 weeks followed by itraconazole p.o. for 6–12 months
Candidiasis	
oropharyngeal	Fluconazole for 5–14 days or nystatin for 14 days or clotrimazole troche for 7–14 days
systemic	Fluconazole p.o. or i.v. for 14–28 days or amphotericin B i.v. for 14 days

Continued

Table 20.19 Continued

Infection	Drug of choice
Chromomycosis	Itraconazole for 18 months
Coccidioidomycosis	Fluconazole for 12–18 months
	Alternative: itraconazole for 12–18 months
Cryptococcosis	
Non meningeal:	Amphotericin B until response then fluconazole p.o. for 8 weeks or fluconazole for 8 weeks
Meningitis:	Amphotericin B plus flucytosine for 6 weeks
chronic suppression	Fluconazole
	Alternative: amphotericin B
Histoplasmosis	
pulmonary or non CNS	Itraconazole
CNS involvement	Amphotericin B
	Alternative: itraconazole
chronic suppression	Itraconazole
Mucormycosis	Amphotericin B
	No dependable alternative
Paracoccidioidomycosis	Itraconazole for 6 months
	Alternative: ketoconazole 6–18 months
Pseudallescheriasis	Surgery plus itraconazole
Sporotrichosis	Itraconazole

Table 20.20 Antifungal therapy

Agent (trade name)	Dosage
Amphotericin B (Fungizone)	1 mg test dose, followed after 4 h by 0.25 mg/kg i.v. Increase dosage each day by 0.25 mg/kg to a maximum of 1 mg/kg per day given as a single daily infusion. For most systemic infections, a total dose of 30 mg/kg is required. When combined with flucytosine, the daily dose is 0.3 mg/kg
Amphotericin B lipid complex (Abelcet, ABLC)	5.0 mg/kg/day
Amphotericin B – liposomal (AmBisome)	3–5 mg/kg/day
Amphotericin B colloidal dispersion (ABCD)	2–6 mg/kg/day
Amphotericin B – cholesteryl (Amphotec)	3–4 mg/kg/day
Clotrimazole	10 mg troche p.o. 5 times per day for 7 days
Fluconazole	i.v.: 12 mg/kg per day div. q.12h
	p.o.: 3–6 mg/kg single daily dose
Flucytosine (Ancobon)	150 mg/kg per day p.o. div. q.6h
Griseofulvin (numerous trade names)	25 mg/kg per day p.o. div. q.24h
Itraconazole	2–5 mg/kg per day p.o. div. b.i.d.
Ketoconazole (Nizoral)	5–10 mg/kg per day p.o. div. q.24h
Nystatin (Mycostatin, Nilstat)	200 000 U (2 ml) p.o. q.i.d. for 6–12 days

Table 20.21 Therapy for common parasitic infections

Infection	Drug	Dosage
Amebiasis (*Entamoeba histolytica*) – see Chapter 10		
Amebic meningoencephalitis		
Naegleria fowleri	Amphotericin B	1 mg/kg per day i.v. plus intraventricular for 30 days
Acanthamoeba	Unknown	
Ancylostoma duodenale	(see hookworm)	
Angiostrongyliasis		
Angiostrongylus cantonensis	Mebendazole	100 mg b.i.d. for 5 days
Angiostrongylus costaricensis	Thiabendazole	75 mg/kg per day in 3 doses for 3 days (maximum 3 g/day)
Anisakiasis (*Anisakis*)	Surgical or endoscopic removal	
Ascariasis (*Ascaris lumbricoides*)	Albendazole	400 mg 1 dose
	Mebendazole	100 mg b.i.d. for 3 days
	or	
	Pyrantel pamoate	11 mg/kg single dose (maximum 1 g)
Babesiosis (*Babesia microti*)	Clindamycin	20–40 mg/kg per day in 3 doses for 7 days
	plus	
	Quinine	25 mg/kg per day in 3 doses for 7 days
Balantidiasis (*Balantidium coli*)	Tetracycline	40 mg/kg per day in 4 doses for 10 days (maximum 2 g/day)
	Alternative:	
	Metronidazole	35–50 mg/kg per day in 3 doses for 5 days
Baylisascariasis (*Baylisascaris procyonis*)	Diethylcarbamazine or levamisole or fenbendazole	
Blastocystis hominis infection	Metronidazole	35–50 mg/kg per day in 3 doses for 10 days
Capillariasis (*Capillaria philippinensis*)	Mebendazole	200 mg b.i.d. for 20 days
	Alternative: albendazole	200 mg b.i.d. for 10 days
Chagas' disease	(see trypanosomiasis)	
Clonorchis sinensis	(see fluke infection)	
Cryptosporidiosis (*Cryptosporidium parvum*)	Paromomycin and/or azithromycin	500–750 mg t.i.d. 600 mg/day
Cutaneous larva migrans (creeping eruption)	Thiabendazole	Topically and/or 50 mg/kg per day in 2 doses (maximum 3 g/day) for 2–5 days
	or	
	Ivermectin	150 µg/kg p.o. for one dose
Cyclospora cayetanensis	Trimethoprim/sulfamethoxazole (TMP/SMX)	1 double strength tablet b.i.d. for 7 days
Cysticercosis	(see tapeworm infection)	
Dientamoeba fragilis infection	Iodoquinol or	40 mg/kg per day in 3 doses for 20 days
	Paromomycin	25–30 mg/kg per day in 3 doses for 7 days
	or	
	Tetracycline	40 mg/kg per day in 4 doses for 10 days (maximum 2 g/day)
Diphyllobothrium latum	(see tapeworm infection)	
Dracunculus medinensis (guineaworm) infection	surgical removal	
	Alternative: thiabendazole	50–75 mg/kg per day in 2 doses for 3 days
Echinococcus	(see tapeworm infection)	

Continued

Table 20.21 Continued

Infection	Drug	Dosage
Entamoeba histolytica (see Chapter 10)		
Enterobius vermicularis (pinworm infection)	Albendazole or	400 mg p.o., single dose; repeat in 2 weeks
	Mebendazole or	single dose of 100 mg; repeat after 2 weeks
	Pyrantel pamoate	11 mg/kg single dose (maximum 1 g); repeat after 2 weeks
Fasciola hepatica	(see fluke infection)	
Filariasis		
Wuchereria bancrofti,	Ivermectin plus	100–440 µg/kg, single dose
Brugia malayi	Albendazole	400 mg, single dose
	Alternative:	
	Diethylcarbamazine	Day 1: 1 mg/kg p.o., after meal
		Day 2: 1 mg/kg t.i.d.
		Day 3: 1–2 mg/kg t.i.d.
		Days 4–21: 6 mg/kg per day in 3 doses
Loa loa	Diethylcarbamazine	Day 1: 1 mg/kg p.o., after meal
		Day 2: 1 mg/kg t.i.d.
		Day 3: 1–2 mg/kg t.i.d.
		Days 4–21: 9 mg/kg per day in 3 doses
Mansonella ozzardi	Ivermectin	25–200 µg/kg, single dose
Mansonella perstans	Mebendazole	100 mg b.i.d. for 30 days
Tropical pulmonary eosinophilia (TPE)	Diethylcarbamazine	6 mg/kg per day in 3 doses for 21 days
Onchocerca volvulus	Ivermectin	150 µg/kg single oral dose, repeated every 6–12 months
Flukes (hermaphroditic infection)		
Clonorchis sinensis (Chinese liver fluke)	Praziquantel	25 mg/kg per day for 3 doses
Fasciola hepatica (sheep liver fluke)	Bithionol	35–50 mg/kg on alternate days for 10–15 doses
Fasciolopsis buski (intestinal fluke)	Praziquantel or Niclosamide	75 mg/kg per day in 3 doses for 1 day for weight 11–34 kg: 2 tablets (1 g) for > 34 kg: 3 tablets (1.5 g)
Heterophyes heterophyes (intestinal fluke)	Praziquantel	75 mg/kg per day in 3 doses for 1 day
Metagonimus yokogawai (intestinal fluke)	Praziquantel	75 mg/kg per day in 3 doses for 1 day
Nanophyetus salmincola	Praziquantel	60 mg/kg per day in 3 doses for 1 day
Opisthorchis viverrini (liver fluke)	Praziquantel	75 mg/kg per day in 3 doses for 1 day
Paragonimus westermani (lung fluke)	Praziquantel	75 mg/kg per day in 3 doses for 2 days
Giardiasis (see Chapter 10)		
Gnathostomiasis (*Gnathostoma spinigerum*)	Surgical removal plus Albendazole	400 mg p.o. daily or b.i.d. for 21 days

Continued over

Table 20.21 Continued

Infection	Drug	Dosage
Hookworm infection (*Ancylostoma duodenale*, *Necator americanus*)	Albendazole or Mebendazole or Pyrantel pamoate	400 mg single dose 100 mg b.i.d. for 3 days 11 mg/kg per day (max. 1 g) for 3 days
Hydatid cyst (see tapeworm infection)		
Hymenolepsis nana (see tapeworm infection)		
Isosporiasis (*Isospora belli*)	TMP/SMX	40 mg TMP/200 mg SMX/kg per day q.i.d. for 10 days then 20 mg TMP/100 mg SMX/kg per day b.i.d. for 3 weeks
Leishmaniasis (*L. mexicana*, *L. tropica*, *L. major*, or *L. braziliensis*, *L. donovani–Kala–azar*)	Stibogluconate sodium or Meglumine antimoniate or Amphotericin B	20 mg/kg div. b.i.d. i.v. or i.m. for 20–28 days 20 mg/kg div. b.i.d. for 20–28 days 0.25–1 mg/kg by slow infusion daily, or every 2 days, for up to 8 weeks
Lice infestation (*Pediculus humanus*, *P. capitis*, *Phthirus pubis*)	1% permethrin or 0.5% malathion pyrethrin with piperonyl butoxide Lindane Ivermectin	Topically Topically Topically 200 μg/kg single dose p.o.
Loa loa	(see filariasis)	
Malaria, treatment of (*Plasmodium falciparum*, *P. ovale*, *P. vivax* and *P. malariae*) All *Plasmodium* except chloroquine-resistant *P. falciparum*)		
Oral	Chloroquine phosphate	10 mg base/kg (maximum 600 mg base), then 5 mg base/kg at 24 and 48 h
Parenteral	Quinidine gluconate or Quinidine dihydrochloride	10 mg/kg loading dose (maximum 600 mg) in normal saline slowly over 1 h followed by continuous infusion of 0.02 mg/kg per min for 3 days maximum 20 mg salt/kg loading dose in 10 ml/kg 5% dextrose over 4 h followed by 10 mg salt/kg over 2–4 h q.8h (maximum 1800 mg/day) until oral therapy can be started
Chloroquine-resistant *P. falciparum*		
Oral	Quinine sulfate plus Pyrimethamine–sulfadoxine (single dose given on last day of quinine)	25 mg/kg per day in 3 doses for 3 days (7 days with doxycycline) < 1 year: 1/4 tablet 1–3 years: 1/2 tablet 4–8 years: 1 tablet 9–14 years: 2 tablets

Continued

Table 20.21   Continued

Infection	Drug	Dosage
	or plus doxycycline	100 mg b.i.d. for 7 days
	or plus clindamycin	20–40 mg/kg per day in 3 doses for 3 days
	Alternatives: mefloquine	< 45 kg, 25 mg/kg single dose
	halofantrine	< 40 kg, 8 mg/kg q.6h for 3 doses
Parenteral	Quinidine gluconate or	Same as for non-resistant stains
	Quinine dihydrochloride	Same as for non-resistant stains
Prevention of relapses (*P. vivax* and *P. ovale* only)	Primaquine	0.3 mg base/kg per day for 14 days
Malaria, prevention in		
Chloroquine-sensitive areas	Chloroquine phosphate	5 mg/kg base (8.3 mg/kg salt) once per week, up to adult dose of 300 mg base
Chloroquine-resistant areas	Mefloquine	15–19 kg: 1/4 tablet
		20–30 kg: 1/2 tablet
		31–45 kg: 3/4 tablet
		> 45 kg: 1 tablet (250 mg) oral once
	or	per week
	Doxycycline	> 8 years of age: 2 mg/kg per day
	or	orally, up to 100 mg/day
	Chloroquine phosphate	as above
	plus	
	Pyrimethamine–sulfadoxine (for presumptive-treatment)	< 1 year: 1/4 tablet
		1–3 years: 1/2 tablet
		4–8 years: 1 tablet
		9–14 years: 2 tablets for self-treatment of febrile illness
	or plus	
	Proguanil (in Africa south of the Sahara)	< 2 years: 50 mg daily
		2–6 years: 100 mg daily
		7–10 years: 150 mg daily
		> 10 years: 200 mg daily and for 4 weeks after exposure
*CDC malaria information: prophylaxis (888)-232-3228 treatment (770)-488-7788		
Moniliformis moniliformis infection	Pyrantel pamoate	11 mg/kg single dose, repeat twice, 2 weeks apart
Roundworm	(see ascariasis)	
Scabies (*Sarcoptes scabiei*)	5% permethrin	Topically, repeat in 1 week
	Alternatives: lindane	Topically
	10% crotamiton	Topically
Schistosomiasis (bilharziasis)		
Schistosoma haemotobium	Praziquantel	40 mg/kg per day in 2 doses for 1 day
S. japonicum	Praziquantel	60 mg/kg per day in 3 doses for 1 day
S. mansoni	Praziquantel	40 mg/kg per day in 2 doses for 1 day
	Alternative: oxamniquine	20 mg/kg per day in 2 doses for 1 day
S. mekongi	Praziquantel	60 mg/kg per day in 3 doses for 1 day
Strongyloidiasis (*Strongyloides stercoralis*)	Ivermectin or	200 µg/kg per day for 2 days
	Albendazole	400 mg daily for 3 days

Continued over

Table 20.21 Continued

Infection	Drug	Dosage
	Alternative: thiabenazole	50 mg/kg per day in 2 doses (maximum 3 g/day) for 2 days
Tapeworm infection – adult (intestinal stage)		
(*Diphyllobothrium latum* (fish), *Taenia saginata* (beef), or	Praziquantel	10 mg/kg single dose
Taenia solium (pork), *Dipylidium caninum* (dog)	Niclosamide	11–34 kg: single dose of 2 tablets (1 g) > 34 kg: single dose of 3 tablets (1.5 g)
Hymenolepsis nana (dwarf tapeworm)	Praziquantel	25 mg/kg single dose
	Alternative: niclosamide	11–34 kg: single dose of 2 tablets (1 g) for 1 day, then 1 tablet (0.5 g)/day for 6 days > 34 kg: single dose of 3 tablets (1.5 g) for 1 day, then 2 tablets (1 g)/day for 6 days
Tapeworm infection, larval (tissue stage)		
Echinococcus granulosus (hydatid cyst)	Albendazole	15 mg/kg per day for 28 days, repeated as necessary
Echinococcus multilocularis	Treatment of choice: surgical excision	
Cysticerus cellulosae (cysticercosis)	Albendazole or	15 mg/kg per day in 3 doses for 8 days, repeated as necessary
	Praziquantel	50 mg/kg per day in 3 doses for 15 days
	Alternative: surgery	
Toxocariasis (see visceral larva migrans)		
Toxoplasmosis (*Toxoplasma gondii*)	Pyrimethamine	2 mg/kg per day for 3 days, then 1 mg/kg per day (maximum 25 mg/kg) for 4 weeks
	plus	
	Sulfadiazine plus	100–200 mg/kg per day for 3–4 weeks
	Prednisone	1 mg/kg/day
	Alternative: spiramycin	50–100 mg/kg per day for 3–4 weeks
Trichinosis (*Trichinella spiralis*)	Albendazole plus Steroids for severe symptoms	400 mg for 14 days
	Alternative: mebendazole	200–400 mg t.i.d. for 3 days, then 400–500 mg t.i.d. for 10 days
Trichomoniasis (*Trichomonas vaginalis*)	Metronidazole	1 dose: 40 mg/kg (max 2 g) p.o. or 15 mg/kg per day orally (maximum 1 g/day) div. b.i.d. for 7 days
Trichostrongylosis	Mebendazole or	100 mg b.i.d. for 3 days
	Albendazole or	400 mg single dose
	Pyrantel pamoate	11 mg/kg single dose (maximum 1 g)
Trichuriasis (*Trichuris trichiura*, or whipworm)	Albendazole or	400 mg single dose
	Mebendazole	100 mg b.i.d. for 3 days

Continued

Table 20.21 Continued

Infection	Drug	Dosage
Trypanosomiasis (*Trypanosoma cruzi*, South American trypanosomiasis, Chagas' disease)	Nifurtimox	1–10 years: 15–20 mg/kg per day in 4 doses for 90 days; 11–16 years: 12.5–15 mg/kg per day in 4 doses for 90 days
	Alternative: benznidazole	5–7 mg/kg per day for 30–120 days
T. brucei gambiense, *T. b. rhodesiene* (African trypanosomiasis, sleeping sickness)	Suramin	20 mg/kg on days 1, 3, 7, 14 and 21
	or	
	Pentamidine isethionate	4 mg/kg per day i.m. for 10 days
Late disease with CNS involvement	Melarsoprol	18–25 mg/kg total over 1 month; initial dose of 0.36 mg/kg i.v., increasing gradually to maximum 3.6 mg/kg at intervals of 1–5 days for total of 9–10 doses
	or	
	Elfornithine	100 mg/kg q.6h i.v. for 14 days then 75 mg/kg p.o. for 21–30 days
	Alternative: tryparsamide	1 injection of 30 mg/kg (maximum 2 g) i.v. q.5d to total of 12 injections; may
	plus	be repeated after 1 month
	Suramin	1 injection of 10 mg/kg i.v. every 5 days to total of 12 injections; may be repeated after 1 month
Visceral larva migrans (Toxocariasis)	Diethylcarbamazine	6 mg/kg per day in 3 doses for 7–10 days
	Alternatives: albendazole or mebendazole	400 mg p.o. b.i.d. for 5 days 100–200 mg b.i.d. for 5 days
Whipworm	(see trichuriasis)	
Wuchereria bancrofti	(see filariasis)	

Index

abdominal infection   184–7
abdominal trauma   187
abscesses (cutaneous)   69
  organisms recovered   69
acetaminophen, loading/maintenance dose
    74
acid-fast stain   91–2
acne, treatment   161
acquired immunodeficiency syndrome
    (AIDS)
  diagnosis   201–2
  prevention   201
  treatment
    gastrointestinal protozoe   211
    lower respiratory tract infections   211
actinomycosis   243
acute aortic insufficiency   3
acute respiratory distress syndrome (ARDS),
    hantavirus-related   12
acute rheumatic fever   3–5
acyclovir   7, 34, 66–7, 191, 210, 234
adenitis   69–70, 161
  cervical   70
  etiology, bacterial   70
  treatment   70
adenopathy   161
  persistent
    approach to   162
    generalized, causes   162
adenovirus   108
albendazole   83, 124
allergy, cutaneous   219–20
Allescheria   171
amantadine   65–6, 107, 111, 211
amebiasis   117–19
  clinical forms   117
  diagnosis   118
  treatment   119
amikacin   143, 173, 211, 234
aminoglycosides, botulism   2
amoxicillin   153–4, 156
  endocarditis   62
  Helicobacter infection   126

otitis media   82
  recurrent   56
pneumococcal sepsis   64
pneumonia   111–13
rheumatic fever   58
salmonellosis   132–3
sinusitis   104
amphotericin B   36, 143, 170–1, 218, 230,
    234
ampicillin   154, 173, 180, 196, 227, 229,
    234
  endocarditis   62
  meningitis   13
  neonatal sepsis   20, 28
  peritonitis   16
  pharyngitis   104
  salmonellosis   132–3
  shigellosis   135
anaerobic cultures   96
anorectal infection   185–6
anthrax   243
antibiotics
  adults, parenteral   240
  classification, in vitro   230
  infants and children, dosages,
    intravenous, intramuscular and oral
    237–40
  neonates
    dosages, daily   234–6
    oral   237
antifungal agents   240–2, 247
antimicrobial therapy   227–53
  adverse reactions   227–9
  allergic reactions, frequency   228
  body surface area   240
  dosages
    adults   233–40
    infants/children   233
    neonates   233
  empiric therapy   227
  prophylactic   55–67
  selection, host factors related   229–32
    compromized host   229–30

hepatic failure   231
   renal failure   230–1
   specific pathogens   240
antiparasitic agents   242
antipyretic therapy   74
antirabies serum   43
antiviral agents   240
appendicitis   184
   antibiotics   185
arbovirus   173
Arcanobacterium hemolyticum   75, 76
Arnold–Chiari malformation   171
Arthus reactions   39
ascariasis   82–3
Aspergillus   181
aspiration pneumonia   113
   organisms causing   113
aspirin
   endocarditis   3
   loading maintenance dose   74
asplenia   64
asthma   106
astrovirus   135
ataxia telangiectasia   215
atelectasis   187
automated reagin test   190–1
azithromycin   62, 111, 120, 191, 193, 209,
      230
azlacillin   143, 218
aztreonam   143, 180, 188, 234

Bacille Calmette–Guerin (BCG)   50–1
Bacillus cereus   123
BACTEC-460 system   96
bacteremia   71
   infants   71
   organisms causing   19
   pneumococcal   71
bacterial infections   25–9
   etiology   26
   group B streptococcal disease, prevention
      26–7
   perinatal risk factors   25
bacteriuria, asymptomatic   154–5
Bacteroides fragilis   69, 177, 183–4
Bacteroides melaninogenicus   69, 183
balanitis   150, 196
   treatment   197

barbiturates, sedation in tetanus   22
bartonellosis   243
benzoyl peroxide (2.5%), topical   161
β-lactamase test   100–1
Bicillin   3
biliary atresia   186
Biocef   154
bismuth subsalicylate   47, 51
   Helicobacter infection   126
bites (animal and human)   70–1
   treatment   71
black widow spider equine antivenin   43
black-dot ringworm   73
bladder
   unstable   152
   washout   85
      interpretation   85
      methodology   85
bladder tap   85
blastomycosis   171
blepharitis   161–2
blood cultures   85–6, 96
   technique   86
      quantitative   86
blood transfusions, infections transmitted
      214
body surface area   240
   antibiotics, dosages   242
   determination scales   241
Bordatella pertusis   105
botulism   1–3, 243
   infant, prevention   3
botulism ABE polyvalent equine antitoxin
      43
brain abscess   167–9
   antibiotic strategies   170
   bacterial organisms, causing   169
   lumbar puncture   168
   management, treatment options   169
   predisposing factors   167
   signs and symptoms   168
   skull, radiographs   168
   treatment   168–9
bronchiolitis   106–7
bronchitis   105–6
bronchopulmonary dysplasia   35
brucellosis   243
burns   181
butoconazole   195

C-reactive protein, elevation   26, 138
caliovirus   135
Campylobacter fetus   119
Campylobacter gastroenteritis   119–20
Campylobacter infection   119–20
   clinical characteristics   119
   extraintestinal manifestations   120
   gastrointestinal manifestations   120
   treatment   120
Candida   36, 168
Candida albicans   36, 109, 196
candidemia   219–20
candidiasis   73
candiduria   160
capreomycin   115
carbenicillin   144, 173
cardiac infections   3–6
cardiac surgery   182–3
cardiopulmonary resuscitation ABC   19
cat-scratch disease   243
catheterization, clean intermittent   159
cefadroxil   62, 143
cefazolin   62, 143, 154, 180, 188, 234
cefepime   218
cefixime   144, 154, 218
cefoperazone   231
cefotaxime   2, 9, 13, 143, 152, 173, 180,
   184–5, 227–8, 234
   neonatal sepsis   20, 28
   peritonitis   16
   pneumonia   113
   salmonellosis   133
cefotetan   196
cefoxitin   186, 188, 196
cefpodoxime   111, 154, 218
cefprozil   111, 154, 218
ceftazidime   154, 218, 234
ceftriaxone   2, 9, 13, 143, 154, 173, 191–2,
   196, 227–8, 230
   meningococcal prophylaxis   15, 63
   neonatal septicemia   20, 28
   peritonitis   16
   pneumonia   113
   shigellosis   135
Cefzil   154
cellulitis   69
   aspirate   85
   buccal   71
   clinical features   72

   clostridia related   179, 182
   facial   71
   orbital   71
   periorbital   71
   treatment   71
Centers for Disease Control and Prevention
   10, 43
   rabies immunoglobulin, recommendations
   42
   Traveller's Health Line   53
central line, quantitative cultures   86
cephalexin   143, 154, 156, 162
cephalothin   173
cerebritis   167–9
cerebrospinal fluid   92
   encephalitis, diagnosis   7
   lumbar puncture   86–7
   meningitis
      bacterial   11–12
      processing   93
   syphilis   32
chalazione   163
chancroid   190–1
chest infection   183–4
chickenpox, AIDS   210
Chlamydia
   culture   99–100
   identification, specimens and tests used
   100
Chlamydia pneumonie   107–9
Chlamydia trachomatis   73, 192–3
   neonatal eye infection   34
chloramphenicol   173, 228–9, 231, 235
   salmonellosis   132–3
   Yersinia infection   136
chloroquine   51–2, 119
cholangitis   186
cholecystectomy   186
cholera, immunization   48, 50
cholesteatoma   80–1
cholestyramine   128
cilastatin   186
ciprofloxacin   120, 144, 191, 196, 211
   meningococcal prophylaxis   15
   shigellosis   135
   traveller's diarrhea   51
   urinary tract infection   57
clarytromycin   62, 111, 120, 165, 209, 211
clavulanate   187

clindamycin   2, 143, 161, 196, 227, 230–1, 235
  abscesses, cutaneous   69
  endocarditis   62
  peritonitis   16
  septicemia   20
  toxic shock syndrome   24
clinical syndromes, therapy   234–5
clostridial myonecrosis   182
Clostridium botulinum   2, 123
Clostridium difficile   128
Clostridium perfringens   123
Clostridium septicum   182
Clostridium tetani   19
clotrimazole   73, 194–5
CNA-LKV biplate   96
coagulase-negative staphylococci   35–6
coccidiodomyeosis   171
collagen vascular disease   5
colon surgery, elective   185
COMBIVIR   206
common cold   76, 103
community acquired pneumonia   108
  patient (in/out), management   112
complement deficiency   215
complement fixation   99
compromized host   229–30
congenital infections   29–34
  clinical manifestations   29
  suspected, laboratory evaluation   30
conjunctivitis   72–3
  etiology and treatment   72
  newborn   34
constipation   159
contiguous osteochondritis   140
  predisposing conditions   141
coral snake equine antivenin   43
coronavirus   135
cortical spinal tract dysfunction   172
Corynebacterium hemolyticum   104
Corynebacterium pseudodiphthericum   1, 4, 6, 75, 92
Coxsackie virus   4–5
cranial nerve palsies   172
creatinine clearance (CrCl)   230–1
CRIXIVAN   207
crotalid polyvalent antivenin   43
croup   8, 104–5
  membranous   1

spasmodic   105
therapy   105
cryotherapy   198
cryptococcosis   171
Cryptococcus   168
cryptococcus neoformans   92–3
culture specimens   1
Curtis syndrome   196
cyclophosphamide   214
cystitis   85
  sexually active   156
cystography   156
cytomegalovirus   5, 29, 33, 126, 174
  prophylaxis   66

decubitus ulcers   162
  treatment   163
dehydroemetine   119
delavirdine   203, 207
Demodex folliculorum   162
dermatophytoses   73
dexamethasone, croup   105
Di George syndrome   215
diaper rash   73
diarrhea   121
dicloxacillin   143
didanosine   203, 206–7
diet, glutamine supplemented   177
dihydration   121
dilution susceptibility testing   100
diphtheria   6, 7
  equine antitoxin   43
diphtheria vaccine   37
diphtheria-tetanus-acellular pertussis vaccine   37, 39
disc diffusion testing   100
discitis   141–2
disease transmission, mechanisms   229
disseminated intravascular coagulation (DIC)   12–13
diverticulitis   129
Donovan bodies   197
doxycycline   51, 120, 161, 180, 192–3, 196, 230
  malaria   51–2
  Yersinia infection   136
dysfunctional elimination syndrome   158

echoencephalography 168
edrophonium 2
ehrlichiosis 163, 243
Eikenella corrodens 70
electrodesiccation 165, 198
electroencephalography 7, 168
  herpes encephalitis 174
electromyographic studies 2
Elimite cream 165
EMLA cream 69
empyema 89, 183
  pneumonia associated, antibiotics 184
encephalitis 6–7
  chickenpox 1
  diagnosis 8
  enteroviral 1
  equine 43, 173
  herpes simplex, acyclovir 7
encephalopathy 6
  differential diagnosis 7
endemic diseases, recommended preventive
    measures 48
endocarditis, bacterial 3, 12, 59–63
  prophylaxis
    dental procedures 60, 62
    gastrointestinal conditions 61–2
    genitourinary conditions 61–2
    related to cardiac conditions 60
    respiratory conditions 61
    special procedures 59, 60–1
endometritis 195
endoscopy 2
endotracheal intubation 2
Entamoeba histolytica 117–18, 186
enteric adenovirus 135
enteric adenovirus gastroenteritis 134
Enterobius 82
Enterococcus 3, 153
enterocolitis, inflammatory 95
enteroviral infection 163
enterovirus 174
epididymitis 196–7
epidural abscess 141
epiglottitis 1, 7–9
EPIVIR 206
Epstein–Barr virus 5, 126
equine western equine encephalitis 43,
    173
erysipelas 243

erythema infectiosum 163
erythrasma 243
erythromycin 161, 163, 191–3, 228–30,
    235
  Campylobacter gastroenteritis 120
  diphtheria 6
  pertussis 65, 105
  pneumonia 111
  respiratory infection, upper 76
Escherishia coli 12, 26, 69, 153, 172, 177,
    184
Escherishia coli infection 121–2
  diarrheagenic, classification 122
ethambutol 114, 165
exanthem subitum 163
exanthematous diseases 162–3
extracorporeal membrane oxygenation
    (ECMO) 4, 11
eye infections, neonatal 34

famciclovir 191
familial Mediterranean fever 186
family travel, restrictions 45
Fanconi's syndrome 229
fecal leukocytes
  gastrointestinal diseases, associated with
    96
  staining procedure 96
fecal specimens 94–5
  evaluation 95
fetal monitoring, internal scalp electrodes
    35
fever
  evaluation, protocols
    continued 75
    initial 74
  neutropenia 217
    management 218
  no aparent source, laboratory studies 73
  occult bacteremia 73–4
  postoperative 187–8
    antibiotic prophylaxis, recommendation
      188
    causes 188
  unknown origin 74
fiber need, daily 159
Filgrastrim 29
fistula-in-ano 186
Fitz–Hugh syndrome 196

fluconazole   36, 144, 170, 195, 218, 235
flucytosine   170–1
fluid exudates, evaluation   97
fluorescent-treponemal antibody-absorption
        test (FTA–ABS)   190–1
fluorodynamic study   156
fluoroquinolones   47
folinic acid   30
food poisoning   122
    clinical aspects   123
    epidemiological aspects   123
FORTOVASE   208
Fournier's gangrene   182
Francisella tularensis   75–6, 104
fungal cultures   98
fungal infections
    central nervous system   169–71
        diagnostic approach   171
        factors predisposing   170
        organisms associated with   171
        tissue reactions   171
    systemic, therapy   246–7
furazolidone   124
Fusobacterium   69

gall bladder disease   186
gallium scanning, osteomyelitis   138
ganciclovir   66–7, 211
Gardnerella vaginalis   194, 196
gas gangrene   243
genital herpes, oral antiviral therapy   191
genital ulcers   189–90
    diagnostic studies   190
genital warts   190, 197
gentomycin   13, 35, 120, 143, 154, 173,
        180, 196, 227–30
    neonatal sepsis   20, 28
Gianotti–Crosti syndrome   163
giardiasis   82, 122–4
    diagnosis   124
    treatment   124
Giemsa stains   92
glomerular filtration rate, normal   231
Go-Lytely   185
gonococcal infections   192
gram stain   91
granulocyte colony stimulating factor   29,
        215
granuloma inguinale   197–8

gray-patch ringworm   73
griseofulvin   73
Guillain–Barre syndrome   1, 2, 9–10, 173
    course   11
    diagnostic criteria   10
    management   11
    onset, factors associated   10

Haemophilus ducreyi   190–1
Haemophilus influenzae   1–2, 78, 85, 92–3,
        104, 107, 145, 187
    type B (Hib)   63–4
    vaccine   8
halothane, inhalational induction in
        epiglottitis   9
Hantavirus pulmonary syndrome   10–11
    related ARDS, management   12
Helicobacter pylori infection   124–6
    clinical diseases associated with   125
    diagnosis   126
    epidemiologic factors   125
helminths   95
hematochesia   119
hepatic abscess   186
hepatic failure, antibiotic dosages   231
hepatitis   126–7
    acute, serologic diagnosis   127
    differential etiology   126
hepatitis A   47, 126
    vaccine   48
hepatitis B   30, 126
    neonates, management   31
    surgery   180–1
hepatitis C   30–1, 127
hepatitis D (delta)   127
hepatitis E   127
herpes encephalitis   174
herpes simplex meningitis   1
herpes simplex virus   29, 33–4, 174
    genital infection   189–90
    prophylaxis   66
histoplasmosis   171
HIVID   206
hookworm   82–3
hordeolum   163
human diploid cell vaccine   14
human immunodeficiency virus (HIV)   29, 31
    bacteremia   209
    exposure in hospital, personnel   212

fungal infection   212
gastrointestinal infections   210
laboratory tests   203
measles   212
prophylaxis   205–9
respiratory infections   209–10
sepsis   209
specific antiviral therapy   202–5
surgery   180–1
tuberculosis   210
varicella-zoster   210–12
human papilloma virus   197
treatment   198
hydrocephalus   171
hyperimmune animal immunoglobulin   43
hyperimmune human immunoglobulin
42, 43, 47
hypogammaglobulinemia   42
X-linked   215

imidazole   194
imipenem   186, 230, 235
imipramine   158
imiquimod   198
Immodium   51
immunizations   37–43
active   37–42
contraindications   39
immunosuppressed patients   40–1
infants, premature   40
routine   37–40, 46
age when provided   46
pasive   42–3
immunocompromised/immunosuppressed
patients
antibiotic synergism   230
prophylaxis   219
vaccination   40–1
immunodeficiency
neonates   213
maturational defects   213
primary   214–16
frequency   215
prophylaxis   219
secondary   216–19
causes, common   216
iatrogenic   213–14
syndromes   215
immunoelectrophoresis, countercurrent   26

immunoglobulin   9, 11, 42
intravenous   9–10
immunologic testing   101
Imovax Rabies   48
impetigo   69, 163, 243
india ink   92–3
indinavir   203, 207
infection control   223–6
hospitalized children, categories   224
isolation policies   223–4
measures   223
infections, pediatric hospital personnel
223
infectious disease emergencies   1–24
infectious mononucleosis   163
influenza A, prophylaxis   65, 107
influenza vaccine   41, 65, 107
indication   41
interferons   198
International Rheumatic Fever Study Group
58
INVIRASE   208
iodoquinol   119, 211
isoniazid   211, 230–1
tuberculosis prophylaxis   65
itraconazole   171
ivermetin   165

Janeway lesions   3
Japanese B equine virus   173
Japanese encephalitis   48, 50
Jc virus   174
joint fluid analysis   145

kanamycin   115, 173
Kawasaki disease   4, 147, 163, 186
Keflex   154
Keftab   154
kerion   73
Kingelle kingae   243
Kirby-Bauer disc diffusion method   100
Klebsiella   122, 153
Klebsiella pneumoniae   110, 113
KOH preparation   73

lacerations   164
Lactobacillus   128, 129
lamivudine   203, 206–7
laryngotracheobronchitis   1, 104–5

latex-particle agglutination   26
Legionnaires' disease   243
leprosy   244
leptospirosis   126, 186
Leucovorin calcium   30
leukemia
    chickenpox   42
    etiology of infection   218
Libman–Sacks syndrome   3
lindane   198
liquid nitrogen freezing   165, 198
Listeria   26
Listeria monocytogenes   12
listeriosis   244
liver abscesses   119
loperamide   47, 57
Lorabid   154
Loracarbet   154
Ludwig's angina   164, 244
lumbar puncture   2, 86
    brain abscess   168
    technique   87
lung aspiration   86
    needle aspiration   87
LVAD   4
Lyme arthritis   146
Lyme disease   147
lymphogranuloma venereum   192

MacConkey plate   96
magnetic resonance imaging
    brain abscess   167
    encephalitis   7
    osteomyelitis   138
    septic arthritis   145
malaria   51–3
    chemoprophylaxis   46, 53
    prevention, antibiotic regimen   52
Mantou skin test, positive, definition   50,
    65–6, 116
measles   163
measles–mumps and rubella vaccine   37, 46
meatal irritation   150
mebendazole   83
meclocycline   161
mediastinitis   183
mefloquine   47, 51, 52
Meibomian gland   163
melioidosis   244

meningitis   1, 11–12
    complications   14
    etiology   12
    management   13
meningococcal vaccine   47, 49
meningococcemia   12–13, 163
    contacts, high risk   14
    diagnosis, laboratory   14
    prophylaxis, antibiotics   15, 63
    treatment   14
meningococcemid   12
meningococcus   49, 63
meningoencephalitis, viral   173–5
    complications   185
    signs and symptoms   174
    viruses associated   174
meningomyelocele   86
Menomune-A/C/Y/W-135   48
meropenen   218, 230, 235
mesenteric adenitis   186
methenamine mandelate   156
methicillin   173, 235
methylene blue stain   91–2
metronidazole   119, 124, 143–4, 180, 186,
    188, 193, 196, 199, 211, 235
    Helicobacter infection   126
    pseudomembranous colitis   128
mezlocillin   143, 187–8, 218, 235–6
miconazole   73, 195
micro-organisms (specific), therapy for
    defined clinical syndromes   243–5
microhemagglutination-*Treponema pallidum*
    test   190–1
microimmunofluorescence methodology
    100
middle ear fluid, aspiration   89
miliaria   163
minimum bactericidal concentration (MBC)
    100
minimum inhibitory concentration (MIC)
    100
minocycline   229–30
    meningococcal prophylaxis   63
missionary families   45–6
Mobiluncus   194
Mollaret's meningitis   174
molluscum contagiosum   164
Moraxella catarrhalis   1–2, 76, 104
Moraxella lacunata   162

Morbidity and Mortality Weekly Report   39
mucormycosis   169
mumps   4–5
mupirocin ointment   163
muscle relaxants, non-depolarizing, tetanus
    22
myasthenia gravis   2
Mycobacterium avium   205
Mycobacterium pneumoniae   106, 108–9
Mycobacterium tuberculosis   65, 70, 165
myocarditis   1, 4
myositis   164

nafcillin   2, 173, 227–30, 236
    osteomyelitis   143
    pneumonia   113
    respiratory infections, upper   76
    toxic shock syndrome   24
nalidixic acid   57, 156
    shigellosis   135
nasopharyngitis   76
necrotizing enterocolitis   184–5
needle aspiration   86
    lung   87
Neisseria gonorrhoeae   73, 75, 76, 190, 192
    neonatal eye infection   34
Neisseria meningitidis   4–5, 12, 63–4
nelfinavir   203, 207
neonatal infections   25–36
neonatal sepsis
    bacterial etiology   27
    clinical manifestations   26
    early vs. late onset, common features   25
    intrapartum antimicrobial prophylaxis
        28
    management   27–9
    suspected, management   28
nephrolithiasis   152
neurogenic bladder dysfynction   159
neuromuscular blocking agents, amino-
    glycosides   2
neutropenia   216–18
    fever   217–18
    secondary to immunosuppressive
        chemotherapy   217
nevirapine   203, 207
Nezelof syndrome   215
nitric oxide, inhaled   11
nitrofurantoin   57, 156, 231

Nocardia   91, 168
nocardiosis   244
norfloxacin
    shigellosis   135
    urinary tract infection   57
normal saline, wet mount   92–3
NORVIR   207
norwalk viruses   134–5
Norwegian scabies   165
nosocomial infections   35–6
nystatin   73, 195

occult blood guaiac method   95
ofloxacin   193, 196
omphalitis   34
onychomycosis   73
operative procedures, classification   178
orchitis   197
ornidazole   124
oropharyngeal infection   74–5
Osler nodes   3
osteomyelitis
    etiologies, specific   139
    hematogenous   137–40
        bacterial etiology   139
        bone involvement, site   138
        diagnosis   137–8
        roentgenographic diagnosis   140
        signs and symptoms   138
    non-hematogenous   140
    pelvic   140
    subperiosteal, aspiration   87
    treatment   142–4
        antimicrobial   143–4
        duration   144
        simplified   142
    vertebral   141
otitis externa   75
    treatment   76
otitis media   55–6, 108
    acute   77
        management, algorithm   78
    bacteremia, predisposing infection   71
    chronic suppurative   80
        management, algorithm   81
    definitions   75–6
    etiology, infants and children   77
    fusion, with   75, 77–80
        management, algorithm   79

microbiology   76–7
neonates   82
    etiology   82
prevention   80–2
recurrent, antibiotic prophylaxis   56
oxacillin   2, 173, 180, 227–8, 230, 236
    osteomyelitis   143
    pneumonia   113
    toxic shock syndrome   24
oxolinic acid   57
oxybutinin   158

p24 antigen   31
Palivizumab   35
pancarditis   4
paracentesis   15
parainfluenza virus   108
paramomycin   119
parasites   95
    detection   96
parasitic infections   82–3
    common, treatment   83
    manifestations   82
    therapy   248–53
paraspinous abscess   141
paromomycin   211
Pasteurella multocida   70
patellar osteochondritis   140
Pediculis capitis   162
Pediculis pubis   162
pediculosis pubis   198
pelvic inflammatory disease   189, 195–6
    therapy   196
penicillin   143, 188
    allergy and desensitization   231–33
    bacteremia   71
    diphtheria   6
    G   180, 236
        rheumatic fever   57–8
        tetanus treatment   22
    pneumococcal sepsis   64
    respiratory infections, upper   76
    syphilis   31
    V
        pharyngitis   104
        rheumatic fever   57–8
pentamidine isethionate   211
Peptococcus   184
pericardial fluid   95

pericardiocentesis   87–8
pericarditis   5
perinephric abscess   160
peritoneal fluid   95, 97
peritoneal tap   88
peritonitis   13–14, 184
    bacteriology   15
    diagnosis, laboratory   15
    forms   15
    pelvic   195
    signs and symptoms   15
    treatment   16
peritonsillar abscess   76
permethrin   198
    cream (5%)   165
pertussis   65, 105
pertussis vaccine   37
    acellular/wholecell, discontinuation   40
    contraindications   39–40
petrolatum ointment   198
phagocytosis   215
pharyngitis   70, 74, 76, 103–4
phytohemagglutination (PHA) skin test
    220
pinworm   82–3, 95
piperacillin   143, 218, 236
plague   244
plasmapheresis   9–11, 175
Plasmodium falciparum   51
pleocytosis   15
pleural empyema   113–14
pleural fluid   95, 97
pneumatosis cystoides intestinalis   185
pneumococcal vaccine   187
Pneumococcus   64
Pneumocystis carinii   110, 205
pneumonia   107–13, 188
    afebrile, infancy   107
    antimicrobial therapy   111
    antiviral therapy   111–13
    aspiration   113
    chest roentgenograms   109–10
    clinical appearance   109
    coliform, neonates   108
    common pathogens, age groups   108
    diagnosis, laboratory   110
    diagnostic evaluation   109
    etiology   108–9
    necrotizing   113

presumed bacterial, empiric antimicrobial therapy   113
pneumothorax, lung aspiration   86
podofilox   198
podophyllin   165, 198
polio virus   4
polymerase chain reaction   31, 174
polyvalent gas gangrene equine antitoxin   43
postpericardiotomy   5
potassium hydroxide (KOH), wet mount   92, 93
prednisone   161, 175, 211
premature infants, vaccination   40
primaquine   52
progressive bacterial synergistic gangrene   182
propantheline   158
Propionibacterium acnes   161
Proteus   153
Proteus mirabilis   110, 113
Proteus vulgaris   75
protozoa   95
pseudomembranous colitis   127–9
   clinical/laboratory findings   128
   treatment   128
Pseudomonas   153, 172, 181
   intravenous drug abusers   141
   osteochondritis   140
Pseudomonas aeruginosa   75, 80, 110, 113, 218
pulmonary abscess   183
pulmonary hypertension   11
puncture wounds   164
pyelonephritis   85
   parenteral antibiotics   154
pyrantel pamoate   83
pyrazinamide   211
pyrethrin   198
pyrimethamine   230
pyrimethamine/sulfadoxine   51–2
pyuria (without bacteriuria), causes   151

Q fever   244
quinacrine   124

rabies   14–16
   diagnosis   17
   management, postexposure   83
      onset, factors affecting   16
      prophylaxis   83
      symptoms   17
rabies vaccines   41–2, 49–50
   FDA approved   42
rape   198–9
rapid plasma reagin (RPR) test   190
rashes, classification   163
Reiter's syndrome   147
renal abscess   160
renal failure, antibiotic dosages   230–1, 232
RESCRIPTOR   207
respiratory infections
   lower
      childhood AIDS, differential diagnosis and treatment   211
      viruses causing   106
   upper
      etiologic agents and treatment   76
      etiology   103
respiratory syncytial virus   35, 76, 106, 108
RETROVIR   206
Reye syndrome   173
rheumatic fever   57–9
   prophylaxis duration, American Heart Association Recommendation   59
   recurrent, chemoprophylaxis   58
rhinoviruses   103, 108
ribavirin   35, 211
   aerosolized   12
   pneumonia   111
Rickettsia rickettsii   4, 16
rifabutin   209, 230
rifampin   12, 35, 165, 173, 211, 229–30, 236
   meningococcal prophylaxis   15, 63
rimantadine   107, 211
   influenza   65
ritonavir   203, 207
Rocky Mountain spotted fever   4, 12, 16–17, 163
   differential diagnosis   18
   laboratory studies   18
   treatment   18
rotavirus   135
   gastroenteritis   134
      clinical aspects   129
      signs and symptoms   130
rotavirus vaccine   37

Roth spots   3
rubella   4, 29, 33, 163
rubella virus   29

Sabourand agar   98
Saccharomyces boulardii   129
salicylates   147
salicylic acid   165
Salmonella   45, 123
Salmonella gastroenteritis
    characteristics   131
    symptoms and laboratory findings   131
    treatment, indications   132
Salmonella typhi   131
salmonellosis   130–2, 186
    enteric fever   132
    factors associated with   131
    focal infections   130
    treatment   133
salpingitis   195
saquinavir   203, 208
scabies   164–5
scalded skin   163
scalp abscess   35
scarlet fever   163, 186
scrofula   165
seizures   171–2
selective IgA deficiency   215
sepsis   1, 2, 17–19
    clinical findings   19
    effects on organ systems   19
    management   20
    meningitis   11–12
    pneumonia, neonates   110
    postsplenectomy   187
        pneumococcal   64
    shock, treatment   21
    syndromes, associated commonly   19
    unknown source, initial antibiotic therapy   19, 20
septic arthritis   144–7
    differential diagnosis   146
    etiology   146
    joint involvement   144
    special considerations   147
septic shock
    progression   20
    see also sepsis
serologic testing   101

severe combined immunodeficiency   215
sexual abuse   198–9
sexually transmitted disease
    classified by pathogen   190
    clinical presentation   189
    etiology   180
    male   196–7
    prevalence   29
Shenton's line   144
Shigella   45
Shigella gastroenteritis   133
    signs and symptoms   133
shigellosis
    complications   134
    treatment   135
shunt infections   171–3
    antibiotics   173
    bacterial organisms associated   172
sickle cell disease
    bone infarction   137
    pneumococcal bacteremia   71
Sin Nombre virus   10
sinergistic necrotizing cellulitis   182
sinusitis   103, 104
    acute   104
small bowel infection   184
snake bites   83–4
    treatment
        emergency   84
        in-hospital   84
soft tissue infection   181
solumedrol   175
splenectomy   187
splenic trauma   187
stains   91–2
Staphylococcus aureus   1–2, 3–5, 12, 69, 80, 109, 122–3, 140, 145–6, 153, 162–3, 172
    neonatal eye infection   34
    toxic shock syndrome   21
Staphylococcus epidermidis   35, 102, 146, 172
    neonatal   3
Staphylococcus intermedius   70
stavudine   203, 206–7
steeple sign   105
    epiglottitis   8
Stevens–Johnson syndrome   229
Streptococcus faecalis   63

Streptococcus pneumoniae 3, 5, 12, 64, 72, 82
Streptococcus pyogenes 75
Streptococcus viridans 3
streptomycin 114–15
  respiratory infections, upper 76
strongyloidiasis 82–3
subdural tap 88–9
sulfametoxazole 51
sulfisoxazole 154, 156, 192
  meningococcal prophylaxis 63
  otitis media 82
    recurrent 56
  urinary tract infections 57
sulphadiazine 30
  rheumatic fever 58
Suprax 154
surgical infections
  general principles 177, 179–80
  prophylaxis 177–8
surgical procedures, recommended
    antimicrobial prophylaxis 180
swimmer's ear 75
syndrome of inappropriate antidiuretic
    hormone secretion (SIADH) 13, 171, 175
synovial fluid 95
  evaluation 97
  examination 97
syphilis 29, 31–2, 190–1
  congenital, treatment 32
  serology testing 191
  therapy 191
systemic lupus erythematosus (SLE) 3, 5

technetium bone scan 137–8
Tensilon 2
terconazole 195
tetanus 19–21
  clinical manifestations 22
  neonatal 20, 22
  prophylaxis 37–9
  treatment 22
tetanus immunoglobulin 39
tetanus toxoid 39
tetracycline 120, 161, 231
  tetanus 22
  yersinia infection 136
thalassemia 187

thiabendazole 83, 211
thoracentesis 89
thrush 73
ticarcillin 20, 143, 154, 186–7, 218, 228–9
tinea capitis 73
tinea corporis 73
tinea cruris 73
tinea pedis 73
tinidazole 124, 194
tipconazole 195
tobramycin 20, 143, 154, 180, 236
tolnaftate 43
tonsillitis 70, 74, 76
TORCH 29
toxic shock syndrome 21–4
  clinical manifestations 23
  diagnosis, criteria 23
  increased risk, factor associated 24
  laboratory abnormalities 24
  staphylococcal, incubation period 22
  supportive intensive care 24
  treatment 24
toxocariasis 82–3
Toxoplasma gondii 29–30
toxoplasmosis 29, 163
  treatment 30
tracheitis, bacterial 1–2
tracheostomy, epiglottitis 9
transplant recipients 220–1
transplantation, timetable for infection 221–2
travel medicine 45–54
travel vaccines 46–51
traveler's diarrhea 51, 121, 245
Treponema pallidum 104, 190
trichloroacetic acid 165, 169
Trichomonas vaginalis 192–3, 196
trichomoniasis 193
Trichophyton rubrum 73
trichuriasis 82
trimethoprim/sulfametoxazole 51, 143, 154, 156, 180, 208, 228–9
  E. coli infection 121
  otitis media 56
  pneumococcal sepsis 64
  salmonellosis 132, 133
  shigellosis 135
  sinusitis 104
  urinary tract infections 57
  yersinia infection 136

trophozoites   95
5-TU-PPD   116
tuberculin skin testing   50–1
tuberculosis   64–5, 114–16, 174
   high risks, immediate and annual skin
      testing   115
   prophylaxis   65
   screening   50–1
      infants and children   114–16
      treatment, recommended   114–15
tubo–ovarian abscess   195
tympanocentesis   89
   diagnostic   82
tympanomastoid surgery, indications   81
Typhin Vi   48
typhoid fever   47–9, 131, 132, 186
typhoid vaccine (oral)   47
typhoid Vi   48
typhus   163
Tzanck test/preparation   34, 98–9, 198

uremia   5
ureter
   duplication   152
   ectopic   152
   obstruction   152
urethritis   150
   non-gonococcal   192–3
Ureuplasma urealyticum   110, 192–3
urinary tract infections   56–7, 149–60
   American Academy of Pediatrics,
      recommendations   150
   bacterial etiology   153
   culture diagnosis, criteria   151
   diagnosis, criteria
      clinical criteria   149
      laboratory testing   149–51
   factors predisposing   152
   initial febrile, evaluation algorithm   158
   localization   153
   lower   157–9
   persistent   156
   radiographic evaluation, indication
      156–7
   recurrent   155–6
      antibiotic prophylaxis   57
      long term management   155–6
   risk factors   152–3
   screening tests   151

symptoms, causes in absence of
   bacteriuria   150
   treatment   153–4
urinary tract obstruction   159–60
urine
   bacterial cultures   95
   examination and analysis   94
   specimens, collection   150–1

vaccination, routine   37–42
   schedule   37
   side-effects, local   39
   vaccines available in the United States   38
vaccines
   travel   46–51
      age limitations and chemoprophylaxis
         47
      scheduling, time before travel   53
      supplies   53–4
vaginosis   194
valacyclovir   66–7, 191
vancomycin   13, 143, 172–3, 218, 228, 230,
      236
   endocarditis   62
   nosocomial infections   35
   pneumonia   113
   pseudomembranous colitis   128
   septicemia   20
   toxic shock syndrome   24
Vantin   154
Vaqta   48
varicella   173
varicella-zoster hyperimmune globulin
      (VZIG)   33, 42, 210
   use, guidelines   43
varicella-zoster virus   32–3, 174
   post-natal exposure, management   33
Veneral Disease Research Laboratories
      (VDRL) test   190
ventilation, assisted   11
ventricular tap   89–90
ventriculitis   171–3
ventriculoperitoneal shunt, aspiration   90
verrucae   165
vesicoureteral reflux   56, 152, 157
   grading   159
Vibrio parahaemolyticus   123
VIDEX   206
Vincent's angine   245